CLINICAL ASPECTS OF NEUTRON CAPTURE THERAPY

BASIC LIFE SCIENCES

Ernest H. Y. Chu, Series Editor

The University of Michigan Medical School
Ann Arbor, Michigan

Alexander Hollaender, Founding Editor

Recent volumes in the series:

Volume 37 GENETIC ENGINEERING OF ANIMALS: An Agricultural Perspective
Edited by J. Warren Evans and Alexander Hollaender

Volume 38 MECHANISMS OF DNA DAMAGE AND REPAIR: Implications for Carcinogenesis and Risk Assessment
Edited by Michael G. Simic, Lawrence Grossman, and Arthur C. Upton

Volume 39 ANTIMUTAGENESIS AND ANTICARCINOGENESIS MECHANISMS
Edited by Delbert M. Shankel, Philip E. Hartman, Tsuneo Kada, and Alexander Hollaender

Volume 40 EXTRACHROMOSOMAL ELEMENTS IN LOWER EUKARYOTES
Edited by Reed B. Wickner, Alan Hinnebusch, Alan M. Lambowitz, I. C. Gunsalus, and Alexander Hollaender

Volume 41 TAILORING GENES FOR CROP IMPROVEMENT: An Agricultural Perspective
Edited by George Bruening, John Harada, Tsune Kosuge, and Alexander Hollaender

Volume 42 EVOLUTION OF LONGEVITY IN ANIMALS: A Comparative Approach
Edited by Avril D. Woodhead and Keith H. Thompson

Volume 43 PHENOTYPIC VARIATION IN POPULATIONS: Relevance to Risk Assessment
Edited by Avril D. Woodhead, Michael A Bender, and Robin C. Leonard

Volume 44 GENETIC MANIPULATION OF WOODY PLANTS
Edited by James W. Hanover and Daniel E. Keathley

Volume 45 ENVIRONMENTAL BIOTECHNOLOGY: Reducing Risks from Environmental Chemicals through Biotechnology
Edited by Gilbert S. Omenn

Volume 46 BIOTECHNOLOGY AND THE HUMAN GENOME: Innovations and Impact
Edited by Avril D. Woodhead and Benjamin J. Barnhart

Volume 47 PLANT TRANSPOSABLE ELEMENTS
Edited by Oliver Nelson

Volume 48 HUMAN ACHONDROPLASIA: A Multidisciplinary Approach
Edited by Benedetto Nicoletti, Steven E. Kopits, Elio Ascani, and Victor A. McKusick

Volume 49 OXYGEN RADICALS IN BIOLOGY AND MEDICINE
Edited by Michael G. Simic, Karen A. Taylor, John F. Ward, and Clemens von Sonntag

Volume 50 CLINICAL ASPECTS OF NEUTRON CAPTURE THERAPY
Edited by Ralph G. Fairchild, Victor P. Bond, and Avril D. Woodhead

---

CLINICAL ASPECTS OF NEUTRON CAPTURE THERAPY

Edited by
Ralph G. Fairchild, Victor P. Bond, and Avril D. Woodhead
Brookhaven National Laboratory
Upton, New York

Technical Editor
Katherine Vivirito
Brookhaven National Laboratory
Upton, New York

PLENUM PRESS • NEW YORK AND LONDON

Library of Congress Cataloging in Publication Data

Clinical aspects of neutron capture therapy / edited by Ralph G. Fairchild, Victor P. Bond, and Avril D. Woodhead: technical editor, Katherine Vivirito.
p. cm. – (Basic Life Sciences; v. 50)
Based on a workshop held Feb. 1-2, 1988, at Brookhaven National Laboratory, Upton, N.Y.
Includes bibliographies and index.

DOI 10.1007/978-1-4684-5622-6
1. Boron-neutron capture therapy – Congresses. 2. Cancer – Radiotherapy – Congresses. I. Fairchild, Ralph G. II. Bond, Victor P. III. Woodhead, Avril D. IV. Series.
[DNLM: 1. Boron Compounds – therapeutic use – congresses. 2. Neoplasms – radiotherapy – congresses. 3. Neutrons – congresses. W3 BA255 v.50 /
QZ 269 C64105 1988]
RC271.R3C56 1989
616.99'40642 – dc19
DNLM/DLC 88-37219
for Library of Congress CIP

Proceedings of a workshop on Boron Neutron Capture Therapy, held February 1-2, 1988, at Brookhaven National Laboratory, Upton, New York

A Division of Plenum Publishing Corporation
233 Spring Street, New York, N.Y. 10013

PREFACE

Since Locher first suggested Boron Neutron Capture Therapy (BNCT) in 1936, this theoretically ideal system has intrigued investigators. Unfortunately, the first clinical trials between 1951-1961 were not successful. However, they served to implant firmly the seed of BNCT, the growth of which has been carefully nurtured at a number of locations world-wide. This fact is attested to by the ongoing clinical trials in Japan as well as by the presence of researchers from active groups in the ten countries represented at this Workshop.

In 1983 and 1985, the first and second international biannual symposia on BNCT were held, in response to a resurgence of interest in this field. In 1986, the DOE sponsored a workshop on NCT, in large part directed toward evaluating the national effort and the various neutron sources available within the United States. It now seems likely, because of various factors including improved neutron beams and boron delivery systems which have made the modality more attractive, that clinical trials will be initiated in the United States within the next few years. This 1988 special workshop, interspersed between the biannual international symposia, represents an effort to seek ideas and advice on the clinical aspects of BNCT, from all those diverse groups with a national commitment to this project. Our purpose is to facilitate our endeavor to incorporate the best procedures and techniques in the upcoming clinical trials. It is understood that because of the initial inability to effect a successful outcome for BNCT, there will be less tolerance for failure in this second attempt within the United States. Further, such a possible failure would have negative effects on other national or international efforts as well. Thus it is incumbent upon every one concerned to incorporate the best approach that can be devised collectively among those present at this workshop.

Special thanks are given to the moderators, L.E. Feinendegen, B. Larsson, S. Rockwell and A. Wambersie, for the skill with which they conducted the working sessions, and worked toward consensus on these difficult questions. They devoted a substantial amount of time and effort to the preparation of these summaries.

Questions to be Considered

The following questions were developed as suggested topics for discussion during the Workshop, and for specific consideration by the working groups. These groups used the questions in an effort to develop a consensus in areas of particular importance to possible clinical applications.

1. Dose Fractionation

1.1 Should US trials copy Hatanaka's exposure schedule (i.e. 4-8 hour irradiation times at a fluence rate of about 10^9 n/cm^2-sec)?

1.2 What are the advantages and disadvantages of a single protracted vs. a single acute (<5 min) irradiation?

1.3 Are protracted irradiations, because of possible benefits from repair of low-LET damage in normal tissue, beneficial for thermal beam irradiations?

1.4 Are protracted irradiations, because of possible benefits from repair of low-LET damage in normal tissue, beneficial for epithermal beam irradiations?

1.5 Would 2-4 fractions be beneficial because of selective repair to normal tissue for thermal or for epithermal beam irradiation?

1.6 Of what significance is radiation damage to blood vessels in normal tissue or in tumor tissue?

2. Blood-Brain Barrier (BBB)

2.1 Does the BBB break down following a single acute "high" dose?

2.2 If the BBB does break down, would boron then "leak" through to irradiate excessive amounts of normal tissue?

2.3 If 2-4 fractions were delivered in 2-4 days, would a BBB break-down be significant and harmful?

2.4 Will malignant cells protected by the BBB preclude successful NCT?

2.5 Can malignant cells protected by the BBB be reached by multiple fractions?

3. Glioblastoma

3.1 Should Hatanaka's compound delivery schedule (30-80 mg ^{10}B/kg of $Na_2B_{12}H_{11}SH$ infused into the carotid or vertebral artery during 1-2 hours, 16 hours prior to irradiation) be followed?

3.2 Should the pharmacokinetics of $Na_2B_{12}H_{11}SH$ be investigated as a function of: mode of administration (i.a.; i.v.; p.o.); length of administration (1 to 12 hours); time between end of administration and irradiation (3 to 24 hours); amount of boron administered (30 to 300 mg/kg)?

3.3 Of what quality (absolute concentrations in tumor, blood, brain and other intervening tissues, such as meningis, concentration ratios) should the pharmacokinetic data of an optimized administration be before clinical trials are feasible?

3.4 Would the dimer $Na_4B_{12}H_{11}S_2B_{12}H_{11}$ be more advantageous than the monomer $Na_2B_{12}H_{11}SH$?

3.5 Is the dimer toxicity prohibitive relative to that of the monomer?

3.6 What significance, if any, with respect to clinical trials, should be attached to the failure to date to demonstrate biological efficacy in animals, of either monomer or dimer?

4. Other Compounds and Tumors

4.1 In view of the evidence demonstrating biological efficacy in various test systems (cells, small and large animals), should p-boronophenylalanine be used in initial clinical trials with malignant melanoma?

4.2 Would melanoma metastatic to brain be a viable system in which to initially evaluate NCT in humans?

4.3 For any compound considered for clinical use,should biological efficacy be demonstrated in animals?

4.4 Are there better compounds over the immediate horizon (i.e., boronothiouracil or phenothiazines, monoclonal antibodies, porphyrins)?

The following working groups were formed to consider the above questions, as well as others evolving during the discussions.

Optimization of Radiation Dose Delivery

A. Wambersie and
L.E. Feinendegen, Moderators

H.L. Atkins
J. Archambeau
V.P. Bond
R.V. Dorn
K.R. Durrant
R.G. Fairchild
R.A. Gahbauer
P. Gavin
M.L. Griebenow
W. Harkness
J. Hopewell
H. Madoc-Jones
A.G. Meek
Y. Ryabukhin
J.H. Spickard
F. Tovarys
F. Wheeler
L. Wielopolski
R.C. Zamenhof

Tumor Compound and Compound Delivery Systems

S. Rockwell and
B. Larsson, Moderators

B.J. Allen
R.F. Barth
J.A. Coderre
D. Gabel
J.D. Glass, Jr.
J.H. Goodman
O. Harling
D.D. Joel
S.B. Kahl
S.R. Marano
Y. Mishima
S. Packer
L.E. Reinstein
J.L. Russell, Jr.
D.N. Slatkin
A.H. Soloway
W.H. Sweet
G. Tyson

<u>Workshop Co-Chairmen</u>
R.G. Fairchild
V.P. Bond

Ms. Bernice Armstrong and Ms. Gloria Jackson provided invaluable assistance in typing these proceedings.

CONTENTS

DOSE RATE AND THERAPEUTIC GAIN

R.G. Fairchild

Medical Department
Brookhaven National Laboratory
Upton, NY 11973

INTRODUCTION

There is a consensus that previous difficulties encountered in U.S. clinical trials of NCT resulted from the use of inorganic compounds showing no tumor selectivity, and the use of thermal neutron beams which are known to have poor penetration in tissue (HVL ≈ 1.8 cm). Consequently, normal surface tissues were over-exposed, while viable tumor remained at depth. Since then, these problems have been largely circumvented through the development of epithermal neutron beams with better tissue penetration, and the synthesis of various boronated biomolecules which demonstrate tumor selectivity.

POSSIBLE PROBLEMS IN NCT

Until unqualified success has been finally achieved, it may be anticipated that additional unforeseen problems will be encountered. Because of this, every effort must be made to optimize conditions in advance, in hopes that such possible problems will not cause failure.

A number of new compounds have shown tumor specificity and uptake adequate for therapy in biological test systems (cell culture, and animal tumor models). These include the various forms of sulfhydryl boron hydride monomer (BSH), dimer (BSSB), dimer monoxide (BSOSB), boronated phenylalanine (BPA), boronated porphyrins (BP), boronated thiouracil (BTU) and dihydroxyboryldeoxyuridine (DBDU). Clearly much work needs to be done to insure that the correct compound is aligned with the right tumor, and that dose delivery is optimized (ie., the pharmacokinetics are exhaustively studied to insure that the maximum tumor uptake and normal tissue clearance is achieved).

In addition to the above gross distribution, it is well known that the intracellular distribution of boron is of prime importance. For example, the hamster V-79 cell line is commonly used as an example of mammalian tumor cells; it has been shown that for a uniform B concentration, within and without the cell ~ 10% of the effective (nuclear) dose comes from boron external to the cell, while ~45% comes from each of the cytoplasmic and nuclear locations.[1,2] Thus for example if a boron compound remains extracellular, as indeed may be the case to a significant extent for antibodies and perhaps BSH, ~10 times as much boron will be needed as for a uniform distribution. Clearly, data on the cellular distribution of prospective therapeutic agents are vital for a realistic prediction of their biological efficacy.

A potential trouble spot in the treatment of brain tumors is the possibility that individual malignant cells may well exist up to a few mm beyond the boundaries of overt tumor, and that these cells may be protected by the blood-brain-barrier (BBB). If such cells are prevented from incorporating boron compounds, they may initiate regrowth. These problems are important, and will be addressed in part by the tumor-compound working group.

It is the main aim of this paper to address the problems which may be encountered due to possible dose-rate effects.

DOSE RATE EFFECTS

Past and current experience with low LET X and γ-rays has shown that repair contributes significantly to observed biological effects. For example, typical normal tissue tolerance for a single high-dose-rate exposure is ~2000 rad, while for the standard regimen of 30 fractions over 6 weeks, the tolerance is 6000 rads. For continuous low-dose rate exposures encountered with permanent implant brachytherapy, tolerance may go up to 18,000 rads.[3,4] While repopulation stimulated by bio-feedback mechanisms clearly contributes to the recovery of normal tissues, repair of sublethal damage, with a $T_{1/2}$ of ~ 1/2 hour, is known to be a major factor.

One of the prime factors contributing to the resurgence of interest in NCT over the past few years, has been the extensive clinical experience of Hatanaka in the therapy of brain tumors. Approximately 100 treatments have been administered since 1968, in which 1 hour infusions of $Na_2B_{12}H_{11}SH$ have been followed by an 18 hour wait, and then a 4-8 hour irradiation (mainly at the Musashi Reactor outside Tokyo; thermal neutron flux density ~10^9 n $cm^{-2}sec^{-1}$). While definitive controlled experiments remain to be completed, it is reported that survival has been significantly extended.[5] Clinical irradiations have also been initiated for the treatment of superficial melanoma using similar irradiation times, as described by Mishima in this Workshop. In view of the short $T_{1/2}$ for repair of low-LET damage relative to the 4-8 hour irradiation times, the possibility exists that repair may significantly increase the tolerance of normal tissue to the photon component of the mixed radiation field. Conventional therapy tries to exploit this parameter by the usual fractionation procedures. BNCT perhaps offers a unique potential for advantage in that the mixed radiation field provides an unbalanced mixture, with the tumor being dosed predominantly with high-LET radiation from the $^{10}B(n,\alpha)^7Li$ reaction. Since the latter component is known to show little or no repair, a situation then exists in which fractionated irradiation would produce an increased therapeutic gain, due to selective repair of normal tissue.

THERAPEUTIC GAIN

Dosimetric measurements have been made at the Brookhaven Medical Research Reactor in an anthropomorphic phantom, in which the various beam components have been resolved (i.e., the dose from gamma rays, the $^{14}N(n,p)^{14}C$ reaction, and fast neutron recoils, or γ, N and H respectively). The components as generated by a thermal neutron beam and a "pure" 2 keV epithermal beam, incident on a phantom head are shown in Fig. 1 and 2. Results are shown in terms of the biologically effective dose (rads x RBE)[6,7]. Information provided by Archambeau in this Workshop indicates that the effective gamma dose can be reduced by 50% by delivering it in a few (one to three) fractions. Assuming a reduction of 50%, the effective dose to normal tissues (no B content) can in principle be reduced by 25 and 40% for a thermal and epithermal neutron beam respectively, as shown in Fig. 3 and 4.

The guiding principle of radiation therapy is that normal tissues are irradiated to their tolerance levels, in the hope that the concomitant tumor dose will be adequate for control. Given this procedure, a 50% reduction in effective gamma dose

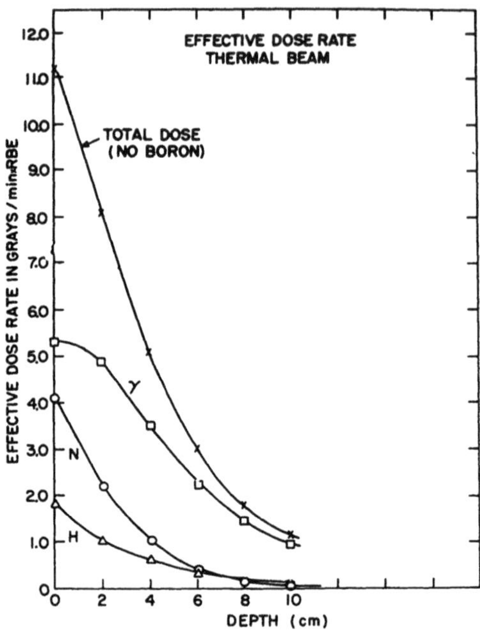

Fig. 1. Biologically effective dose rate (rad x RBE) in a tissue equivalent phantom head, as measured with an incident thermal neutron beam.

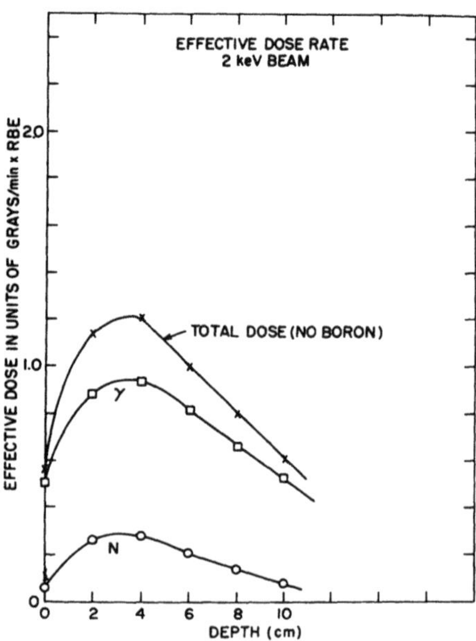

Fig. 2. Biologically effective dose rate (rad x RBE) in a tissue equivalent phantom head, as measured with an incident 2 keV neutron beam.

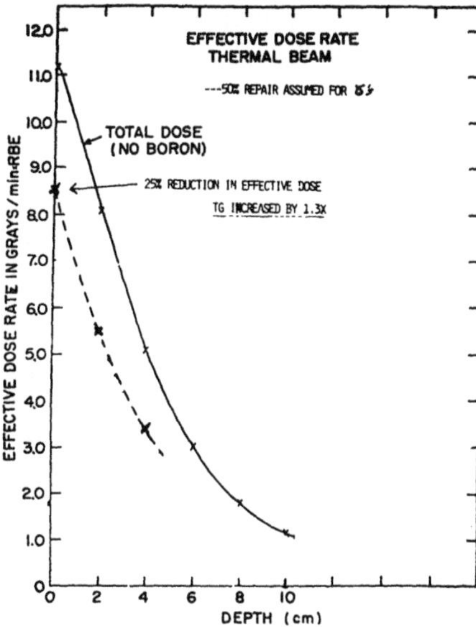

Fig. 3. Biologically effective dose rate (rad x RBE; dashed line) obtained from the thermal neutron beam in Fig. 1, by reducing the γ-component by 50% because of repair.

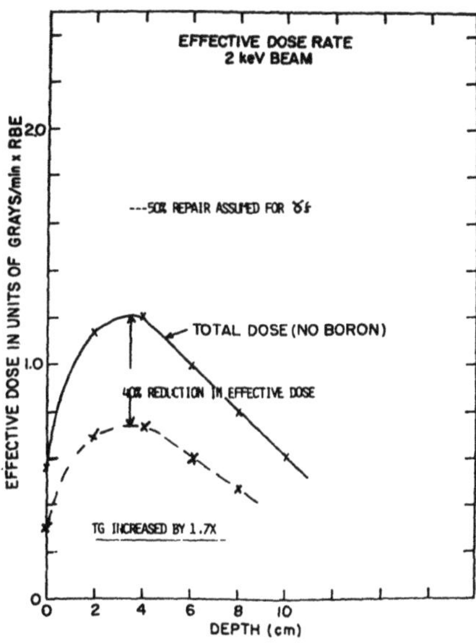

Fig. 4. Biologically effective dose rate (rad x RBE; dashed line) obtained from the incidence 2 keV beam in Fig. 2, by reducing the γ-component by 50% because of repair.

would produce an increase in therapeutic gain (TG) by a factor of 1.3 for a thermal beam, and 1.7 for the epithermal beam.

DISCUSSION

It is generally accepted that a 10% increase in TG will produce a significant increase in local control (it is thought that a 1% increase in tumor dose will produce a 2% increase in tumor control). Straightforward considerations indicate that TG's for BNCT can be increased by factors of 1.3 and 1.7 (thermal and epithermal beams, respectively) through the delivery of therapeutic irradiations in a few fractions. Such increases in therapeutic gains are multiplicative, so that for example, if NCT produces a TG of 2 for a single therapy dose with an epithermal beam, a fractionated application may increase this to 3.4.

The field of clinical NCT is not well understood. Apparent good results may be due to a variety of causes which have yet to be properly identified; one of these causes may be the effect of repair with the thermal beam employed for the 4-8 hour irradiations carried out in Japan. As clinical trials are initiated in the U.S., we would be well advised to ensure that all parameters have been optimized to the best of our ability, in hope of avoiding pitfalls which may as yet not even have been identified.

REFERENCES

1. T. Kobayashi and K. Kanda, Analytical calculation of boron -10 dosage in cell nucleus for neutron capture therapy, Radiat. Res. 91:77 (1982).
2. D. Gabel, S. Foster, and R. G. Fairchild, The Monte-Carlo simulation of the biological effect of the $^{10}B(Nn\alpha)^{7}Li$ reaction in cells and tissue and its implication for boron neutron capture therapy, Radiat. Res. 111:14 (1987).
3. B. J. Hall, "Radiobiology for the Radiologist," Harper and Rowe, New York (1986).
4. B. S. Hilaris, ed., "Handbook of Interstitial Brachy-therapy", Publishing Science Group Inc., Criton, MA (1975).
5. H. Hatanaka, ed., "Boron Neutron Capture Therapy for Tumors," Nishimura Co., Ltd., Japan (1986).
6. R. G. Fairchild and L. J. Goodman, Development and dosimetry of an "epithermal" neutron beam for possible use in neutron capture therapy. II. Absorbed dose measurements in a phantom man, Phys. Med. Biol. 11:15 (1966).

7. R. G. Fairchild and V. P. Bond, Current status of ^{10}B-neutron capture therapy: Enhancement of tumor dose viabeam filtration and dose rate, and the effects of these parameters on minimum boron content: A theoretical evaluation, Int. J. Radiat. Oncol. Biol. Phys. 11:831 (1985).

SWINE SKIN: A MODEL TO EVALUATE DOSE RECOVERY FROM DIFFERENT RADIATIONS

J. O. Archambeau

Department of Radiation Biology
Loma Linda University
Loma Linda, California 92354

INTRODUCTION

Unacceptable scalp and facial skin reactions were produced during the first clinical trials of neutron capture therapy. These complications resulted because the half-value layer (HVL) of thermal neutrons in tissue is small (about 1.8 cm), and the boron-10 partition between the blood/skin and cancer located several centimeters below the surface was poor. As a consequence, when a therapeutic dose was delivered to the cancer at depth, the dose from the adventitious gamma, fast-neutron and capture radiations to the skin exceeded the limits of tolerance.[1]

A swine skin model was selected to quantify the tissue dose response produced by the thermal neutron beam, adventitious radiations and boron-10 radiations used in the BNL clinical trials. This model was chosen because the irradiation geometry, anatomy with a subcutaneous fat layer, histology and known response to irradiation all approached that found in humans.

The study quantified the parameters in the swine skin at gross,[2-4] histologic,[5-9] morphologic,[5,7] cytologic,[5,6] and kinetic[6,8,10-14] levels and also simulated the radiation changes.[12,13,15-17] The gross and histologic dose response to single-dose fractions of thermal neutrons, degraded fission neutrons (epithermal beam) and X rays, the dose response to multiple dose fractions of X rays, and the $^{10}B(n,\alpha)^{7}Li$ reaction were compared.[4,5] These post-clinical studies confirm the dose distribution from the $^{10}B(n,\alpha)^{7}Li$ reaction and accompanying adventitious radiations.

This paper lists the absorbed doses at which 50% of the irradiated fields were not healed (ED-50), the dose ratios, and the dose recovery values obtained in the post-clinical studies. The model will be used to obtain a preclinical appraisal of the dose distribution expected to be produced in humans using the optimized epithermal neutron beams on skin containing a range of boron-10 concentrations from compounds of clinical interest.

MATERIAL AND METHODS

Immature female Yorkshire (white-skinned) swine, 3 to 5 months of age and weighing 30 to 70 kg, are purchased from local vendors and maintained in communal pens and fed 2 to 2 1/2 pounds of a standard growth mash.[1-3] All animals appeared in good health and were growing when irradiated.

The animals were irradiated to circular fields of 10-cm diameter on the shoulder, flank and ham. In some animals the flank field is omitted. The evolution, time-course, dose-dependence of the extent of epilation, and degree of erythema were determined, as well as the presence of a moist reaction, the area involved and completeness of healing.

Parameters

Erythema is an inconsistent finding and cannot be scored effectively when only two or three fields are used on each animal. The extent of epilation is estimated by the time of occurrence and the completeness of loss. The principal change measured is whether or not the moist reaction occurs. A moist reaction is defined as the loss of sufficient epidermis to permit loss of serum and crust formation, abrasion, ulceration, or necrosis. If a moist reaction occurs, the area of the field involved is determined using a plastic grid look-through, or is measured planimetrically on photographs. The time of onset, the maximal field involvement, and the time of maximal or complete healing are noted.

If a moist reaction is produced, it involves an increasing area of the field reaching a maximum area within 21-25 days. With few exceptions, the reaction heals partially or completely within 36 days. The field then remains intact or breaks down again before 49 days have elapsed. The second moist reaction does not heal except from the edge.

Whether or not the field is healed at 49 days is determined. The parameter used to characterize the dose response is the dose at which 50% of the fields are not healed within 49 days, that is, the ED-50.[2]

Table 1. Dose Contribution of Thermal Neutron Beam[4]

Component	Rad/MW-min	%
Gamma	143.0	68.6
$^{14}N(n,P)^{14}C$	47.4	22.8
H	18.0	8.6
Total	208.4	100.0

The RBE for the different radiations or mixed beams is obtained using 250 kVp X rays as a standard. The RBE of the principal radiation in mixed beams is determined by subtracting the contribution from adventitious radiations. The dose contributions from the adventitious radiations of various beams at the Brookhaven Medical Research Reactor[4] (MRR) are listed in Tables 1, 2 and 3. The elemental content of skin is given in Table 4.[4,8]

The degree of dose recovery (DQ) is estimated by:

$$DQ = \frac{(ED\text{-}50)_n - (ED\text{-}50)_1}{n-1}$$

where ED-50 (n) is the absorbed dose at which 50% of the fields are not healed following multiple equal dose fractions, (ED-50[1]) is the dose response following a single dose fraction; n is number of dose fractions.

RESULTS

The complete results are available in the original publications. The focus here is on those produced by 250 kVp X rays and thermal neutrons. These will be the predominant radiations studied in the preclinical trials that will be conducted to evaluate the new optimized epithermal neutron beams and partition of new boron-10-containing compounds.

The time of occurrence of events in the evolution of a moist reaction for X rays, thermal neutrons, degraded fission neutrons, and the $^{10}B(n,\alpha)^7Li$ reaction are listed in Table 5.[4] The time of evolution of the moist reaction is essentially the same for all reaction. The ED_{50} for selected radiations and the dose response ratio compared with X rays are listed in Table 6.[4] The isoeffect dose response for

Table 2. Dose Contribution of Degraded Fission Neutron Beam 4

Component	Rad/MW-min	%
Fn	28.4	67.0
Gamma	13.6	32.1
$^{14}N(n,P)^{14}C$	0.4	0.9
Total	42.4	100.0

fast neutrons is shown in Table 8.[18-22] The RBE for thermal neutron capture reaction for tissue nitrogen, $^{14}N(n,p)^{14}C$ is estimated as 2.7. The RBE for degraded fission neutrons is estimated to be 3.6.

The RBE for $^{10}B(n,\alpha)^{7}Li$ reaction could not be determined because of uncertainties in measuring boron concentration.[4] The ED-50 ratio with X ray was 2.2 for the mixed beam. The dose response occurred over a range calculated for humans. Delivering the total dose in six fractions over a period of 12-16 days did not increase the dose tolerance.

Table 3. Dose Contribution of Microgram Boron-10/gram; $0 = 4.2 \times 10^{12}/cm^2$ (4)

Component	Absorbed Dose (Rad)	%
Gamma	317.9	29.1
$^{14}N(n,P)^{14}C$	105.4	9.6
H	39.9	3.6
$^{10}B(n,\alpha)^{7}Li$	630.4	57.7
Total	1093.6	100.0

Table 4. Elemental Analysis of Swine Skin[8]

Wet Weight (%)	H (%)	N (%)	H_2O (%)
Whole	9.7	5.8	63.2
Epidermis	10.1	3.7	76.0
Dermis	8.9	5.6	58.6
Fat	11.3	0.7	16.8
Hair	7.4	13.6	10.7

The X ray dose response to single- and multiple-dose fractions is displayed in a reciprocal total-dose, dose-fraction isoeffect plot in Fig. 1. The alpha/beta ratio (a/B ratio) of 221 rad is in agreement with data from other sources (Table 8).[16,18-22] The range of dose recovery values following multiple dose schedules is listed in Table 9.[16]

The change in dose response in one study[23] evaluating the changes produced by continuous irradiation was measured using an arbitrary scoring system. The dose at which the isoeffect was produced increased as the dose rate decreased using cesium (^{137}Cs), radium (^{226}Ra) gamma and Californium (^{252}Cf) neutron gamma mixed beam (Figure 2).

Table 5. Time Course of Moist Reaction[4]

Radiation	First Seen (Day)	Maximal Healed (Day)
X Ray		
Shoulder	17.5±0.6	36.0±1.0
Ham	20.8±0.8	38.0±1.3
Thermal Neutrons	18.2±0.9	43.7±1.6
Degraded Fission Neutrons	20.0±1.6	38.0±2.5
$^{10}B(n,\alpha)^{7}Li$	15.2±0.7	45.3±1.3

DISCUSSION

Model

The swine skin is a suitable model for preclinical studies. The skin dose responses for different radiations and different time dose responses for different radiations and different time dose schedules are available, and the gross and histologic parameters are quantified. The radiobiologic and cell kinetic characteristics of the epidermis, dermis and microvasculature also are known.[2-17]

The experimental approach can be varied to simulate various beam compositions or boron distribution. The use of different thicknesses of tissue-equivalent-bolus will permit evaluation of the beam composition at different depths in normal tissue. When data are available for humans, the results are similar to those measured for swine.[1]

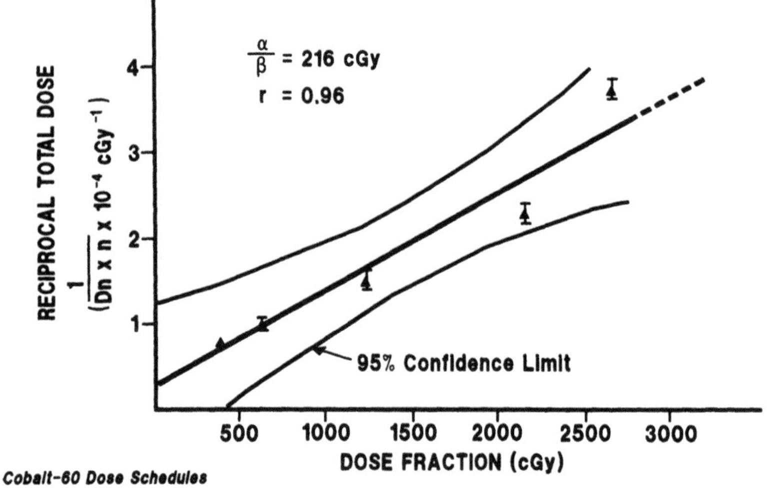

Fig. 1. Reciprocal total dose-dose fraction isoeffect curve for swine skin 50% effect using the daily irradiation schedules listed in Table 9. The alpha/beta ratio is 221 rad for the best fit line. The total dose is increased by a factor of 4.38 when the daily dose fraction is 356 rad given in 30 daily dose fractions.

Table 6. Swine, 50% Effective Dose [4]

Radiation*	Dose (Rad)	Ratio	"RBE"
X Ray			
Shoulder	2273±103	--	--
Ham	2278±141	--	--
Thermal Neutrons	1469±107	1.5±.3	2.7
Degraded Fission Neutrons	944±109	2.7±.3	3.6
$^{10}B(n,\alpha)^{7}Li$	1100±112	2.2	

*Single dose fractions

Dose Response

An arbitrary scoring system is used frequently to assess the skin's response to irradiation. The degree of erythema, dry desquamation and area of the field involved with a moist reaction are assigned incremental, unit scores. It is not certain that the average score within each unit-increment relates to a fixed population isoeffect.

When this scoring system is used instead of the ED-50 to determine the skin dose response, there is a poor dose-dependent

Table 7. Swine Dose Response[18-22]

Radiation	Schedule	Isoeffect	Ratio
Fast Neutron			
42 MeV, d-Be	Single	Average Score	1.4-1.6
		Necrosis	1.3
		Contraction	1.5
50 MeV, d-Be	2x/wk x 6 1/2 wk	Average Score	< 2
		Contraction	2.2-2.6
	4-5x/wk x 6 1/2 wk	Average Score	< 2.5
		Contraction	3.1-3.4

Table 8. Swine Skin Dose Response 16,18,19,21,22

Isoeffect	Alpha/Beta Ratio (RAD)
ED-50[16]	221
Contraction[21,22]	305
Necrosis[18,19]	220-360

relationship between severity of the reaction (score) and dose. The principal difficulty is knowing what the epidermal and microvascular population changes are when represented by a unit incremental score correlating erythema, dry desquamation, moist reaction, mauve discoloration, and necrosis. If such subjective and non-parametric scoring techniques are to be used, they should be evaluated using non-parametric statistical techniques.[21,22]

Dose Recovery

Operationally, when the total X ray or gamma dose (low-LET) is divided into equal dose fractions and given at intervals of 6 hours, 24 hours, or daily for prolonged periods, the total dose required to produce the isoeffect is increased.[3,16] When continuous gamma irradiation is used, the dose required to produce the isoeffect is increased as the dose rate is decreased.[23] The dose difference between schedules represents the increment of dose response (injury) that was recovered over the period of irradiation.

The gain in normal tissue dose tolerance is 1.38 when the total dose is given in two equal dose fractions separated by 24 hours and increases to 4.38 when 30 equal daily fractions are given over a period of 40 days (Table 9).[16] The gain in dose tolerance is 1.29 when the total dose is given in a period of 10 hours of continuous irradiation[23] using cesium or radium moulds and compared to a single-dose fraction.

The 1.29 and 1.38 gains reflect the dose recovery represented by the repair of sublethal injury and cell redistribution. The 4.38 value also includes the dose recovery that results from epidermal repopulation.[10]

These data suggest that as the total time of the neutron beam irradiation is increased or as the total dose is divided into equal increments given at intervals (greater than 6 hours), the normal tissue dose tolerance to low-LET radiations will be increased (Table 9). Data from the literature reviewing the tissue response obtained using multiple dose fractions of fast neutrons and the data obtained in the study evaluating multiple fractions of the $^{10}B(n,\alpha)^{7}Li$ reaction indicate that little or no dose recovery will occur.[4,18-22] As a consequence, a therapeutic gain of an amount similar to the gain in normal tissue tolerance should be present for neutron capture therapy of cancer containing boron 10.

CONCLUSION

The review of the data indicate that extended periods of multiple fractions of neutron irradiation are indicated to increase the dose response of normal tissue (skin) by a factor of 1.14,1.29, or 1.38 or more for low-LET, adventitious gamma radiation. The dose fractionation schedule required will depend on the relative dose contribution from boron-10 reaction and other high-LET adventitious radiations.

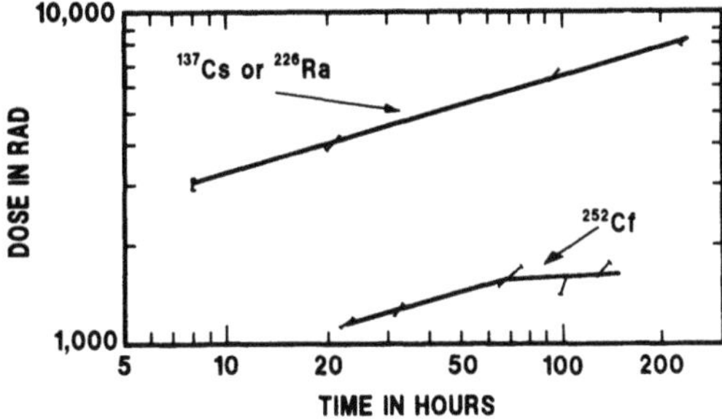

Fig. 2 Log-log total dose-length of irradiation isoeffect curve for swine skin arbitrary scoring using continuous cesium or radium gamma irradiation and californium mixed beam radiations. The best fit linear approximation has a slope of 0.29 for the gamma radiation indicating that dose recovery is occurring during irradiation as the dose rate decreases. The response to continuous mixed beam high-LET neutron and low-LET gamma irradiation has a similar slope up to 70 hours, after which there is little change as the dose response from the high-LET neutron radiation predominates.

Table 9. Swine Skin Dose Recovery

Time-Dose[a] Schedule	Isoeffect	Isoeffect[b] Dose Dose (RAD)	Dose[c] Recovered (RAD)	Gain in Tissue[d] Tolerance by Fractionation
Single	50% non-heal	2437±89	--	1.00
2 in 6 hr	50% non-heal	2794±92	357	1.15
2 in 24 hr	50% non-heal	3360±86	923	1.38
5 in 4 d	50% non-heal	4761±366	581	1.95
30 in 40 d	50% non-heal	10670	284	4.38

a Time-dose schedule: single or equal exposures separated by interval of 6 hr, 24 hr, daily for 5 days, or daily except weekends.

b Dose required to produce isoeffect.

c Average dose (DQ) recovered: $DQ = D^n - D^1/(N-1)$. Dn is dose required to produce isoeffect when n equals daily (except weekends) dose fractions are used. D^1 is dose required to produce isoeffect as a single dose fraction. N is number of dose fractions.

d Gain in normal tissue dose tolerance by fractionation = D^n/D^1.

REFERENCES

1. J. O. Archambeau, The effect of increasing exposures of the $^{10}B(n,\alpha)^7Li$ reaction of the skin of man, Radiology 94:187 (1970).

2. J. O. Archambeau, G. R. Mathieu, H. J. Brenneis, K. Thompson, and R. G. Fairchild, The response of the skin of swine to increasing multiple exposures of 250 kVp X rays, Radiat. Res. 36:299 (1968).

3. J. O. Archambeau, G. R. Mathieu, H. J. Brenneis and K. H. Thompson, The response of the skin of swine to increasing multiple exposures of 250 kVp X rays, Radiat. Res. 37:141 (1969).

4. J. O. Archambeau, R. G. Fairchild, H. J. Brenneis, The response of the skin of swine to increasing absorbed doses of radiation from a) thermal neutron beam; b) degraded fission neutron beam; and c) the $^{10}B(n,\alpha)^7Li$ reaction, Radiat.Res. 45:145 (1971).

5. J. O. Archambeau, R. G. Fairchild, and H. J. Brenneis, Response of the skin of swine to increasing absorbed doses of the $^{10}B(n,\alpha)^{7}Li$ reaction: histologic and cytologic changes, Radiat. Res. 45:137 (1971).
6. J. O. Archambeau, G. W. Bennett, J. J. Abata, and H. J. Brenneis, Response of swine skin to acute single exposures of X rays: quantification of epidermal cell changes, Radiat. Res. 79:298 (1979).
7. J. O. Archambeau, A. Ines, and L. F. Fajardo, Response of swine skin microvasculature to acute single exposures of X rays: quantification of endothelial changes, Radiat. Res. 98:37 (1984).
8. J. O. Archambeau, and G. W. Bennett, Quantification of morphologic, cytologic and kinetic parameters of unirradiated swine skin: a histologic model, Radiat. Res. 98:254 (1984).
9. J. O. Archambeau, A. Inex, and L. F. Fajardo, Correlation of the dermal microvasculature morphology with the epidermal and endothelial population changes produced by X ray single exposures of 1700, 2300 and 2700 R in swine skin. Int. J. Radiat. Oncol. Biol. Phys. 11:1639 (1985).
10. J. O. Archambeau, D. Hauser, and R. M. Shymko, Basal cell proliferation in swine skin during a course of daily irradiation given five days a week for six weeks (6000 rads), Int. J. Radiat. Oncol. Biol. Phys., in press (1988).
11. G. M. Morris, and J. W. Hopewell, Changes in the cell kinetics of pig epidermis after repeated daily doses of X rays, Brit. J. Radiol. 19:34 (1986).
12. G. M. Morris, and J. W. Hopewell, Pig epidermis: a cell kinetic study, Cell Tissue Kinet 18:407 (1985).
13. R. M. Shymko, D. L. Hauser, and J. O. Archambeau, Lack of correlation between basal cell survival and gross response in irradiated swine skin, Int. J. Radiat. Onco. Biol. Phys. 10(7):1079 (1984).
14. R. M. Shymko, D. L. Hauser, and J. O. Archambeau, Field size dependence of radiation sensitivity and dose fractionation response in skin. Int. J. Radiat. Oncol. Biol. Phys. 11(6):1143 (1985).
15. J. O. Archambeau and G. R. Mathieu, Comparison of the observed results of irradiation with those expected from an idealized model. Radiat. Res. 40:285 (1969).
16. J. O. Archambeau, 1987, Relative radiation sensitivity of the integumentary system, dose response of the epidermal, microvascular and dermal populations, in: "Advances in Radiation Biology", Academic Press, New York.
17. J. O. Archambeau and R. M. Shymko, Tissue population configuration as a dose response modifier, Int. J. Radiat. Oncol. Biol. Phys., in press (1988).

18. R. J. Berry, G. Wiernik, and T. J. S. Patterson, Skin tolerance to fractionated X irradiation in the pig: how good a predictor is the NSD formula? Brit. J. Radiol. 47:185 (1974).
19. R. J. Berry, G. Wiernik, T. J. S. Patterson, and J. W. Hopewell, Excess late subcutaneous fibrosis after irradiation of pig skin, consequent upon the application of the NSD formula, Brit. J. Radiol. 47:277 (1974).
20. J. W. Hopewell, D. W. H. Barnes, D. T. Goodhead, J. F. Knowles, G. Wiernik, and C. Young, The relative biological effectiveness of fast neutrons (42 MeV leads to Be) for early and late normal tissue injury in the pig. Int. J. Radiat. Oncol. Biol. Phys. 8:2077 (1982).
21. H. R. Withers, H. D. Thames, D. Hussey, B. L. Flow, and K. A. Mason, Relative biological effectiveness (RBE) of 50 MV (Be) neutrons for acute and late skin injury, Int. J. Radiat. Oncol. Biol. Phys. 4:603 (1978).
22. H. R. Withers, H. D. Thames, B. L. Flow, and K. A. Mason, The relationship of acute to late skin injury in 2- and 5-fraction/week gamma-ray therapy, Int. J. Radiat. Oncol. Biol. Phys. 4:595 (1978).
23. H. L. Atkins, R. G. Fairchild, and J. S. Robertson, Dose-rate effects on RBE on californium and radium reactions of pig skin. Radiology 103:439 (1972).

NEUTRON CAPTURE THERAPY IN SUPPORT OF OTHER RADIATION TREATMENT

Borje Larsson

Department of Radiation Sciences
Uppsala University
Box 535, S-751 21 Uppsala, Sweden

INTRODUCTION

Neutron capture therapy (NCT) appears potentially useful, not only as a treatment modality per se, but also as an adjuvant in the context of established clinical measures to control pathological growth. Since the probability of local control is a steep function of absorbed dose, even a modest specific exposure of neoplasms by such techniques would significantly increase the chances of cure. Such a prospect seems most natural in fast neutron therapy [1,2,3] where slow neutrons are automatically available in the target area. As a promising alternative, it would be possible to combine the use of protons or heavier ions with a booster therapy based on boron compounds and intermediate-energy neutrons.[4] Such a situation would be particularly relevant when there are needs both for the precision of heavy charged-particle beams--permitting tailored 3-dimensional dose plans for the treatment of structures visible by computerized imaging methods--and for the particular features of NCT that also aim at eradication of invisible but suspected microsopic growth in larger anatomical regions.

A conceived combination of accelerated heavy particles and moderated spallation neutrons is attractive from a practical standpoint, in the research phase, because it can be realized in one and the same environment, i.e., a high-current cyclotron or linear accelerator facility. This is a technical reason why NCT and allied problems have been made part of the biomedical program for the 200 MeV Gustaf Werner cyclotron in Uppsala.[5] More important, at this time, is the scientific motive that cell-seeking boron compounds are very useful models for other nonradioactive or radioactive, targeting pharmaceuticals designed for diagnosis or therapy in various types of neoplastic disease. Boron compounds can be detected by sensitive track-etch techniques, at the microscopical level.[6] Because ^{10}B is stable, there is the additional possibility of labelling with radionuclides to permit a coordinated macroscopic study by positron or single photon emission tomography.[7]

The basic and applied NCT research program in Sweden has otherwise the same immediate goals as those of other groups interested in this field: (1) Development of non-reactor sources of intermediate-energy neutrons; (2) development and tests of boron compounds with selectivity for neoplastic cells; (3) design of treatment protocols that favor high uptake in pathological structures and low exposure to the reaction products of neutron capture in critical healthy structures; and (4) improved knowledge of the radiobiological aspects of NCT. Noteworthy aspects of this work will be briefly reviewed here below, with reference to published material or developments in progress. The headings PHYSICS, PHARMACOLOGY, PHYSIOLOGY, AND RADIOBIOLOGY are used to signify the mentioned four research efforts.

It should be noted that the Studsvik R2-0 reactor facility provides a special heavy-water moderated thermal beam dedicated to this program.[8] This resource is being used whenever thermal neutrons are required for the experiments, for neutron capture radiography or for neutron irradiation of cell cultures or experimental animals.

PHYSICS

The applied physics project is focused on the development of an accelerator-based spallation source for neutron capture therapy by intermediate-energy ("epithermal") neutrons, as described in a separate report in these proceedings.[5] In this context the choice of target-moderator configuration is being addressed, as well as techniques of neutron spectroscopy and dosimetry. The project is run in close collaboration with the Paul Scherrer Institute, in Villigen, Switzerland.

PHARMACOLOGY

In neutron capture therapy, the aim is to induce, by neutron irradiation, a curative amount of alpha and ^{7}Li tracks through the cellular nuclei of the neoplastic target structures. At present, we therefore devote much effort to the development of quantitative measuring techniques for determination of boron localization in cells, tumor spheroids, and tissues at the microscopic level.[9] At the same time the distribution of boron in tumor models is studied by gross quantitative autoradiography.[10] Of special interest are boronated amino acids, melanin precursors, porphyrins, and various receptor-seeking antibody or growth factor derivates. Most of this work is made within the framework of interdepartmental or international collaborations.[11] The various boron preparations are tested in single cell culture, tumor spheroids, or animal models with murine or human cell lines (usually derived from glioma, colorectal carcinoma or melanoma).

PHYSIOLOGY

Through the above-mentioned and other contacts with the international community of boron chemists and drug-targeting specialists, we hope to eventually identify boron compounds that would qualify for pre-therapeutic realistic tests in animal models or humans (at diagnostic dosage). In order to meet the clinical requirements for optimization of injection and irradiation protocols, routines are now being developed for boron determination in biopsy and blood specimens. Labeling with radionuclides for positron emission tomography can be applied also, when so decided, since the proper experience and apparatus are now available (cf. ref. 5).

In NCT--more than in conventional radiotherapy--the therapeutic ratio will be dependent on physiological factors. This is evidently so because the boron concentration in various structures is the factor that decisively determines the probabilities for eradication of pathological cells, and for healthy tissue damage. It is well understood that it is not only the boron concentration, but also the localization of the disintegrating boron atoms in relation to cellular nuclei, that determines the biological effect.[11] These observations have inspired us to elucidate the uptake of boron-labeled antibodies of growth factors in target cells. The aim is to outline the microscopic behavior of the boron load in terms of cellular storage or elimination, under <u>in vitro</u> as well as <u>in vivo</u> conditions. A special place in this project is given to tumor spheroids that are used to study the transport of receptor-seeking compounds in aggregated cell structures and the behavior of the boron load at the cellular level.[12]

In a project, aiming at improved conditions for injection of therapeutic drugs, boron compounds have been injected intraarterially in combination with digestible starch particles (Spherex^{R}) that increase the period of drug occupancy in the vascular tree of the target region.[13] The results obtained in model studies with radioactive substances indicate that the tumor-blood ratio can be favorably affected by such strategies, particularly in the case of drugs that easily penetrate the blood-tumor barrier.[14]

RADIOBIOLOGY

The study of the effects of neutron capture reactions in living systems requires pure beams of slow neutrons, since the presence of fast neutrons and gamma rays make interpretation uncertain. Our initial radiobiological experiments were made with a beam of cold neutrons available at the end of a neutron beam guide at the high-flux reactor of Institut Laue-Langevin (ILL) in Grenoble, France.[14] In this way, and by combining the results with survival curves obtained at different boron concentrations at Brookhaven, it was possible to arrive at seemingly reliable values for the RBE in V79 cells, of the neutron capture reactions in boron and nitrogen.[15] Although the quality of the ILL cold neutron beams for the study of neutron capture is unsurpassed, it was decided, for reasons of convenience, to establish a useful experimental situation also in Sweden, at the Studsvik R2-0 reactor. Also here the relative content of fast neutrons is now very low. The gamma ray contamination from the reactor core is higher than in Grenoble but, with current modification of the beam channel, the dose associated with reactor gamma rays is likely to be less than 10 percent of the neutron capture dose in irradiated target cells and tissues. Experiences from preliminary experiments with cell cultures and animal tumor show the usefulness of this new thermal neutron facility that permits uniform irradiation at a fluence rate of up to $10^{10}\ n_{th} \cdot cm^{-2} \cdot s^{-1}$ in fields 20 cm in diameter.

CLINICAL IMPLICATIONS

Our plans call for the construction of a prototype intermediate-energy neutron source, for tests of NCT, adjuvant or *per se*. The clinical interest is primarily focused on vascular malformations, in the CNS and elsewhere, when irradiation could be performed by relatively small neutron fields, 4-8 cm in diameter, by cross-fire, and in single or few fractions. Boron would have to be bound to large molecules that do not penetrate the endothelial cells or basal membranes of the blood vessels. There are two options. One is the use of blood-boron dextrane, that would deliver an undiscriminated neutron capture dose to the entire vascular endothelium.[14] Another is the use of boronated substances, still of large molecular size, but with affinity for the endothelial cells. Both alternatives are being subjected to development, for evaluation in animal model experiments, with a view towards use of NCT as adjuvant to stereotactic radiation treatment with protons and photons.

In a longer perspective, depending on the outcome of the present search for efficient tumor-seeking boron compounds, there are also plans for the use of adjuvant NCT for treatment of malignant brain tumors, colorectal carcinomas and melanomas. The aim of the main conventional treatment should be curative, and the NCT dose fraction should not be expected to influence the therapeutic ratio in a negative direction. The selection of cases is an important problem, and factors such as the degree of local spread and probability of distant metastases have to be given careful consideration. From an ethical standpoint, the use of such NCT as an adjuvant to other, established types of radiation therapy is an attractive concept.

REFERENCES

1. F. M. Waterman, F. T. Kurchnir, L. S. Skaggs, D. K. Bewley, B. C. Page, and F. H. Attix, The use of ^{10}B to enhance the tumor dose in fast neutron therapy, Phys. Med. Biol. 23:592 (1978).
2. B. Larsson, Boron in fast neutron therapy? Implications of present research with slow neutrons, Strahlentherapie 160:129 (1984).
3. V. Lorvidhaya, S. Na Chiangmai, T. Vilaithong, S. Wanwilairat, N. Chawapun, O. Sornsuntisook, W. Wangpreedalertkul, Y. Anusri, and B. Larsson, Neutron treatment of cervical carcinoma - an experimental approach, Paper No. 15-6 presented at the 3rd Int. Conf. on Neutron Capture Therapy, Bremen, FRG, 1988.
4. H. Conde, E. Grusell, B. Larsson, E. Ramstrom, T. Ronnqvist, O. Sornsuntisook, S. Villa, J. Crawford, H. Reist, B. Dahl, and N. G. Sjostrand, Status report on the development of a spallation neutron source for neutron capture therapy, in: "Proc. of Workshop on Neutron Capture Therapy", Brookhaven, 1988, in press.
5. B. Larsson, Biomedical program for the converted 200 MeV synchrocyclotron at the Gustaf Werner Institute, Radiat. Res. 104: 310 (1985).
6. B. Larsson, D. Gabel, and H. G. Borner, Boron-loaded macromolecules in experimental physiology: tracing by neutron capture radiography, Phys. Med. Biol. 29:361 (1984).
7. B. Larsson, Labelled macromolecules for studies of cellular receptors in vivo, Medical Applications of Cyclotron III, Ann. Univ. Turkuensis D:17:87 (1987).
8. B. Larsson, O. Sornsuntisook, G. Ericson, E. Johansson, K. Skold, B. Nilsson, and M. Fantini, Neutron microradiography for cell-seeking boron compounds, in: "Neutron Radiography", Proc. 2nd World Conf., D. Riedel, ed., Paris (1986) p. 497.
9. J. Carlsson, G. Ericson, E. Grusell, B. Larsson, G. Possnert, F. Wikstrom, S. Na Chiangmai, O. Sornsuntisook, B. Stenerlov, and P. Stromberg, Developments in microradio-

graphy of charged particle tracks. Paper No. 9-5, presented at the 3rd Int. Conf. on Neutron Capture Therapy, Bremen, FRG, 1988.
10. D. Gabel, H. Holstein, B. Larsson, L. Gille, G. Ericson, D. Sacker, P. Som, and R. Fairchild, Quantitative neutron capture radiography for studying the biodistribution of tumor-seeking boron-containing compounds, Cancer Res. 47: 5451 (1987).
11. D. Gabel, R. G. Fairchild, B. Larsson, K. Drescher, and W. R. Rowe, The bioloical effect of the $^{10}B(n,\alpha)^{7}Li$ reaction and its simulation by Monte Carlo calculations, in: "Proceedings of 1st Int. Symp. on Neutron Capture Therapy", R.G. Fairchild and G. L. Brownell,eds., U.S. Government Printing Office (1984) pp. 128-133.
12. J. Carlsson and B. Larsson, Boron-loaded antibodies and slow neutrons: Status report from experiments on biological models II, Studies of antibody penetration in cellular spheroids, in: "Neutron Capture Therapy", ed. H. Hatanaka, Nishimura Co. Ltd., Niigata (1985), p. 359.
13. B. Larsson, J.Carlsson, H. Borner, J. Forsberg, A. Fourcy, and M. Thellier, Biological studies with cold neutrons, An experimental approach to the LET problem in radiotherapy, in: "Progress in Radio-oncology II", ed. R. H. Karcher, Raven Press, New York (1982), p. 151.
14. L. E. Lorelius, A. R. Benedetto, R. Blumhardt, H. W. Gaskill, J. L. Lancaster, and H. Stridbeck, Enhanced Drug Retention in VX2 Tumours by use of Degradable Starch Microspheres, Inv. Radiology, 19:212-5 (1984).
15. D. Gabel, R. Fairchild, B. Larsson, and H. G. Borner. The relative biological effectiveness in V79 Chinese hamster cells of the neutron capture reactions in boron and nitrogen, Radiat. Res. 98: 307 (1984).

RESEARCH ON NEUTRON CAPTURE THERAPY IN THE USSR

Yuri Ryabukhin

World Health Organisation
Geneva, Switzerland

INTRODUCTION

Research on neutron capture therapy in the USSR began in 1964 at the Research Institute for Medical Radiology, Obninsk (Ryabukhin, 1965). At that time the American trials were generally qualified as unsuccessful, but we were optimistic as ways for improvements and new approaches were coming to light (Ryabukhin, 1970a, 1970b). Towards 1975 prime knowledge in physics, pharmacology and radiobiology had been accumulated (Ryabukhin, 1972a, 1973a; Ivanov, 1974). It was realized that inherent to NCT is a variety of modalities as to the type and location of the tumour, the energy and source of neutrons, the nature and transportation of the nuclide-carrying agent (NCA), etc. Thus, it became likely that some modalities would turn out to be clinically feasible.

At the end of the 70s, studies of borane derivatives began at the All-Union Oncological Research Centre, Moscow. These studies were stimulated by the clinical trials in Japan. Still, neutron capturing nuclides (NCN) other than ^{10}B are regarded as promising.

Research was aimed at clinical trials that could ensure sufficient safety, convenience and conclusiveness. Hence, new requirements emerged (Ryabukhin, 1987), such as the pre-clinical modelling of NCT in big animals and the monitoring of tumour response to each fraction of NCT. Usual requirements are also to be met, that is:
tailoring neutron beams with an adequate intensity and energy,
choosing NCNs and finding suitable NCAs,
physical and radiobiological planning including adoption of tentative RBEs and time-fractionation regimen,
selecting tumours as candidates for NCT, and
developing techniques for monitoring NCNs in vivo.

NEUTRON PHYSICS

Reasons For Study

An optimal energy of incident neutrons had to be defined and determined in dependence upon the concentration of NCN chosen, the target depth, the beam diameter, etc. Limitations of NCT with regard to the target depth had to be identified.

Results

The optimal energies were determined on the basis of two criteria. First, a given difference between the average target dose and the highest normal tissue dose must be achieved at the minimal NCN concentration in the tumour (Ryabukhin, 1966). Secondly, the difference of dose between neighbouring tumourous and normal cells must be maximal at given concentrations of NCN in these cells (Zaichik et al, 1971a). The energies optimal for both criteria, as well as the required concentrations of NCN, sharply rise with the depth. It was recognized that NCT can be feasible only at depths less than 7-8 cm provided that broad beams of neutrons with energies not greater than 50-100 keV could be applied and NCN concentrations of tens of ug/g or more could be achieved. If a cross dimension of a neutron beam is less than 5-10 cm, the depth limit will have to be further cut back because necessary absolute concentrations of NCN are difficult to achieve except for the shallow depths (Ivanov et al, 1973a). The adverse "beam diameter effects" arise because the smaller the diameter is the less is the thermal fluence/concomitant dose ratio (Ryabukhin and Ivanov, 1973; Ivanov et al., 1975).

First clinical trials using intermediate neutrons will be carried out at a nuclear reactor. There are a few reactors available and a biomedical facility has been already set up at one of them (Zherbin et al., 1975). In the long run a clinically designated accelerator should be designed. A 2.5 MeV proton accelerator with a lithium target was considered feasible (Stepanenko et al., 1975).

Thermal, "cold" and "hot" neutrons are suitable for superficial tumours such as melanoma. For tumours at natural or surgically made cavities in the body, thermal and cold neutrons might also be applied (Ryabukhin, 1981). Especially attractive seems the idea of transporting such neutrons through a full-reflection guide to a clinical room beyond the reactor building. The guide could be jointed with a tube inserted into the cavity. The tube can be lined with a full-reflection layer for minimizing irradiation of surrounding normal tissues. The dose distribution over the target could be improved with an "adjuster" which scatters and absorbs neutrons. The reactor PIK (Erykalov et al., 1983), being completed in Gatchina, would be well suited for intracavitary NCT. Cancers of the oral cavity, uterus, colon and rectum seem suitable for such treatment.

DOSIMETRY

Reasons For Study

An ample set of techniques had to be available. Each beam should be described in terms of the energy spectrum, the flux density of neutrons, and the dose rate of accompanying gamma-rays. In planning both experimental and clinical NCT procedures the distribution of different dose components must be known.

Results

The following techniques were investigated to be used for characterisation of the beam:
combination of chemical ferrosulphate and thermoluminescent alumosilicate dosimeters for separate determination of doses from gammas and neutron collisions (Ryabukhin et al., 1969), and ^{6}Li-nitrocellulose films and copper discs for measurements of the thermal neutron fluence (Zaichik et al., 1973).

The former combination was found to be convenient also for phantom measurements (Ivanov et al., 1973b; Ryabukhin et al., 1973). The chemical yield depends on the spectrum (Ryabukhin, 1972b) which is best determined by computational methods. Spectrometric measurements such as with fission detectors. (Keirim-Marcus et al., 1973) were used for verifying the computations. Computations are indispensible to determine the dose distribution in experimental objects and in the patient. Using Monte Carlo techniques Ivanov et al. (1969, 1973c, 1974, 1975) calculated dose distributions and integral doses in body-simulating objects.

PHARMACOLOGY: LITHIUM-6

Reasons For Study

Depending on the tissue, lithium seems to be recognized by cells as a substitute for either sodium or potassium so that suitable pairs "tumour-critical normal tissue" are likely. In particular, the applicability of Li for NCT of soft tissue sarcomata and their metastases deserved investigation. The sodium-potassium pump mechanism should favour a more homogeneous distribution of lithium over the tissue. Lithium salts are permitted for clinical use in psychiatry.

Results

Among normal tissues, muscles had positive uptake against the concentration gradient, i.e. K-like behaviour, and liver and skin had negative uptake against the gradient, i.e. Na-like behaviour (Letov et al., 1970a). A radiation-induced fibrosarcoma and the

Walker carcinosarcoma in the rat did not show any active transport of Li (Letov et al., 1970b). However, it was demonstrated by neutron activation autoradiography that lung metastases of the latter tumour took up lithium to concentrations 2-3 times higher than the surrounding lung tissue (Zaichik et al., 1971b). Lithium was retained in the metastases for a time sufficient for NCT, i.e. longer than an hour. The distribution of Li appeared essentially homogeneous at the tissue level on neutron autoradiographs of normal tissues and the whole body (Zaichik et al., 1972). By contrast, the distribution in the tumourous tissue varied greatly.

Using regional perfusion with a lithium salt solution through legs of the dog, Levin et al. (1972) achieved concentrations of Li as high as over 100 mg/kg with no toxic side-effects.

PHARMACOLOGY: GAMMA-EMITTING NCNs (^{113}Cd, $^{155/157}Gd$)

Reasons For Study

Incorporation into tumour cells is not an obligatory requirement for such NCNs. Hence, even mechanical means may be used for delivering a NCN to a tumour lesion or post-surgery tumour bed. Striking differences in concentrations of Cd among some normal tissues implied the possibility of NCT of metastases. Highly selective Cd accumulation in a metastasis of hypernephroma to the lung was observed (Boekelman, 1968). There were a number of observations on cytotoxic effects of Cd compounds. The chemical versatility of Cd and Gd offers hopes for finding a suitable tumour-seeking NCA.

Results

No transplantable tumour showed selective accumulation of Cd (Ryabukhin et al., 1967; Krasnoshchekov et al., 1971). Nevertheless, Vasileva and Ryabukhin (1973) showed that some inorganic compounds of Cd retarded the growth of sarcomata in rats. Cadmium- or Gd-based moulds and cavity fillings could be easily made (Ryabukhin, 1973a). Naidenov and Raiskaya (1973) demonstrated deposition of Cd and Gd colloids in lymphatic nodules of the dog.

PHARMACOLOGY: BORON-10

Reasons For Study

Data obtained in the USA and Japan pointed to selective uptake of mercaptoboranes in brain tumours and also in murine melanomata. In searching for boron carriers applicable for many tumours, a number of carboranes and mercaptoboranes had to be synthesized and brought in to toxicological and pharmocokinetic studies.

Results

Mercaptoundecahydrododecaborane (MHB) injected i/p was selectively taken up by melanoma B-16 in the mouse (Spryshkova et al., 1980). After a week of daily injections, the ratio "tumour-tissue" achieved 39, 3.2, 12 and 1.4 for blood, skin, muscle and bone, respectively. None of 13 dicarboranes investigated had a definitely advantageous distribution. Moreover, toxicity of carborane monomer analogs of MHB was higher than that of MHB (Spryshkova et al., 1981). Oligomers had a lower toxicity. Boron seemingly incorporated into the cell nucleus and mitochondria. Shabalkin et al.(1985) showed that MHB induced transient cell proliferation and differentiation in the peripheral area of melanoma B-16. Thus, it is likely that resting melanocytes could be involved into the cell cycle after each administration of MHB during fractionated NCT.

Skoropad and Ryabukhin (1967) discussed the possibility of loading antibodies with boron, and estimated a required number of boron atoms per antibody to be not less than 1000.

RADIOBIOLOGY

Reasons For Study

It was not known what RBE should be ascribed to neutrons and the disintegration products of ^{6}Li and ^{10}B. No data were available on biological effects of internal irradiation from gamma-emitting NCNs. Suitable end-points were needed to be applied in vivo because end-points in vitro would hardly be informative enough for experimental NCT and even less for clinical NCT. Given an average NCN concentration, the response of a tumour cannot be accurately predicted due to a particular NCN distribution among and in the cells, and variations of RBE from tumour to tumour. Hence, the response should be monitored between fractions so that the initially chosen regimen could be altered for the rest of the course. As to the modelling before clinical trials of NCT, it was not clear whether experiments on NCT of small animals only would be adequate.

Results

A concept of tentative RBE was used (Ryabukhin et al., 1987). The tentative RBEs are to be replaced by "therapeutically derived" RBEs after each series of NCT trials in animals or humans. A "standard irradiation isoeffective dose" of 10 Gy per fraction was thought likely in future clinical trials of NCT. Given this dose, Ryabukhin (1972a) figured out tentative RBE values of 5.2 and 3.5 respectively for the disintegration products of ^{6}Li and ^{10}B in the connective tissue, on the assumption that the intracellular concentrations were equal to the average ones for that tissue.

Corrections can be made to allow for differences between these concentrations. A relatively high value of 4.1 was figured out for broad spectrum neutrons used in experiments on NCT. Neutrons with energies below 0.35 MeV contributed half the absorbed dose. For the N (n,p) reaction, we arrived at a tentative RBE value of 3.0.

Having studied effects of intermediate neutrons, Obaturov (1987) concluded that elastic collisions which become dominant below a neutron energy of 2 keV may have an RBE as high as 20-60. Thus, the 2 keV neutrons do not appear as advantageous as thought before.

Intralymphatic administration of Cd or Gd colloids resulted in such high concentrations in lymphatic nodules of the dog that these nodules could absorb thermal neutrons in a "black hole" manner (Ryabukhin, 1972a). Irradiation in an intermediate neutron beam completely destroyed these nodules. Conversion electrons in the case of Gd may significantly contribute to the dose.

The change of tumour volume in time provides a relatively simple opportunity for evaluating the tumour response to irradiation in vivo (Spryshkova et al., 1986). Once lethally damaged cells have died out, the volume undergoes retardation which may depend exponentionally on the dose. That was observed after X-ray irradiation of B-16 melanoma in the mouse. Then this end-point was used to compare effects of a thermal beam alone, the capture reaction on boron delivered as MHB, and X-rays. At "standard irradiation isoeffective doses" of about 10 Gy, RBE values turned out to be 3.9 and 1.9 for the nitrogen and boron capture, respectively. These results are preliminary and more data is needed about the intracellular contents of nitrogen and boron in B-16 to review our suprising findings.

Feinendegen, Porschen and other researchers showed in numerous experiments that radioiodine-labelled IUdR can be used to assess cell loss and suppression of DNA synthesis that are important for monitoring the tumour response. It should be noted that IUdR can be labelled with different iodine radioisotopes to distinguish between responses to successive fractions. Following this line (Ryabukhin, 1984) we studied in vivo the kinetics of the radioiodine label in melanoma B-16 and sarcoma-180 after irradiation followed by injection of IUdR. Using a simplified model for IUdR metabolism, Ryabukhin et al. (1986) estimated levels of radioiodine retention in these tumours after different doses. The reduced retention is thought to reflect suppression of DNA synthesis. For practical reasons, it may be enough to measure the drop of radioactivity at the initial segment of the kinetic curve (Spryshkova et al., 1986). The tumour responses to X-ray irradiation assessed by the indices of volume retardation and DNA synthesis suppression appeared to correlate quite well with each other. RBE values for the nitrogen and boron reactions estimated from the latter index, turned out to be 3.8 and 2.3, respectively. Again, these values should be regarded as preliminary.

In our experiments with thermal neutron beams, small animals could be easily protected against irradiation of large portions of their body so that the animals could be followed-up for a time. For the modelling of NCT of deep-seated tumours using Li and intermediate neutrons, the small animals including rats were found inadequate (Ryabukhin et al., 1973; Letov et al., 1976). The contribution of the capture on Li to the biologically isoeffective dose in a 5-cm diameter beam was only 20% or less. The contribution could be increased by enlarging the irradiation area but this led to premature radiation death of rats. Therefore, it was only in the Walker carcinosarcoma but not in the radioresistant fibrosarcoma that some effect of neutron capture on ^{6}Li could be observed.

ELEMENTAL CONTENTS OF TISSUES

Reasons For Study

Irradiation with neutrons may do more harm than good if NCN concentrations and their distribution over tissues and time are not adequate. Concentrations of native elements such as hydrogen and nitrogen in specific tissues are also important. It was necessary to evaluate analytical means for measuring concentrations of hydrogen, nitrogen and especially those of NCN. There are significant individual variations in NCN concentrations and in their distribution. Therefore, such analytical means were sought that NCN concentrations for each procedure of NCT could be measured.

Results

A technique was developed for estimating average concentrations of ^{6}Li in vivo by radiometry of ^{18}F produced in a secondary reaction. The technique was demonstrated for extremities of the rabbit (Kalashnikov, 1972).

Borisov and Naidenov (1986) developed a prompt gamma technique for estimating ^{10}B in vivo in tumours of the mouse, so that boron could be followed-up during a few days.

Any results on average concentrations of Li or B should be supplemented by an investigation on the contents of these NCNs in the cells of interest. Neutron autoradiography techniques were mastered for this purpose (Ryabukhin and Zaichik, 1972).

Average concentrations of nitrogen were determined in biopsy samples by activation with fast neutrons from a reactor (Ryabukhin, 1967) and by photoactivation (Ryabukhin, 1973b). A technique based upon activation of indium by epicadmium neutrons scattered in the sample, turned out to be satisfactory for the determination of average concentrations of hydrogen. Enhanced concentrations of nitrogen and hydrogen were revealed, for example, in samples of osteogenic sarcoma as compared with normal bone tissue (Kalashnikov et al., 1973). Until their concentrations are known at the cellular level, it is questionable whether these findings really imply an enhanced tumor dose, or even an outlook for "nitrogen" NCT .

CONSIDERATIONS ON FUTURE DEVELOPMENTS

The first clinical goal seems to be NCT of melanoma with the use of MHB as a "universal" NCA applicable also for other tumours. Thermal neutrons can be available at three reactors, at least. Techniques for the determination of boron in vivo should be tried in big animals and in patients who would be candidates for NCT. A few of IUdR-based techniques for monitoring the tumour response between fractions should be tested and compared with clinical observations. Melanin-related agents could be used at a later stage.

Trials should be performed for NCT of osteosarcoma in dogs using MHB or a Li-salt administered by regional perfusion. Intermediate neutrons can be available for such experiments at two reactors, at least. Contingent on the results obtained, clinical trials could be discussed. In case of successful NCT of primary osteosarcoma, NCT could be extended to its metastases in the lung and other organs.

NCT of brain tumours is accounted as prospective, but its implementation depends on the availability of a source of intermediate neutrons in the vicinity of a specialized medical institution.

Intracavitary NCT with guides of cold or thermal neutrons looks a good prospect for the treatment of colorectal, gynaecological and oral cavity tumours. Various boron-carriers including antibodies, as well as fillings containing gamma-emmitting NCNs could be tried. The reactor PIK (Erykalov et al., 1983) seems to be the most suitable for this NCT modality.

From weighting its advantages and disadvantages, NCT has to be given, as a rule, in fractions. The decisive advantage is a greater assurance that in the end the tumour will be eradicated and normal tissues spared. This consideration is especially important at initial phases of trials and, therefore, all the potential for monitoring the tumour response between fractions should be utilized. Advantages from the radiobiological viewpoint are the greater repopulation of normal tissues and the redistribution of tumour cells with regard to their ability for taking up NCNs. An important advantage is that the minimum flux density required for NCT is reduced proportionally to the number of fractions.

The disadvantages seem to be:

difficulties in increasing the number of therapeutic procedures,
decrease in efficiency of the boron reaction due to the statistical fluctuations of disintegrations,
accumulation of chemical toxicity of NCN after each fraction, and additional expenditures for a costly NCN agent and procedures.

It may be concluded that the scientific and technological base created in the USSR holds good prospects for putting NCT into clinical practice.

REFERENCES*

Boekelman, W., 1968, Opneming van cadmium door niercarcinomen bij mens en dier, Ned.T.Geneesk., 112:1511.

Borisov, G. I., and Naidenov, M. G., 1986, A direct method for controlling tissue and equivalent doses from thermal neutron irradiation, Byull. Izobr., N35, 23 Sept.:1.(R)

Erykalov, A. N., Kondurov, I. A., Konoplev, K. A., Krasotsky, Z. K., Petrov, Yu. V., Sumbaev, O. I., and Trunov, V. A., 1983, "Research Potentialities of the PIK Reactor," Leningrad Institute of Nuclear Physics, preprint 852, Leningrad.(R)

Ivanov, V. N., 1974, "Theoretical and Experimental Studies on the Dose Distribution for Neutron Capture Therapy," Ph. D. Degree, Moscow.(R)

Ivanov, V. N., Ryabukhin, Yu. S., Parfenov, E. N., and Ignatev, U. V., 1969, Calculations of tissue doses from broad neutron beams with a Monte Carlo technique, Med. Radiologiya, 14, N3:47.(R)

Ivanov, V. N., Ryabukhin, Yu. S., Ivanova, L. F., and Parfenov, E. N., 1973a, "Nuclide Concentrations Needed for Neutron Capture Therapy with Finite Diameter Beams," VNIIMI, Moscow.(R)

Ivanov, V. N., Ryabukhin, Yu. S., Letov, V. N., and Ivanova, L. F.,1973b, Dosimetrie der Neutronenbündel eines Reaktors bei strahlentherapeutischen Unterssuchungen, Radiobiologia Radiotherapia (Berlin), 14:557.

Ivanov, V. N., Parfenov, E. N., and Ryabukhin, Yu. S., 1973c, Calculations of tissue doses for oblique incidence of neutrons, Med. Radiologiya, 18, N2:54.(R)

Ivanov, V. N., Ivanova, L. F., Parfenov, E. N., and Ryabukhin, Yu. S., 1974, Integral absorbed doses in neutron capture therapy, Med. Radiologiya, 19, N1:50.(R)

Ivanov, V. N., Ivanova, L. F., Parfenov, E. N., and Ryabukhin, Yu. S, 1975, Tissue doses due to irradiation with neutron beams, Atomnaya Energiya, 39:360.(R)

*The references in Russian are marked with (R).

Kalashnikov, V. M., 1972, Calculation of an effective cross section for the ^{18}F production in biological tissues saturated with lithium during neutron capture therapy, in: "Summary Reports at the Conference of Young Scientists and Specialists," Research Institute for Medical Radiology, Obninsk.(R)

Kalashnikov, V. M., Litvitsky, A.M., Ryabukhin, Yu. S., and Khrushchev, V. G., 1973, Photoactivation analysis of nitrogen and phosphorus in normal tissues and tumours of the bone, in: "Summary Reports at the All-Union Seminar on the Use of Accelerators for Elemental Analysis," Moscow.(R)

Keirim-Marcus, I. B., Kraitor, S. N., Popov, V. I., Ivanov,V.N., Ryabukhin, Yu. S., and Efimov, I. A., 1973, Use of new dosimetric methods for radiobiological research at reactor radiation beams, in: "Dosimetry in Agriculture, Industry, Biology and Medicine,"IAEA, Vienna.(R)

Krasnoshchekov, G. P., Ryabukhin, Yu. S. and Vasileva, N. A., 1970, Incorporation of ^{109}Cd into an ascitic hepatoma, Med. Radiologiya, 15, N12:46.(R)

Letov, V. N., Ivanov, V. N., Ryabukhin, Yu. S., Uspensky, V. A., and Gorvat, F. Yu., 1970a, Incorporation of Li^6 into tissues, organs and transplanted tumours of rats, Med. Radiologiya, 15, N11:50.(R)

Letov, V. N., Ivanov, V. N., Ryabukhin, Yu. S., Uspensky, V. A., and Gorvat, F. Yu., 1970b, A study of the lithium distribution for normal rats and rats with the Walker carcinosarcoma, Med. Radiologiya, 15, N12:12.(R)

Letov, V. N., Ryabukhin, Yu. S., and Ivanov, V. N., Experimental research on ^6Li neutron capture therapy, in: "Extrapolation from Radiobiological Experiments to Man," Moscow, 1976.(R)

Levin, Yu. M., Nikitina, P. G., and Ryabukhin, Yu. S., 1972, Perfusion of the dog extremity with lithium chloride in connection with its use in neutron capture therapy, Med. Radiologiya, 17, N6:29.(R)

Naidenov, Yu. P., and Raiskaya, T. N., 1973, Saturation of lymphatic nodules with ^{113}Cd, a neutron capturing nuclide, in: "Radiation and Organism," Obninsk.(R)

Obaturov, G. M., 1987, Outcome of studies on biological effects of neutrons, Med. Radiologiya, 32, N9:20.(R)

Ryabukhin, Yu. S., 1965, Some new ways for neutron capture therapy, in: "Summary Reports of the First Conference of Institute for Medical Radiology," Obninsk.(R)

Ryabukhin, Yu. S., 1966, The optimal energy of incident neutrons in neutron capture therapy, Med. Radiologiya, 11, N6:9.(R)

Ryabukhin, Yu. S., 1970a, The status and future for neutron and neutron capture therapy, Med. Radiologiya, 15, N5:74.(R)

Ryabukhin, Yu. S., 1970b, Neutron capture therapy of malignant tumours, Med. Radiologiya, 15, N8:81.(R)

Ryabukhin, Yu. S., 1972a, "Nuclear Reactions and Activation

Induced by Reactor Neutrons, for Medical Purposes," D. Sci. Thesis, Leningrad.(R)
Ryabukhin, Yu. S., 1972b, Application of the standard ferrosulphate dosimeter for reactor radiations, in: "Dosimetry and Radiation Induced Processes in Dosimetric Systems," Tashkent.(R)
Ryabukhin, Yu. S., 1973a, Medical applications of nuclear reactions induced by reactor neutrons, in: "Radiation and Organism", Obninsk.(R)
Ryabukhin, Yu. S., 1973b, Photonuclear activation analysis in medicine, in: "Summary Reports at the All-Union Seminar on the Use of Accelerators for Elemental Analysis," Moscow.(R)
Ryabukhin, Yu. S., 1981, Prospects in research on neutron capture therapy, in: "Prospects in the Use of Basic Facilities at JINR for Biological Research", Dubna.(R)
Ryabukhin, Yu. S., 1984, The problem of individualized monitoring for tumour and normal tissue responses during radiation therapy, Strahlentherapie, 160:678.
Ryabukhin, Yu. S., 1987, Problems of neutron capture therapy, in: "Proceedings of the 8th International Congress of Radiation Research," vol. 2, E. M. Fielden, J. F. Fowler, J. H. Hendry, and D. Scott, eds., Taylor and Francis, London.
Ryabukhin, Yu. S., and Ivanov, V. N., 1973, Thermal neutron fluxes in a tissue-like phantom irradiated with finite diameter neutron beams, Med. Radiologiya, 18, N1:51.(R)
Ryabukhin, Yu. S., and Zaichik, V. E., Neutron activation autoradiography in medicine, in: "Radiation Medicine," Moscow, 1972.(R)
Ryabukhin, Yu. S., Baranova, F. S., Vasileva, N. A., Uspensky, V. A., and Filin, E. V., 1967, Experimental neutron capture therapy, in: "Radiation and Organism", Obninsk.(R)
Ryabukhin, Yu. S., Tkachenko, V. V., Bologova, G. S, Vakhlakova, T. V., Obaturov, G. M., and Vasilev, A. G., 1969, Chemical and thermoluminescent dosimetry of neutron beams at a fast reactor, Med. Radiologiya, 14, N8:66.(R)
Ryabukhin, Yu. S., Letov, V. N., and Ivanov, V. N., 1973, On the possibility of extrapolation from results of experimental neutron capture therapy research to the clinics, Med. Radiologiya, 18, N7:41.(R)
Ryabukhin, Yu. S., Sevastyanov, A. I., and Spryshkova, R. A., 1986, Effect of X-ray irradiation on the IUdR label kinetics in a tumour, Med. Radiologiya, 31, N9:35.(R)
Ryabukhin, Yu. S., Chekhonadsky, V. N., and Sushikhina, M. A., 1987, The concept of isoeffect dose in radiation therapy, Med. Radiologiya, 32, N4:3.(R)
Shabalkin, I. P., Spryshkova, R. A., and Serebryakov, N. G., 1985, Cell population kinetics in transplantable B-16 melanoma after administration of ^{10}B-enriched mercapto-undecahydrododecaborane, Med. Radiologiya, 30, N11:32.(R)

Skoropad, Yu. D., and Ryabukhin, Yu. S., 1967, The possibility of using antibodies as carriers for neutron-capturing nuclides in NCT, Med. Radiologiya, 12, N6:53.(R)

Spryshkova, R. A., Bratsev, V. A., and Shabalkin, I. P., 1980, The use of dimercaptoborane derivatives for neutron capture therapy, Med.Radiologiya, 25, N11:46.(R)

Spryshkova, R. A., Karaseva, L. I., Bratsev, V. A., and Serebryakov, N. G., 1981, Toxicity of functional derivatives of polyhedral carboranes, Med.Radiologiya, 26, N6:62.(R)

Spryshkova, R. A., Sevastyanov, A. I., Naidenov, M. G., Ryabukhin, Yu. S., and Serebryakov, G. N., ^{125}I-Iodoxyuridine and the response of experimental tumours to irradiation, 1986, Med. Radiologiya, 31, N9:40.(R)

Stepanenko, V. F., Ivanov, V. N., Kononov, V. N., and Stavissky, Yu. Ya., 1975, On the use of an intermediate energy neutron source like the accelerator KG-2.5 for neutron capture therapy, in: "Summary Reports at the All-Union Seminar on Problems in the Development of Radiotherapeutic Facilities," Moscow.(R)

Vasileva, N. A., and Ryabukhin, Yu. S., 1973, Toxicity of Cd compounds and their effects on transplantable sarcomata as related to the possibility of using Cd for neutron capture therapy, in: "Radiation and Organism", Obninsk.(R)

Zaichik, V. E., Ivanov, V. N., and Ryabukhin, Yu. S., 1971a, Local dose inhomogeneity in neutron capture therapy, Med. Radiologiya, 16, N8:63.(R)

Zaichik, V. E., Krasnoshchekov, G. P., Letov, V. N., and Ryabukhin, Yu. S., 1971b, Quantitative autoradiography of ^{6}Li in lung metastases of the Walker carcinosarcoma, Med. Radiologiya, 16, N2:47.(R)

Zaichik, V. E., Stepanenko, V. F., and Ryabukhin, Yu. S., 1972, Zur quantitativen Neutronenaktivierungs-Autoradiographie von ^{6}Li in Biopräparaten mit Hilfe von Nitrozellulosefilm, Radiobiologia Radiotherapia (Berlin), 13:691.

Zaichik, V. E., Ivanov, V. N., Kalashnikov, V. M., Ryabukhin, Yu. S., and Stepanenko, V. F., 1973, Thermal neutron flux measurements in neutron capture therapy, Atomnaya Energiya, 34:393.(R)

Zherbin, E. A., Ivanov, V. N., Luchnik, N. V., Efimov, I. A., Zeinalov, E. I., Obaturov, G. M., and Shalin, V. A., 1975, Experience in constructing neutron biomedical beams and prospects for their use, Med. Radiologiya, 20, N7:52.(R)

BNCT PROJECT IN CZECHOSLOVAKIA

J. Burian[1], I. Janku[2], J. Kvitek[3], V. Mares[4], Z. Prouza[5], F. Spurny[6], K. Sourek[7], B. Stibr[8], and O. Strouf[8]

1Institute of Nuclear Resesarch, Czechoslovak Atomic Agency, Prague
2Institute of Pharmacology, Czechoslovak Academy of Sciences, Prague
3Institute of Nuclear Physics, Czechoslovak Academy of Sciences, Prague
4Institute of Physiology, Czechoslovak Academy of Sciences, Prague
5Institute of Biophysics and Nuclear Medicine, Faculty of Medicine, Charles University, Prague
6Institute of Radiation Dosimetry, Czechoslovak Academy of Sciences, Prague
7Neurosurgical Clinic, Faculty of Medicine, Charles University, Prague
8Institute of Inorganic Chemistry, Czechoslovak Academy of Sciences, Prague

INTRODUCTION

In Czechoslovakia, a multidisciplinary research group for BNCT of human brain gliomas has been constituted in 1980. Mercaptoborane compound has been synthesized suitable for clinical use. The configuration of a thermal neutron beam with appropriate parameters has been created using the 10 MW VVR-S research reactor and proved experimentally. The realization of a technical project for a clinical pilot study could be expected by 1992. The project has been sponsored by the Czechoslovak Academy of Sciences and Faculty of Medicine, Charles University in Prague.

In the multimodality treatment of malignant gliomas the methods and the long-term results in Czechoslovakia do not differ substantially from those reported in other countries. The mean survival of our patients does not exceed 12 months, and the quality of the post-operative life is still far from satisfactory. This situation motivated neurosurgeons to look for a more efficient treatment of malignant brain gliomas.

Boron Neutron Capture Therapy (BNCT) seemed to us to be the most attractive method, not only because of its theoretical radiobiological advantages and selectivity, but also for its availability in Prague.

The first practical contacts with clinical BNCT were made during a visit to Hatanaka in Tokyo in 1978.[1,2,3] In 1980 we formed a research group, getting together a broad spectrum of workers. The preliminary goal of our multidisciplinary group was to reproduce and verify Hatanaka's procedure using mercaptoborane and the source of appropriate thermal neutrons at the Research Reactor in Rez near Prague. Simultaneous research into the new boron compounds and later into alternative radiation techniques with epithermal neutrons should form the basis for further progress in the clinical use of BNCT.

BORON COMPOUNDS-CHEMISTRY, PHARMACOLOGY, BIOLOGY

A six-step synthesis of $Na_2{}^{10}B_{12}H_{11}SH$ from $^{10}B(OH)_3$, shown in Fig. 1, was developed as an alternative to the recently published procedure.[3]

Typically the total yield from the process is in the range of 23-25% (based on $^{10}B(OH)_3$ used) and the isotopic purity of the product is 97%. Steps (ii)-(iv) are the subject of three Czechoslovak patents[4-6] and steps (v) and (vi) represent a modification of the earlier method of Tolpin et al.[7]

$^{10}B(OH)_3$ →(i)→ $^{10}B(OR)_3$ —(ii)→ $Na^{10}BH_4$ →(111) $Et_3N^{10}BH_3$ —(iv)→ $Na_2{}^{10}B_{12}H_{12}$ —(v)→ $Na^{10}B_{12}H_{11}$ · NMMBT (vi)→ $Na_2{}^{10}B_{12}H_{11}SH$

Fig. 1. The synthesis of $Na_2{}^{10}B_{12}H_{11}SH$.

Reagents:
(i) etherification with $MeOC_2H_4OC_2H_4OH$;
(ii) Na, Al, H_2 higher pressures, elevated temperature;
(iii) Et_3N, $CO_2(g)$, $Na^{10}BH_4$, 230-250°C;
(iv) NMMBT (N-methyl-=2-mercaptobenzthiazol);
(vi) NaOH

Of potential interest for NCT seem to be the C-substituted derivatives of the closo-$(1\text{-}CB_{11}H_{12})^-$ anion. These were prepared[8-10] according to Figs. 2 and 3.

For studying biological effects, Na^+ $(1\text{-}Me_2N\text{-}1\text{-}CB_{11}H_{11})^-$ and Na^+ $(1\text{-}MeNH\text{-}1\text{-}CB_{11}H_{11})^-$ salts were prepared by treatment of the last two species with NaOH. Other C-substituted derivatives of $(1\text{-}CB_{11}H_{12})^-$ were prepared[10] as in Fig. 3.

To determine the small amount of $Na_2B_{12}H_{11}SH$ in tissue for neutron capture therapy two independent analytical methods were examined: colorimetry and emission spectrometry. The first was a modification of the Soloway-Messer method[11,12] based on 1:1 complex of boric acid and 1,1'-dianthrimide with absorption maximum at 620 nm. In the oxidation step, sodium persulfate was used instead of the dangerous 90% hydrogen peroxide. The dynamic range of the method is 0.8-8 μg B for $B(OH)_3$, the regression coefficient being above 0.99. This extremely versatile method gives results for twenty samples within 2.5 hours. The effect of interference of biological matrix on sensitivity as well as the accuracy of the method is discussed. The method has been used in a preliminary pharmacological study on mice and rabbits.

The second method - emission spectrometry - has a linear dynamic range 0.05-6.7 μg B for $Na_2B_{12}H_{11}SH$ in murine tissue (brain, blood, kidney, liver). The method avoids the necessity to convert $Na_2B_{12}H_{11}SH$ to boric acid: a biological sample (8-25 mg) is decomposed on the electrode and directly analyzed. The line for boron at 249,773 nm and the line at 259,254 nm of germanium (internal standard) are evaluated in terms of the difference of

$B_{10}H_{14}$ —(i)⟶ $(B_{10}H_{13}CN)^{2-}$ —(ii)⟶ $7\text{-}H_3N\text{-}7\text{-}CB_{10}H_{12}$ ⟶

—(iii)⟶ $7\text{-}Me_3N\text{-}7\text{-}CB_{10}H_{12}$ —(iv)⟶ $1\text{-}Me_2NH\text{-}1\text{-}CB_{11}H_{11}$ ⟶

—(v)⟶ $1\text{-}MeNH_2\text{-}1\text{-}CB_{11}H_{11}$

Fig. 2. Preparation of C-substituted derivatives of closo-$(1\text{-}CB_{11}H_{12})^-$ anion.

Reagents:
(i) KCN, H_2O;
(ii) concd. HCl;
(iii) Me_2SO_4; NaOH:
(iv) Et_3NHB_3, 200°C;
(v) CH_2O, K_2CO_3, I_2.

corrected values P. This parameter and the logarithm of boron concentration have a linear relation with regression coefficients higher than 0.97 for all tissues studied. The method does not suffer from the negative influence of biological matrix and thus can be used for checking of the routine colorimetric method.

The most sensitive quantitative method for determination of boron is based on the detection of prompt alpha particles from $^{10}B(n_{th},alpha)^{7}Li$ nuclear reaction. Originally, this technique was developed for boron determination in semiconductors.[13] Thin slices or liquid suspensions of biological materials are deposited into thin Al foils and dried. The samples are analyzed in a vacuum chamber, situated in a horizontal neutron beam from a VVR-S research nuclear reactor. Thermal neutron flux at the sample is $1.4 \times 10^{8}\ s^{-1}.sm^{-2}$. Alpha particles are registered by a semiconductor surface-barrier detector connected with standard spectrometric chain. The resulting spectra of alpha particle energy are stored in the memory of ND-66 multichannel analyzer and evaluated on computer. Typical measuring time is several tens of minutes per sample, for samples with total boron content higher than 10^{14}at.$^{10}B.cm^{-2}$. Boron distribution over the sample can be mapped subsequently by shielding different parts of the sample. With time, this technique of boron analysis was steadily improved, so that the current detection limit is as low as 10^{11} at.$^{10}B.cm^{-2}$. A further substantial decrease of the detection limit is expected in the future, when a neutron guide about 5 m in length will be put into operation.

At present, we are preparing alpha autoradiography combined with the computerized image analysis of tissue sections.

The pharmacological studies of acute toxicity revealed the LD_{50} as 308 mg/kg in mice for i.v. injection. The sub-acute toxicity of mercaptoborane was tested in mice for i.v. doses of 50,100 and 150 mg/kg for 7 days. No sub-acute toxicity was found except for slight leucopenia in 150 mg/kg dose. No neurotoxic effects of the mercaptoborane were found in mice, either after i.v. injection of 100 mg/kg or after intraventricular instillation of 20 μg per mouse.

In the preclinical biological studies we examined the cell and tissue uptake of mercaptoborane into biopsies of human brain tumor, and into animal and human cells grown in cultures by using neutron-induced nuclear reaction. It was found that the uptake of the drug into tumor biopsies *in vitro* is higher than in the samples of the normal surrounding brain parenchyma.[14] Studies on cultures of several types of cell (normal and tumorous animal and human cells) showed that the uptake of mercaptoborane is more intense in cells growing at higher rate. Further, the rate of the uptake of ^{10}B was, in general, faster than its release from the cells previously exposed to ^{10}B[14,16]. Recently we started to irradiate rats injected with mercaptododecaborane, as well as human glioma cells in cultures to test the irradiation conditions in TK 12 channel.[15,16]

NEUTRON BEAM CONFIGURATION AND DOSIMETRY

The studies were performed on the reactor VVR-S in the Nuclear Research Institute in Rez. This research tank-type reactor is usually exploited on 5-6 mW power. For NCT the graphite-thermal column was used in two configurations (Fig. 4).

The vertical channel TK 12 was modified for irradiation of mice. With bismuth filters the thermal neutron flux of 3.10^9 n/cm^2 was obtained with gamma-to-neutron ratio about 5%.

The moderating and shielding layers (graphite, heavy water, lead and bismuth) were placed in the empty space of the thermal column (Fig. 5). The design was made by use of transport codes ANISN and DOT and verified by direct measuring. The thermal neutron flux was 5.10^8 n/cm^2/s when the reactor power was 30 kW.

We used the following dosimetric methods and detection systems.

Phantom, optimizing (shielding configurations) measurements are performed by the following methods:

- distribution of a thermal neutron flux density, activation of a sandwich of foils (Au, Au+Cd)[17];
- gamma-dose - a system of TL detectors differing in neutron sensitivities (^{7}LiF, Al_2O_3, $CaSO_4$:Dy)[18];
- neutron dose - Czechoslovak Si diode.[19]

$1\text{-}Me_2NH\text{-}1\text{-}CB_{11}H_{11}$ —(i)⟶ $1\text{-}Me_3N\text{-}1\text{-}CB_{11}H_{11}$ ⟶

—(ii)⟶ $(1\text{-}CB_{11}H_{12})^-$ —(iii)⟶ $(1\text{-}HS\text{-}1\text{-}CB_{11}H_{11})^-$

$(1\text{-}CB_{11}H_{12})^-$ —(iv)⟶ $(1\text{-}HOCO\text{-}1\text{-}CB_{11}H_{11})^-$

Fig. 3. Preparation of C-substituted derivatives of $(1\text{-}CB_{11}H_{12})^-$

Reagents: (i) Me_2SO_4, NaOH;
(ii) Na/NH_3(l);
(iii) LiBu, S;
(iv) LiBu, CO_2

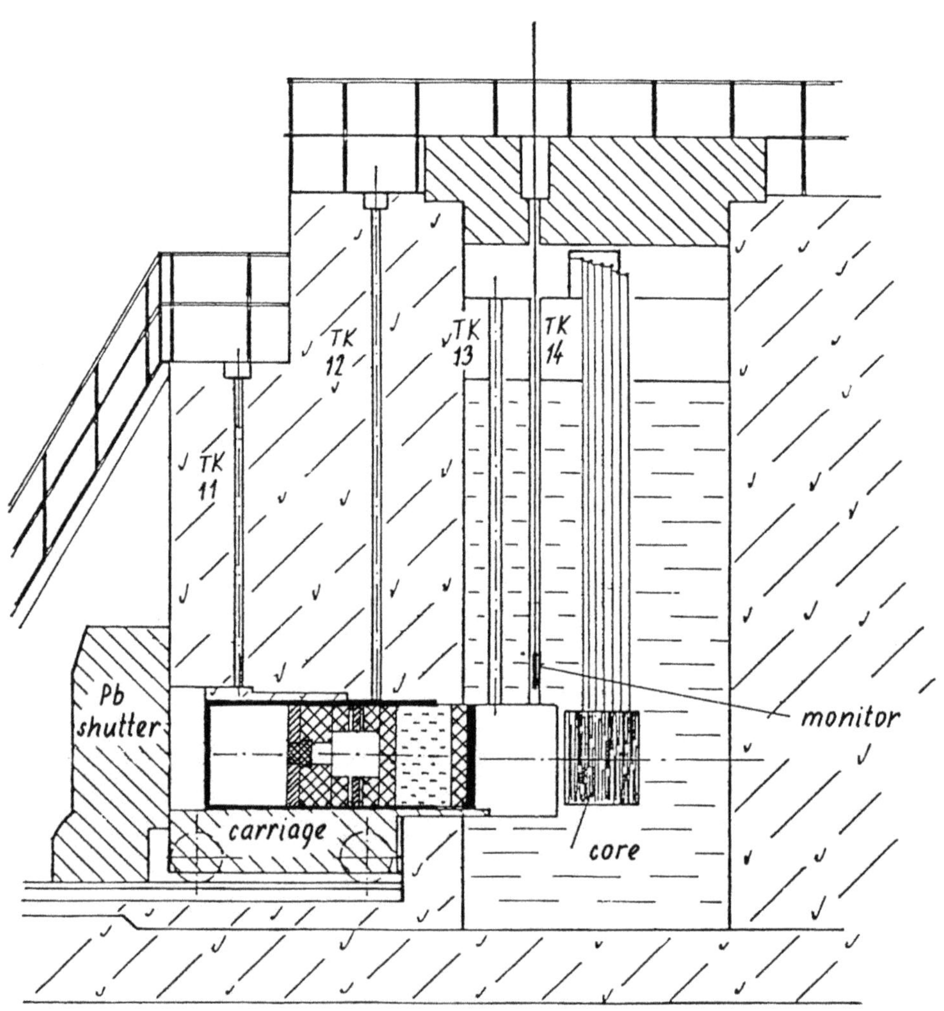

Fig. 4. Experimental situation on the reactor VVR-S.

The use of the activation detectors represents the classical method which is sufficiently sensitive and precise for the given purpose (activities of Au-foils are measured by the absolutely calibrated gamma spectrometer CANBERRA with the GeLi detector).

The TLD system was checked in many radiation fields. Sensitivities of the particular detectors to different types of radiations were determined, which made it possible to determine the neutron dose by correcting the observed sensitivities to mixed radiation fields (in the given case to thermal neutrons, on the basis of data gained from Au-detectors).

The quick and easy determination of neutron dose is done by the Czechoslovak Si-diode. Simultaneously, the developed diode exhibits the sensitivity ≈1 V/Gy and it is practially kerma-equivalent for neutrons with energies above 100 keV (the sensitivity to gamma-rays, expressed in kerma, is by three orders of magnitude lower).

All three methods provide local information and fully comply with the aim - a scanning of model fields and phantom measurements.

To estimate neutron energy distribution, the moderation method (Bonner spectrometer) was used. The ^{6}LiI crystal connected with a one-channel analyzer serves as a detector. The spectrum unfolding is carried out with the help of the program SAND II and the program BAY[20] which is based on the method of the conditional probability. The BAY provides mean values of dosimetric quantities and their confidence intervals.

Moreover, pair ionization chambers (Al+argon, tissue-tissue, a sensitive volume of about 1 cm^3, which have been tested extensively[21], are available. They make it possible to determine tissue kerma of both gamma rays and of fast neutrons. However, their use is limited by their sensitivity (≈1 μGy/h).

Monitoring of nuclear reactor power is ensured by:

- the BF_3 proportional counter covered by the Cd-filter;
- the semiconductor detector DTN with the ^{6}LiI radiator placed in the polyethylene sphere having the diameter 50.8 cm (with the Cd-filter).

A dynamical measurement during biological experiments (when monitoring the power as mentioned above) was performed at an object, using the thermal neutron detector based on the Si-detector with the ^{6}LiI converter. Almost directionally

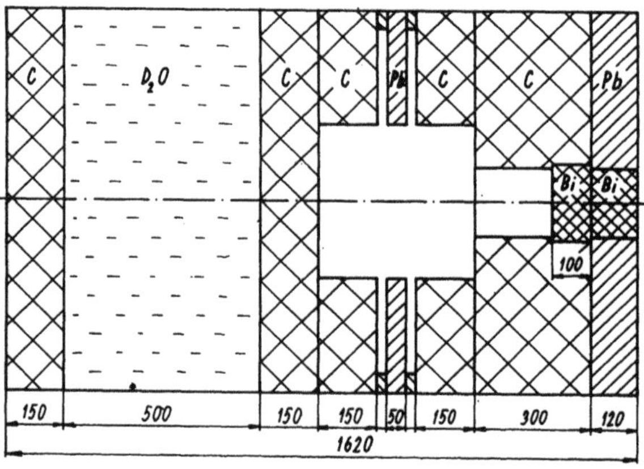

Fig.5. Moderating and shielding layer - variant (c)

independent measurement of thermal neutron flux densities greater than 10^2 $cm^{-2}s^{-1}$ is achieved in this way[22]. The sensitivity of the detector to gamma rays and to fast neutrons is three orders of magnitude lower (expressed in kerma).

PROSPECTS FOR THE CLINICAL USE OF BNCT IN CZECHOSLOVAKIA

Taking into account the theoretical and technical problems, the realistic goal of the individual steps for the BNCT is:

1. A clinical pilot study of the distribution and pharmcological properties of mercaptoboron in humans 1989
2. Microdistribution of boron in human gliomas, brain tissue and blood vessels.................... 1990
3. Realization of a technological project for the clinical use of BNCT in malignant glioma.... 1991.

The wider use of BNCT in clinical cases of malignant gliomas cannot be expected before 1995, because of the long-term followup needed after the first procedures. Theoretical as well as technical failures would postpone the clinical use much more; moreover, new developments in oncology could make the BNCT completely out of date. Nevertheless, in the present situation, BNCT presents the most attractive way of treating malignant tumors. A concentrated, well-planned research effort that is internationally focused seems to be the best way to prove or to realize the concept of BNCT in a relatively short time.

REFERENCES

1. H. Hatanaka and W. H. Sweet, Slow-neutron capture therapy for malignant tumours. Its history and recent development. in: Biomedical Dosimetry, International Atomic Energy Agency, 147-178, Vienna (1975).
2. F. Tovarys, Lecba mozkovych nadoru zachytem tepelnych neutronu na boru. Cas. Lek. ces., 29:118 (1979).
3. M. Komura, K. Aono, K. Nagasawa, and S. Sumimoto, Chem. Express 2:173 (1987).
4. B. Casensky and J. Machacek, Czech. Pat. 187046.
5. J. Plesek, B. Stibr, E. Drdakova, and T. Jelinek, Czech. Pat. Appl. PV 8695-84.
6. J. Plesek, B. Stibr, and E. Drdakova, Czech. Pat. 238254.
7. E. I. Tolpin, G. R. Wellum, and S. A. Perley, Synthesis and chemistry of mercaptoundecahydro-closo-dodecaborate (2-), Inorg. Chem. 17:2867 (1978).

8. J. Plesek, T. Jelinek, E. Drdakova, S. Hermanek, and B. Stibr, A convenient preparation of 1-$CB_{11}H^-{}_{12}$ and its C-amino derivatives, Collect. Czech. Chem. Commun. 49:1559 (1984).
9. J. Plesek, T. Jelinek, and B. Stibr, Unusual demethylation of 1-dimethylamine-1-carba-closo-dodecaborane (11), Polyhedron 3:1351 (1984).
10. T. Jelinek, J. Plesek, S. Hermanek, and B. Stibr, Chemistry of compounds with the 1-carba-closo-dodecaborane (12) framework, Collect. Czech. Chem. Commun. 51:819 (1986).
11. A. H. Soloway and J. R. Messer, Anal. Chem. 36:433 (1964).
12. A. Kaczmarczyk, J.R. Messer, and C. E. Pierce, Rapid method for determination of boron in biological materials, Anal. Chem. 43:271 (1971).
13. J. Cervena, V. Hnatowicz, J. Hoffman, Z. Kosina, J. Kvitek, and P. Onheiser, The use of neutron induced reaction for boron profiling in Si, Nucl. Instr. and Meth. 188:185 (1981).
14. V. Mares, M. Baudysova, J. Kvitek, J. Sykorova, J. Cervena, J. Vacik, V. Hnatowicz, and Z. Kunc, Uptake of $Na_2B_{12}H_{11}SH$ in cell lines and human biopsies. in: "Molecular Basis of Neural Function," S. Tucek et al., eds., E.S.N., Prague, 1978.
15. V. Mares, J. Burian, M. Baudysova, Z. Prouza, and Z. Kunc, Interaction of thermal neutrons and boron-10 in the immature brain, Physiol. Bohemoslov. 36:545 (1987).
16. M. Baudysova, V. Mares, J. Kvitek, J. Cervena, J. Vacik, V. Hnatowicz, and Z. Kunc, Incorporation of $Na_2{}^{10}B_{12}H_{11}SH^{2-}$ used for boron neutron capture therapy into tumor-derived and normal cells, Physiol. Bohemoslov. (in press).
17. Z. Prouza, D. Nikodemova, A. Hrabovcova, J. Kubeckova, H. Solnicka, Jaderna energie 24:6,213 (1978) (Engl.)
18. F. Spurny, R. Medioni, G. Pescayre, and G. Portal, Proc. 3rd Symp. Neutron Dosimetry in Biology and Medicine, Neuherherg, 977, EUR 5848 DE/EN/FR, Luxembourg, 77 (1978) (Engl.).
19. A. Skubal, Z. Prouza, J. Hermanska, Energy and kerma dependence of the Czechoslovak dosimetric Si-diode, Jaderna energie 31:10,371 (1985) (Engl.).
20. J. Hermanska, Z. Prouza, M. Karny, and I. Nemec, Bayes-based dose equivalent estimation using multisphere data, Kernenenergie 30:10,409 (1987).
21. F. Spurny and I. Votockova, Proc. 4th Symp. Neutron Dosimetry,Neuherberg, 1981, EUR 7448 EN, Luxembourg, 327 (1981) (Engl.).
22. J. Huylka, Z. Hrdlicka, Z. Janout, S. Pospisil, Z. Kansky, and Z. Prouza, Merenidistribuce hustolg tokutepelnych neutroni v objektu, modeljicim lidske telo, ponoce polovodicoveho kremikoveho detektoru S ^{6}Li-konvertorem, Jaderna energie 31:10,376 (1985).

PROPOSED CLINICAL TRIAL STUDYING THE PHARMACOKINETICS OF B.S.H.

William Frederic James Harkness

Department of Neurosurgery
The Radcliffe Infirmary
Oxford, U.K.

INTRODUCTION

There has been considerable interest in BNCT at Oxford for several years, which has been facilitated by the proximity of the clinical Departments of Neurosurgery and Radiotherapy as well as the Radiobiology unit and the Atomic Energy Research Establishment at Harwell. Each unit has been collaborating over this time with the end objective of a therapeutic facility at Harwell.

In the Department of Neurosurgery, we are about to embark on a clinical study of the pharmacokinetics of a boron compound. This is a non-therapeutic trial as we cannot offer a neutron facility at Harwell as yet. Full approval of the Ethical Committee has been granted.

Boron Compound

We intend to use $Na_2{}^{10}B_{12}H_{11}SH$ (BSH) as a vehicle for ^{10}B administration. Although this may not be the ideal compound, it has the advantage of having undergone extensive investigation in animals and humans. There also is a well-established source of supply. We are interested in the possibility of using other compounds in the future and developing new compounds.

Patient Selection

The patients who will be included in the trial will be over 18 years of age, with a pre-operative clinical diagnosis of malignant glioma. We shall obtain informed consent from the patient, and they will be free to discuss the trial with their relatives.

We will exclude from the trial patients whose tumors we feel are inoperable. In view of the potential damage to the liver and the possibility of cardiac side effects, we will exclude people with a history of liver or cardiac abnormality and those with abnormal liver enzymes or ECG.

Administration of BSH

The BSH will be given in solution intravenously over approximately four hours with continuous cardiac monitoring. We do not think it is ethically justified to give the compound via the carotid when there is evidence that the intravenous mode is equally effective. Initially, we will be giving a single dose, as the pharmacokinetics need to be studied fully before multiple doses are considered.

The dosages that we intend to give are between 12.5 mg and 50 mg ^{10}B/kg. The assumption has been made that there is a linear relationship between dosage and its concentration by the tumor. Existing data does not appear to support this, but by varying the concentration, we may prove or refute this assumption. Also, it may prove necessary to increase the dose as the trial progresses.

Sampling and Measurement

Blood and urine specimens will be taken at six-hourly intervals after the administration of the BSH to reinforce the existing data on the metabolism of BSH. At surgery, we will take specimens of normal brain, tumor, skin, bone, muscle and CSF. The delay between administration of BSH and surgery will be varied, so that we can gauge the optimal timing for therapy. This knowledge is especially important as data from the radiobiology unit suggests that fractionation over 5 days is desirable, and thus we need to know if a single dose of BSH will be adequate. Before surgery, daily blood tests will be taken to assess hematocrit and liver functions tests, and these parameters will be monitored post-operatively.

Analytical Method

In conjunction with G. Constantine at AERE, Harwell, we plan to analyze the liquid and solid specimens by the solid-state track etch technique. We feel this technique has proven accuracy, and we have made trial runs with standardized boron solutions. We also hope to perform quantitative neutron capture radiography on the histological specimens.

DISCUSSION

Our subjects, unlike those of other groups, will never have undergone previous surgery. It is difficult to predict the mode of entry of boron into the tumors under these circumstances. It may also be argued that it is not a therapeutically meaningful situation, as we intend to irradiate following definitive surgery. However, we are sure that there will be variation in BSH uptake due to individual patient variation and to histological variation of the tumors. For this reason, we hope to study as many patients as is practically and financially possible.

The administered dose of BSH and the sampling time are the two main variables in our trial. As the trial progresses it may be necessary to adjust one or other of these parameters to gain further information.

FRACTIONATION IN BORON NEUTRON CAPTURE THERAPY

K.R. Durrant and J. Hopewell

The Churchill Hospital
Oxford, England

INTRODUCTION

The theoretical basis has been described for the value of BNCT in the treatment of cerebral glioblastoma multiforme.[1] Early clinical trials in the United States showed unexpected and excessive damage to normal brain tissue. Subsequent analysis suggests that this damage was due to high levels of boron in blood at the time of irradiation. After modification of the technique, Hatanaka[2] demonstrated that the method is effective, with 30% of the patients in his study surviving five years. This is a striking result in the treatment of a tumor, where a 95% two-year mortality and 100% five-year mortality can be expected after treatment by conventional photon radiation therapy.[3] It also is clear that some patients tolerated the treatment without gross intellectual damage, although data on normal tissue damage in this series is incomplete.

In both series of patients, irradiation was given as a single dose, mainly because it was necessary to irradiate intraoperatively with reflection of the scalp to avoid excessive damage to superficial normal tissues from the low-energy (thermal) neutrons. Current evidence suggests that epithermal neutron beams could be used more effectively with sparing from excessive superficial tissue damage and more even irradiation of deeper cerebral tissue. This change would allow irradiation without surgery (other than pre-irradiation diagnostic surgery) and, therefore, treatment with fractionated irradiation--the division of the total radiation dose into smaller increments over a period of time. Although this regime would have the advantage of reducing the period that the patient is immobilized during any one treatment session, it would have some disadvantages. Neutron irradiation from reactors is expensive, and during the period of treatment (which would include the time taken to move the patient in and out of the area and to position him, which is a considerable period of time in conventional therapy and would be much longer if a reactor were used), the treatment port would be unavailable to other users, thus increasing the expense as well as the complexity of the irradiation. Further, in centers without preexisting treatment rooms, the extensive shielding used around the patient, including the head, would be subjectively unpleasant and anesthesia may be necessary, entailing multiple inductions and anesthetics, with the attendant risks and complexities. Boron compounds themselves are in short supply. The plasma half-life of these compounds is not known exactly, but it is clear that, with fractionated radiation therapy, considerably more boron will be required for each patient.

The most critical factor in determining optimal fractionation is that of the tolerance of normal tissue (neural and vascular) to this form of mixed radiation and its variation with different types of fractionation. It is essential to avoid the severe damage to normal neural tissue that occurred with some previous attempts at BNCT.

CLINICAL FACTORS

The clinical benefit of fractionation for photon irradiation was established quantitatively by Strandqvist[4], although empirical observations 30 years before had shown that multiple small fractions of radiation treatment could cure a tumor without the high incidence of necrosis of normal tissue, which occurred with radiation in a single fraction. This process led to the general acceptance that for all but a few normal tissues that are particularly radiosensitive, a total dose of 60 Gy (6000 rad) in 30 treatments over 42 days is the maximum dose that can be tolerated by a modest (10 x 10 x 10 cm) volume of normal tissues. For normal adult brain, volumes larger than this should not be irradiated over 40 to 45 Gy (4000 to 4500 rad) in fractionated doses.

RADIOBIOLOGY

Radiobiological data suggest that the main benefit of fractionation therapy with low-LET radiation is the repair of sublethal irradiation damage,[5] most of which takes place within 6 to 24 hours after irradiation. A further factor in reducing radiation damage of normal tissue is repopulation, the regeneration of surviving cells during the intervals between radiation treatment. This process is principally important in rapidly proliferating normal tissue.

PREDICTION OF THE EFFECTS OF NON-STANDARD FRACTIONATION

Neither the radiobiological data nor statistical analysis of clinical data with different fractionation schedules allows an accurate and safe prediction of the effects of new fractionation schedules. In a recent pilot study of accelerated fractionation (multiple treatments per day and shortened overall treatment time), an untoward increased incidence of excessive damage to normal tissue was found, despite theoretical calculations indicating that the dose used was within the normal limits of tissue tolerance. The only safe test of new fractionation schedules is the controlled clinical trial.

BNCT

In BNCT there are three major radiation products: the high-LET alpha particles of the $B(n,\alpha)Li$ reaction, the recoil protons from the incident neutron beam in non-borated tissue, and the low-LET gamma radiation, both from the treatment beam and from that induced in the reaction. Damage from the gamma radiation component is likely to be considerably reduced by fractionation. If a differential concentration of boron between tumor cells, normal nervous tissue cells and blood and endothelial cells is achieved, there would be a ten-fold differential dose to tumor versus normal tissue cells. Most radiation damage of non-borated tissue would arise from gamma radiation with the proton recoil effect dependent upon the energy of the neutron beam.

The most significant difference between neutron and photon irradiation is the greater biological effectiveness of neutrons, associated with the reduction of repairable sublethal damage. These affect both total dose and fractionation. For very high-LET radiation, radiobiological data suggests that fractionation would not reduce radiation damage. However, data for neutron irradiation at c.16 MeV from Hornsey (unpublished) and Hopewell[7] suggest that for both spinal cord and skin, the fractionation of the neutron dose of 4 to 6 fractions results in increased repair of sublethal damage, but that further fractionation would not reduce late radiation damage significantly.

Using the Harwell Pluto reactor with a neutron flux of 5×10^{12}, an estimated dose of 100 Gy to the tumor cells, and a normal tissue dose of 10 Gy from the neutron flux, the dose would ideally be divided into 4 to 6 fractions. Until data is provided to the contrary, this would seem the minimum safe fractionation for giving BNCT in the initial stages of new trials. However, before this it will be necessary to establish firmly the distribution of boron compounds in the tumor, normal brain and blood and their pharmokinetics, the radiation dosimetry of the beams used, and also to do large studies on animal skin to assess the approximate radiation tolerance.

CLINICAL TRIALS

The most important clinical use of BNCT and its ultimate aim is to irradiate patients with glioblastoma multiforme. However, there are considerable uncertainties about the levels of boron compounds in brain tumor cells, normal neural cells and blood vessels that would be obtained and about radiation dosimetry. In view of the previous lethal complications in experimental BNCT for brain tumors, any modified BNCT would be better tested clinically at an anatomical site where radiation toxicity is unlikely to be fatal or to produce severe intellectual damage. The first clinical trials ideally would be carried out in patients with incurable disseminated tumors with multiple accessible lesions whose response to different treatments could be assessed objectively. If the experimental irradiation was used only on limb lesions, it would be possible to safely and accurately evaluate the response of the tumors to different radiation doses at different boron levels using several dose schedules. Such a trial would facilitate the quantitative assessment of the toxicity of this radiation to normal human tissues. It would be essential to use the standard methods used in clinical oncology at this time to assess efficacy and toxicity. These were described in detail[8] and are currently considered the only acceptable form of reporting the results of experimental cancer treatment.

PROPOSAL FOR EARLY CLINICAL TESTING OF BNCT

Introduction

A good test model for BNCT would be the treatment of patients with extensive incurable recurrent or metastatic melanoma of the limbs. Chemotherapy is not very effective, surgery cannot cure patients once the disease has spread, and conventional radiotherapy is of very limited value.

It would be ethically justifiable to request volunteers from patients with this stage of disease to cooperate in a study of BNCT, which may be of palliative value to them. Radiation treatment of tumors on limbs is unlikely to produce lethal complications. Malignant melanomas concentrate some boron compounds. Boron concentrations in tumor and normal tissue can be measured from biopsies taken under general anesthesia given for the BNCT.

Each separate tumor would be measured accurately in two diameters, and then the response to different irradiation doses accurately determined. Similarly, the response of normal tissue (skin, connective tissues, and vasculature) would be assessed using a standard scoring system.[10] The responses of normal tissue and tumor could be related to the known tissue levels of boron, of radiation dose and radiation fractionation. Standard test systems used by RTOG and EORTC would be used.

Objectives of the Trial

1. To assess the response rates of inoperable, recurrent or metastatic malignant melanoma of the limbs at different levels of boron in tissue and blood and increasing fractionated radiation doses in boron neutron capture therapy.

2. To evaluate the side-effect profile of BNCT with dose escalation on the skin, connective tissue and blood vessels.

Selection of Patients

Criteria for Inclusion.

1. Histologically verified malignant melanoma.

2. Radically inoperable disease of limbs (palliative surgery does not exclude).

3. Measurability in two dimensions (WHO criteria).

4. No concomitant or previous irradiation to the sites being assessed.

5. No cytotoxic chemotherapy for the previous 6 weeks.

6. Protocol agreed by local hospital ethical or human science committee.

Criteria for Exclusion.

1. Tumors of head, chest or trunk.

2. Patients with severely reduced pulmonary function (clincal examination, CXR, FVC).

3. Patients with impaired renal function (creatinine clearance less than 50 ml/m).

4. Patients in poor general condition. PF of 4, or Karnofsky <30, unlikely to survive for more than three months untreated.

5. Patients with severe co-existent somatic or psychological disease.

6. Other concurrent or previous malignancy except BCC skin.

Trial Design.

1. Patients can only enter the study and receive randomization after investigation and assessment has confirmed that disease is not curable (possibly other than by amputation).

2. Stratification will be made by the Center.

3. Five daily treatments or five treatments in ten days will be used.

4. Dose escalations of 20%, 40%, 60%, 80% and 100% of a calculated full dose will be used in successive patients, treating three patients at each dose level, unless acute toxicity exceeds a defined level (grade 4).

5. Patients with multiple co-existent lesions can be randomized to receive different escalations of dose for the different lesions after at least three dose-escalations have been tested in earlier patients.

6. The minimum duration of treatment for assessment of tumor response will be four days.

7. The minimum period of observation for assessment of acute toxicity will be four weeks and for assessment of late toxicity, three months.

8. Follow-up will be weekly for six weeks, then monthly for one year.

9. End-points are:

   a. tumor response (WHO criteria)

   b. duration of response

   c. acute toxicity for normal tissue

   d. late toxicity for normal tissues

Therapeutic Regimens

Boron dose required to produce levels in the tumor of approximately 30 μg/g will be used.

Radiation Dose. A maximum tolerance neutron dose of 5×10^{12} is assumed from previous data and will be divided into five doses. Dose increments of 20% of the maximum dose per session will be given with subsequent treatments.

Each dose will be given to the lesion or lesions for assessment with a minimum of 1 cm and a preferred rim of 3-5 cm of apparently normal adjacent skin.

No medication other than 1% hydrocortisone ointment should be applied to the irradiated area.

In the event of severe acute skin toxicity (grade 4), subsequent dose schedules should be one increment lower.

Treatments may be given using full or basal anesthesia if patients desire this because of the nature of neutron shielding that is necessary.

Required Clinical Evaluation, Laboratory Tests, and Follow-Up

Pre-treatment tests include histological confirmation of diagnosis of malignant melanoma, and tests included under criteria for exclusion.

Tumor size will be measured by three observers before the treatment starts, every two weeks until the sixth week, then monthly.

Skin toxicity will be assessed by three observers using WHO/RTOG grades weekly for six weeks, then every six weeks for eight months (weeks 0, 1, 2, 3, 4, 5, 6, 12, 18, 24, 30, 36, 42, 48, 54). The late toxicity system also will be used.

Criteria for Evaluation

WHO/RTOG criteria of tumor response and early and late toxicity will be used.

REFERENCES

1. R. G. Zamenhof, B. W. Murray, G. L. Brownell, G. R. Wellum, and E. I. Tolpin, Boron neutron therapy for the treatment of cerebral gliomas, Med. Phys. 2:47 (1975).

2. H. Hatanaka, K. Amano, S. Kamano, and K. Sano, Clinical experience of boron neutron capture therapy for malignant brain tumors (1968-1985), in: "Neutron Capture Therapy," H. Hatanaka, ed., Nishimura, Tokyo (1986).

3. M. D. Walker, S. B. Green, and D. P. Byar, Randomized comparison of radiotherapy and nitrosoureas for malignant gliomas after surgery. N. Eng. J. Med. 303:1323 (1980).

4. M. Strandquist, Studien ube die Kumulative Wirkung der Roentgenstrahlen bei Fraktionierung. Acta Radiol. (Suppl) 55:1 (1944).

5. M. M. Elkind, H. Sutton-Gilbert, W. B. Moses, T. Alescio, and R. W. Swain, Radiation response of mammalian cells in culture, Radiat. Res. 25:359 (1965)

6. F. Ellis, Dose, time and fractionation: a clinical hypothesis. Clin. Radiol. 20:1 (1969).

7. J. W. Hopewell, D. W. H. Barnes, M. E. C. Robbins, J. M.Samson, J. T. Knowles, and G. J. M. J. van den Aardwig, The relative biological effectiveness of fractionated doses of fast neutrons for normal tissues in the pig. Brit. J. Radiol. (in press).

8. A. B. Miller, B. Hoogstraten, M. Staquet, and M. D. Winkler, Report: results of cancer treatment. Cancer 47:207 (1981).

9. B. J. Allen, J. K. Brown, and B. Harrington, Neutron capture therapy research for malignant melanoma, in: "Neutron Capture Therapy," H. Hatanaka, ed., Nishimura, Tokyo (1986).

10. J. F. Fowler, R. L. Morgan, and J. A. Silvester, Experiments with fractionated x-ray treatment of the skin of pigs. Br. J. Radiol. 36:188 (1963).

DOSE FRACTIONATION IN NEUTRON CAPTURE THERAPY FOR MALIGNANT MELANOMA

B. J. Allen and J. K. Brown

Australian Nuclear Science & Technology Organisation
Lucas Heights Research Laboratories
Private Mail Bag 1
Menai NSW 2234 Australia

INTRODUCTION

Australia is entering a joint clinical trial with Japan for thermal Neutron Capture Therapy of selected patients with superficial local recurrent, local advanced and isolated metastatic malignant melanoma. The para-boronophenylalanine (BPA) compound will be used with a neutron fluence of about 10^{13} neutrons per cm^2 , to be delivered in a single dose. While in the initial trials of NCT, the single dose is a practical procedure, there may be advantages in dose fractionation, and these are considered in this paper.

ANAESTHESIA

In the initial NCT procedure of Mishima et al.[1], the patient was anaesthetised for the duration of the exposure. In this case the tumour was at the back of the head, and the anaesthetic ensured the patient's comfort and immobility of the well defined target area. However, if therapy sessions were short enough and the location of the tumour readily accessible to the neutron beam, then patients might not need to be anaesthesised. The maximum exposure time would depend on the site of the tumour and the patient's comfort, but 15-30 minutes might be considered typical, requiring 6-12 fractions to deliver 10^{13} neutrons per cm^2 at a neutron flux of 10^9 neutrons $cm^{-2}s^{-1}$. Unless a beam shutter was available, run-up and run-down times for the reactor power would add considerably to the total elapsed time.

RADIATION ENHANCEMENT OF MELANISATION

A further, yet unconfirmed, advantage of dose fractionation may lie in the increased melanisation which has been observed in surviving melanoma cells following both high and low LET radiation exposures[2]. BPA and most other melanoma-affined biochemicals target cells synthesising or containing melanin. Stimulation of this condition should improve the efficacy of NCT, particularly with respect to the more amelanotic metastases. Radiation stimulation of melanisation would be more practical than the use of substituted melanotropins or melanin stimulating hormone[3], theophylline[4] or arabinofuranosylcytosine[5], but may be unsuitable because of the time required between fractions for adequate melanisation, if the results of 5-10 days in vitro can be taken as a guide. However, for some compounds such as BPA or decarbonyl thiouracil (B-TU), stimulation of the tyrosinase activity happens on a much shorter time scale[3] and would ensure enhanced uptakes.

INTERNALISATION OF MONOCLONAL ANTIBODIES

A number of melanoma-associated antigens have been identified on the membranes of human melanoma cells, each with receptor densities of about 10^6 sites. Boron-conjugated monoclonal antibodies (MCA) with about 1000 boron atoms are required to saturate the available sites to achieve the required boron loading per cell. However, the effectiveness of boron atoms at the cell membrane is markedly reduced[6] relative to those in the nucleus.

Internalisation of antibodies bound to membrane antigens, with subsequent re-expression of the free antigen, was recently reported[7]. Modulation of the surface membrane of the human melanoma SK-ME128 by ^{111}In-labelled MCA96.5, which recognises the p97 determinant, was examined using direct radioimmunoassay and indirect fluorescent antibody staining. The MCA was internalised within 24 hours, and a second treatment increased the cell-associated activity, while at the same time rendering the cells immunofluorescent again. The p97 antigens underwent endocytosis following exposure to the MCA, and were regenerated and expressed on the cell membrane.

This observation opens up the possibility of pumping boron into a cell in excess of the saturation antigenic density, until boron equilibration is achieved. Neutron capture immunotherapy (NCIT) therefore, could be preferred over immunotherapy with toxins (e.g.ricin), or radioisotopes (e.g.^{125}I) which are limited by critical organ tolerance.

Boron-MCA inoculations could maintain saturated cell capacity, during a course of fractionated therapy. But rejection of the mouse antibody is expected to occur within eight to fourteen days[8] so extended dose fractions with successive antibody inoculations would need to be given within this period.

RADIOBIOLOGY

Critical factors in conventional radiotherapy are the kinetics of reoxygenation, cell cycle redistribution, the repair of sublethal damage, fractionation and repopulation of tumour cells[9] How important are these factors in NCT? The Li and He ions emitted in the boron neutron capture reaction are high LET radiations with dE/dX~100 keV μm^{-1}, with radiobiological properties similar to those for fast neutrons.

Reoxygenation

Hypoxic cells, being starved of oxygen, are inactive and relatively insensitive to low LET radiation and, to a much lesser extent, to high LET radiation. If the oxygen tension across 150 μm of tumour from the vasculature is inadequate, what is the likelihood of boron compounds reaching these hypoxic cells? The transfer of boron carriers to hypoxic regions of the tumour may occur by either passive diffusion, or by active transfer by the microvascular system of the tumour. The former would ensure adequate boron uptakes whereas the latter might not. Experiments with hypoxic cell sensitisers show that passive diffusion can occur[10]. Further, after perilesional injection of BPA, NCT of a highly heterogeneous swine melanoma[11] showed no local recurrence after many months, suggesting that all cells took up adequate concentrations of boron.

The monomer and dimer of $Na_2B_{12}H_{11}SH$ were distributed differently in the viable and necrotic regions of mouse tumours[12], the former showing uptake in necrotic cells while the latter did not. Boron distributions across tumour sections were obtained by neutron radiography. While the monomer and dimer may have different transport mechanisms, the possibility that cells were killed after uptake of the monomer cannot be excluded.

It appears then that slowly metabolising boron carriers can be decoupled from the oxygen tension by diffusing through the extra-cellular space. For systemic boron carriers which are subject to reduced uptake by hypoxic cells, fractionation would be expected to enhance the efficacy of NCT. The results reported by Coderre et al. (this volume) for single and two-dose fractions for NCT of Hardy Passey melanoma support this contention.

Cell Cycle Redistribution

One disadvantage of using large dose fractions in low LET radiotherapy lies in the partial synchronisation of cells in the radioresistant phase of the cell cycle. This is undesirable for slowly proliferating tumours, but could be useful for sparing normal cells. The variation of cell cycle radiosensitivity for high LET radiation is much smaller, and the RBE for normal and malignant cells would be similar. The therapeutic gain, being the ratio of tumour and normal cell RBE, would be close to unity and fractionation would not have a significant effect on the high LET component of NCT.

Sublethal Damage

For low LET radiation, small dose fractions allow repair of sublethal damage in normal cells. This effect is not significant for high LET radiation because of the single-hit characteristic of survival curves. NCT reactor beams give exponential in vitro survival curves as a function of dose, showing the dominance of neutron effects over those of the concomitant gamma dose. The boron capture reaction increases the high LET component even more. However, low LET radiation is the major source of whole body dose, and contributes about half of the RBE dose to the normal cells around a superficial tumour. Fractionation would reduce the damage to these cells.

Fractionation and Tumour Cell Repopulation

Major disadvantages of fractionation are the increased time required for a course of radiation, and the repopulation of tumour cells between dose fractions.

Overall, the aim of radiotherapy should be to deliver the maximum dose tolerated by critical late-responding tissues, in the shortest time consistent with acceptable acute morbidity. Because NCT produces high LET radiation, this aim is probably best achieved by few, rather than many, dose fractions.

ACKNOWLEDGEMENT

The assistance of the US Department of Energy in allowing one of us (BJA) to attend the workshop on Clinical Aspects of Neutron Capture Therapy is gratefully acknowledged.

REFERENCES

1. Proceedings of the Second Japan-Australia Workshop on Neutron Capture Therapy for Malignant Melanoma, to be published in Pigment Cell Research, 1988.
2. D. Barkla, B. J. Allen, J. K. Brown, and M. M. Mountford, Ref. 1.
3. Z. A. Abdel Malek, K. L. Kreutzfeld, M. M. Marwan, M. E. Hadley, V. J. Hruby, and B. C. Wilkes, Prolonged stimulation of 591 melanoma tyrosinase by [Nle^4,D-Phi^7] - substituted α - melanotropins. Cancer Res. 45:4735 (1985).
4. M. L. Steinberg, and J. R. Whittaker, Stimulation of melanotic expression in a melanoma cell line by theophylline. J. Cell. Physiol. 87:265 (1976).
5. T. H. Lee, M. S. Lee, and M. Lee, Effects of α-MSH on melanogenesis and tyrosinase of B-16 melanoma. Endocrinology, 91:1180 (1972).
6. D. Gabel, S. Foster, R. G. Fairchild, Monte Carlo simulation of the biological effect of the $^{10}B(n,\alpha)^7Li$ reaction in cells and tissue and its implication for boron neutron capture therapy, Radiation Res. 111(1):14 (1987).
7. S. Wang, A. L. Lumanglas, J. Silva, V. Ruszala-Mallon, F. E. Durr, Internalisation and re-expression of antigens of human melanoma cells following exposure to monoclonal antibody. Cell Immunology, 106:12 (1987).
8. P. Hersey, Preclinical and phase I studies of monoclonal antibodies in melanoma - application to boron neutron capture therapy of melanoma, Ref. 1.
9. H. R. Withers, H. D. Thames, Jr., L. J. Peters, Biological bases for high RBE values for late effects of neutron irradiation, Int. J. Radiat. Onc. Biol. Phys. 8:2071 (1982).
10. E. J. Hall, "Chemical and Pharmacological Modifiers, Radiobiology for the Radiologist," Harper & Row Publishers, Inc., N.Y. (1978).
11. Y. Mishima, M. Ichihashi, M. Tsuji, M. Ueda, S. Hatta, T. Nakagawa, C. Tanaka, K. Taniyama, T. Suzuki, Prerequisites of first clinical trial for melanoma selective thermal neutron capture therapy, Neutron Capture Therapy Proc. Second Int. Sym., Tokyo, October, 1985, ed., H. Hatanaka, Nishimura, 230 (1986).

THERMAL NEUTRON CAPTURE THERAPY: THE JAPANESE-AUSTRALIAN CLINICAL TRIAL FOR MALIGNANT MELANOMA

B. J. Allen

Australian Nuclear Science & Technology Organisation
Private Mail Bag 1
Menai NSW 2234 Australia

A. S. Coates and W. H. McCarthy

The Sydney Melanoma Unit
Royal Prince Alfred Hospital
Camperdown NSW 2050 Australia

H. Mameghan

Radiation Oncology
Prince of Wales Hospital
Randwick NSW 2031 Australia

Y. Mishima and M. Ichihashi

The Institute for Neutron Capture Therapy
Kobe University Hospital
7-5-1 Kusunoki-cho Chuo-ku
Kobe Japan

MALIGNANT MELANOMA IN AUSTRALIA

Australians of Anglo-Celtic origin are constitutionally unsuited to living in a tropical environment. They suffer not only from weathered skin, solar keratoses, basal and squamous cell carcinomas, but also from an increasing incidence of malignant melanoma[1]. The northern state of Queensland has the highest incidence of melanoma in the world, at 35 cases per 100,000. New South Wales has half that rate, but because of the larger population and centralised nature of treatment, the Sydney Melanoma Unit has the largest case load in the world, with more than 700 new cases each year. Despite early diagnosis and curative surgery in the majority of these patients, there remain a number of patients with locally recurrent or metastatic melanoma which present a therapeutic challenge. Current therapy for these patients is almost always unsatisfactory.

Local recurrence near the excision scar or in the regional lymph nodes is usually managed by further radical surgery. If this is not possible, local control with radiotherapy may be achieved, but more selective destruction of recurrent melanoma and sparing of normal tissues is desirable.

Neutron capture therapy is a promising approach, which has the potential of being selective for melanoma. It may be applied to metastases in superficial areas of the body and perhaps later developed for deep-seated organs such as the brain, lung, bone and liver. The limited penetration of thermal neutron beams that are currently available is quite suited for the treatment of superficial or subcutaneous lesions. Internal metastases, however, would be more effectively treated if an epithermal beam were available.

Patients in Sydney with recurrent or metastatic melanoma may now participate in clinical trials of isolated limb perfusion, levodopa-carbidopa, bleomycin with caffeine, continuous infusion of cisplatin during radiotherapy, and adjuvant immunotherapy with vaccinia melanoma cell lysate in stage 2 or high risk stage 1 melanoma. The large number of patients and the clinical trial expertise available are well suited to the critical clinical evaluation of neutron capture therapy.

AUSTRALIAN-JAPANESE COLLABORATION

Operating within the framework of the bilateral agreement on Science and Technology between Japan and Australia, workshops on NCT for malignant melanoma were held at Lucas Heights in April 1986[2] and Kobe in September 1987[3]. These workshops stimulated national and bilateral collaborative research, and led to a joint clinical trial between the two countries using the reactor facilities and techniques developed by Mishima's group in Japan[4,5,6].

PROSPECTIVE CLINICAL TRIAL

Following the first NCT treatment for melanoma last year in Japan[3], it is planned to treat at least 12 patients during 1988, from Australia and Japan. Patients will be selected from those having evaluable superficial or subcutaneous local recurrence or isolated metastasis. In addition, selected Japanese patients with thick primary acral-lentiginous melanoma or superficially spreading melanoma (>3 mm thick) that have poor prognosis with conventional therapy (surgery plus anti-neoplastic drugs) will be treated with NCT.

Australian patients will be selected from those attending the Sydney Melanoma Unit at Royal Prince Alfred Hospital. They will have no detectable deep-seated distant metastases and should have an estimated life expectancy of at least 6 months. Locally recurrent or advanced melanoma are rare conditions, thanks to the increased awareness of the public and general practitioners and to the more stringent procedures adopted by surgeons.

METHOD

The joint trial will utilise the melanoma seeking ^{10}B compound $^{10}B_1$-boronophenylalanine.HCl ($^{10}B_1$-BPA) synthesised in Japan[4] at a dose level of 200 mg/kg. Administration will be by perilesional injection at 4 cm margin to the tumour, with boron-10 concentrations in the tumour of 20-30 μg 10B per g of tumour, to be determined by prompt analysis of boron neutron capture gamma rays before therapy. A single irradiation of about (1-1.5)x 10^{13} neutrons cm^{-2} at the tumour surface will be applied[3]. The field size of the neutron beam is defined by a ^{6}LiF shield, which absorbs the thermal neutron component. At the Musashi Institute of Technology reactor, the maximum field size is 20 x 20 cm^2. The maximum allowed dose equivalent to normal tissues will be 0.5 Sv and to the eyes 0.15 Sv, as specified in ICRP recommendations.

In the case of recurrent or metastatic melanoma, improved uptakes would result from intralesional injection. However, this method would be inappropriate because of the risk of disseminating malignant cells.

In all cases, the thermal beam will be ideally suited to the shallow nature of the lesions. It is only required that the lesion site should be readily accessible to the horizontal beam from the Musashi Institute of Technology reactor. At that reactor the neutron flux rate is 10^9 neutrons $cm^{-2}s^{-1}$, requiring exposure times of about 2~3 hours for a neutron fluence of 10^{13} neutron cm^{-2}. For this period the patient would be immobilised by anaesthesia.

The BPA compound is taken up by both melanotic and amelanotic melanomas, but retention could be 30% less for the latter[7]. Metastatic melanomas have a tendency to become less melanised, and as a consequence NCT less effective. While heavily pigmented tumours are preferred for the trial, the ultimate aim must be to cause all melanomas to regress. Preclinical results to date suggest that the NCT procedure is effective against lesions with varying degrees of pigmentation[8].

Australian patients must be in good health and spirits to tolerate protracted therapy. After the irradiation, they will return to the Sydney Melanoma Unit for ultimate follow-up.

END POINTS OF CLINICAL TRIAL

Complete local control with acceptable side effects over six months is the critical end point on which the trial is based. On return to Australia, patients will be carefully examined for local and systemic side effects and serial measurements of tumour volume will be made. Skin reaction will be gauged at weekly intervals for one month and then at monthly intervals over 12 months. Skin reaction gradings used are:

- 0 no or mild erythema
- 1 brisk erythema
- 2 dry desquamation
- 3 moist desquamation

Monthly clinical assessments and blood tests will be made to monitor the function of the liver, kidney, bone marrow and lungs. Tumour dimensions will be monitored by clinical as well as CT or MRI measurement of the height, the major diameter and the orthogonal minor diameter. Complete response would be defined according to standard World Health Organisation criteria[9].

ACKNOWLEDGEMENT

We are grateful to the Sydney Melanoma Foundation, the Department of Industry, Technology and Commerce and the Ministry of Education in Japan for their support. The assistance of the US Department of Energy is gratefully acknowledged.

REFERENCES

1. W.H. McCarthy, Malignant Melanoma. Recent Advances in Surgery, Churchill and Livingston, Ch5:87-100 (1982).
2. B.J. Allen, Australian-Japan Workshop on Neutron Capture Therapy for Malignant Melanoma. Cancer Forum, 10.2:64 (1986).
3. Y. Mishima, Second Japan-Australia Workshop on Neutron Capture Therapy for Malignant Melanoma, Kobe, Sept 1987. Papers submitted to Pigment Cell Research.

4. Y. Mishima, Selective thermal neutron capture therapy of cancer cells using their specific functional differentiation. Kyoto University Research Reactor Institute - Technical Report KURRI-TR 195: 1 (1980).
5. Y. Mishima, Selective thermal neutron capture treatment of malignant melanoma using its specific metabolic activity. KURRI-TR 260: 1 (1985).
6. H. Fukuda, T. Kobayashi, T. Matsuzawa, K. Kanda, M. Ichihashi, Y. Mishima, RBE of a thermal neutron beam and the $^{10}B(m,\alpha)^{7}Li$ reaction on cultured B16 melanoma cells, Int. J. Radiat. Biol. 51: 167 (1987).
7. M. Tsuji, M. Ichihashi, Y. Mishima, Selective affinity of ^{10}B-paraboronophenylalanine to malignant melanoma, Japanese J. Derm. 93.7:773 (1983).
8. Y. Mishima, M. Ichihashi, M. Tsuji, M. Ueda, S. Hatta, T. Nakagawa, C. Tanaka, K. Taniyama, T. Suzuki, Prerequisites of first clinical trials for melanoma selective thermal neutron capture therapy. Neutron Capture Therapy. Proc. Sec. Int. Symp. Tokyo, October 1985, Nishimura 230 (1986).
9. A.B Miller, B. Hoogstraten, M. Staquet, A. Winkler, Cancer, 47:207 (1981).

BNCT AND DOSE FRACTIONATION

John L. Russell Jr.

Theragenics Corporation
900 Atlantic Drive
Atlanta, GA 30318

Some portion of the radiation dose received by a patient during BNCT consists of primary and secondary gammas. The biological effect of that portion of the dose will depend upon the time history of the delivered dose. The well-known models for relating time-dose effects to clinical experience, principally those of Orton[1] and Ellis[2] are of questionable value in understanding dose effects in the time regime of a few hours, and for doses of less than tolerance. In order to examine the time-dose effect in the regime of interest to BNCT a simple phenomenological model was developed and normalized to the accepted body of clinical experience. The model has been applied to the question of fractionation of BNCT and the results are presented.

The model is simply a linear healing model with two time constants. In other words, a first hit of radiation is assumed to wound (or potentiate) a cell. Given time, the cell will fully repair itself. If a second hit occurs before the cell has healed, the cell is killed. Apparently, there are two kinds of healing, one which occurs in 30 to 60 minutes, the other in two to four days. A small fraction of the cells will die on the first hit, Figure 2.

The equations describing the model are:

$$\frac{dN_o}{dt} = -\phi\sigma N_o + \lambda_1 N_1 + \lambda_2 N_2$$

$$\frac{dN_1}{dt} = -\phi\sigma N_1 - \lambda_1 N_1 + \alpha\phi\sigma N_o$$

$$\frac{dN_2}{dt} = -\phi\sigma N_2 - \lambda_2 N_2 + \beta\phi\sigma N_o$$

$$N_3 = N_o(0) - N_o - N_1 - N_2$$

Table 1. Cell Kill Computed by Model for Several Standard Time-Dose Schedules

Dose History	Tolerance Dose, Rads	Cell Kill
Single Instantaneous	1,800	0.275
14 Inst., one every 3 days	5,074	0.286
30 Inst. over 6 weeks	6,000	0.271
Continuous for 7 days	6,000	0.275
Exponential 17 days half-life	10,500	0.301

where: $No(0)$ = initial number of normal cells
No = number of normal cells
N_1 = number of group(1) potentiated cells
N_2 = number of group(2) potentiated cells
N_3 = number of dead cells
λ_1 = group(1) decay constant, days^{-1}
λ_2 = group(2) decay constant, days^{-1}
α = fraction of group (0) hits going to group (1)
β = fraction of group (0) hits going to group (2)
$(1-\alpha-\beta)$ = fraction of cells which die with one hit
t = time in days
Φ = radiation dose rate
σ = cross section for one hit

The equations can be solved for a specified history of dose rate vs. time to determine the ratio N3/No(0), the total fraction of cells killed by the course of radiation. By specifying a particular cell-kill fraction as "tolerance," the total dose required to achieve that fraction can be calculated.

The free variables in the equations can be chosen to bring the model into agreement with accepted clinical experience. Table 1 lists five types of radiation history and the corresponding tolerance dose in rads. Also listed is the cell kill fraction predicted by the equations for the following parameters:

$1800\,\Phi\,\sigma$ = (rads/day) (hits/rad)
$\lambda_1 = 30$ days^{-1}
$\lambda_2 = 0.3$ days^{-1}
$\alpha = 0.85$
$\beta = 0.12$

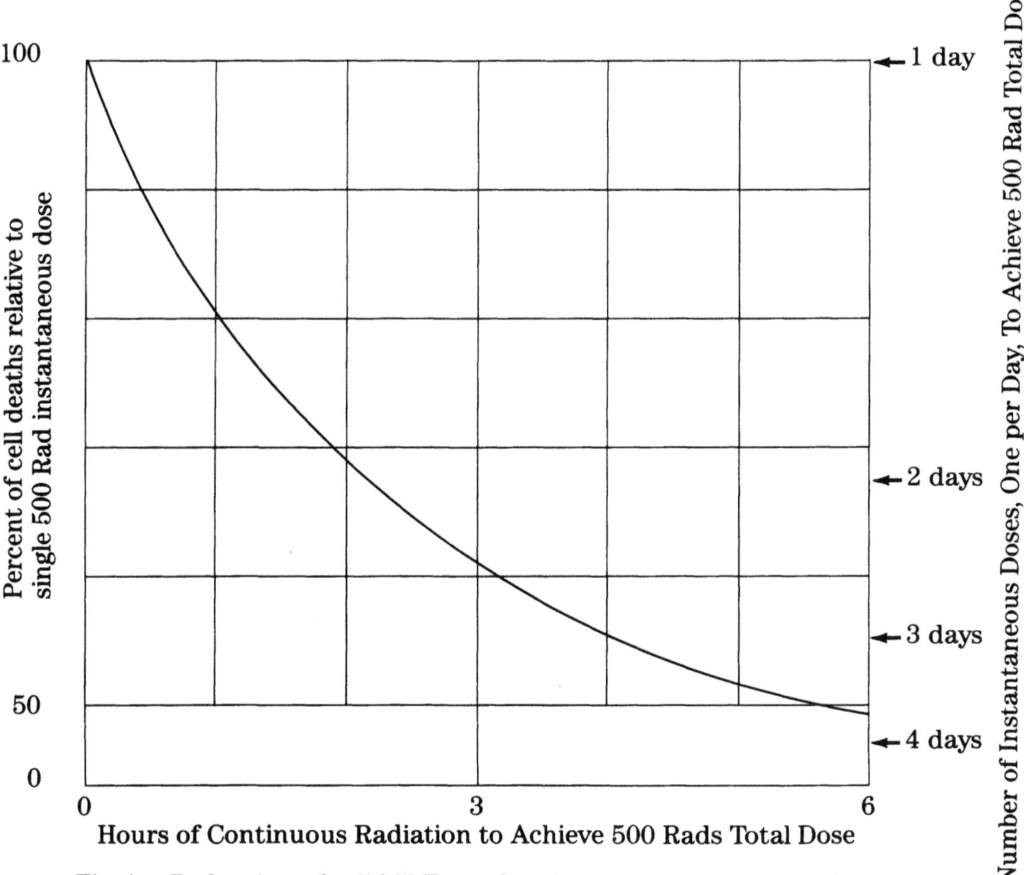

Fig. 1. Reduction of cell kill From fractionating or prolonging Dose

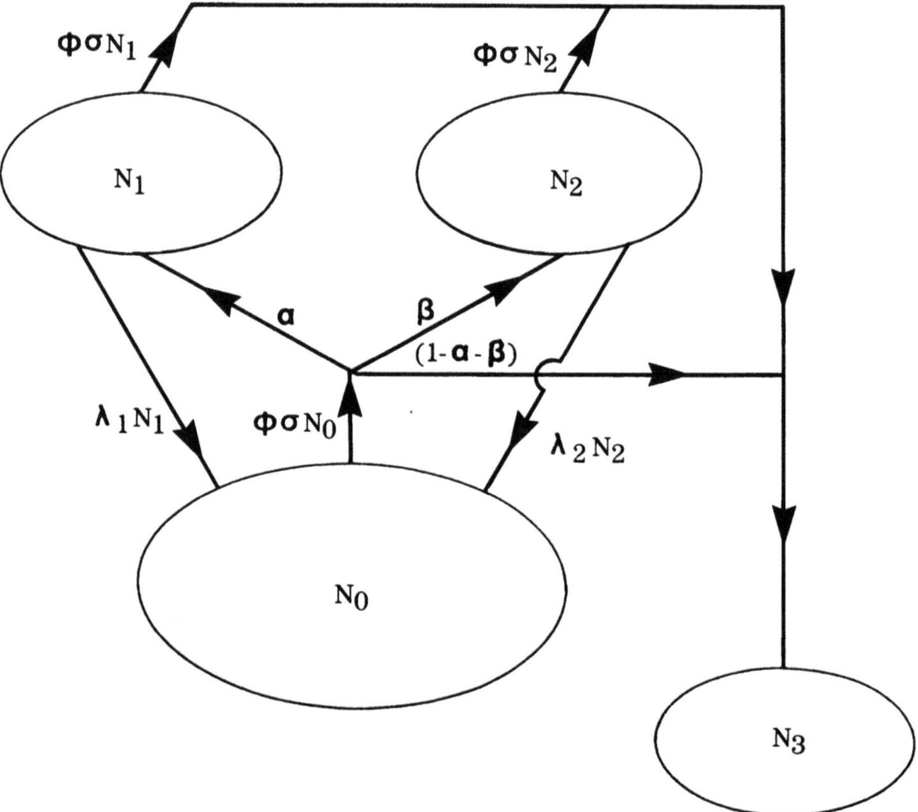

Fig. 2. Representation of radiation dose effect model.

A two time-constant model is the simplest model which can approximate the large body of clinical experience. The chosen parameters are not necessarily the optimum values, but are adequate for the purposes of this note.

To illustrate the effect of fractionation in BNCT, assume that 500 rads of the total dose is from primary and secondary gammas, and that the effect of the rest of the dose is not influenced by dose history. Fractionation has the effect of reducing the normal cell kill from the gammas, while not influencing the cancer cell kill from alpha particles.

The equations were solved for two types of dose history: 1) continuous radiation for the number of hours to deliver 500 rads; and 2) a number of instantaneous doses delivered at one per day to deliver 500 rads total. The cell kill for a 500 rad instantaneous dose is plotted at 100% in Fig. 1, and the reduction in normal cell kill for the various regimes is plotted. Clearly, there is a large benefit to be gained from either fractionation, reduced dose rate or both. Also, there appears to be a diminishing return after about three fractions, or four hours of continuous radiation.

REFERENCES

1. C. D. Orton, Time-dose factors (TDFs) in brachytherapy, Br. J. Radiol. 47:603 (1974).
2. F. Ellis, Fractionation in radiotherapy, in: "Modern Trends in Radiotherapy," T. J. Deeley and C. A. P. Woods, eds., Vol. 1, Butterworth, London (1967).

SOME THOUGHTS ON TOLERANCE, DOSE, AND FRACTIONATION IN BORON NEUTRON CAPTURE THERAPY

Reinhard Gahbauer,[1] Joseph Goodman,[2] and Thomas Blue[3]

Divisions of [1]Radiation Oncology, [2]Neurosurgery, [3]Nuclear Engineering, The Ohio State University, Columbus, Ohio

A general principle in radiation therapy holds that maximum tolerated doses to normal tissue be delivered in the treatment of most tumors, except in those tumors where lower doses are clearly sufficient to accomplish local control.

The question of tolerance in boron neutron capture therapy is clearly complicated or very simple, mainly dependent on the boron compound delivery to tumor (Fig. 1).

Tolerance

- H (n,gamma)D
- N (n,p)^{14}C
- ? incident gamma and neutrons
- Bo concentration in
  - normal brain
  - skin
  - blood

Fig. 1. Tolerance in BNCT.

If every single cancer cell takes up sufficient quantities of boron and at the same time the boron clears normal tissue and blood completely, epithermal neutron doses required will be low and certainly within tolerance. However, this ideal situation has not yet been approached.

In this discussion, it is assumed that an ideal beam, similar to the described 2 KeV beam, is available and will be used to treat the whole brain through bilateral treatment ports.

In this situation, the maximum amount of epithermal neutrons tolerated will depend on the capture gamma and capture high LET dose unavoidably resulting from the procedure. Any incident gamma and neutron dose will further have to be considered. Unique to boron neutron capture therapy, the tolerance very strongly depends on the boron concentration in normal brain, skin and blood. If one first considers the ideal situation of a 2 KeV beam and a compound clearing from normal tissues and blood, the tolerance dose to epithermal beams relates to the maximum tolerated capture gamma dose and capture high LET dose, H (n,gamma)D and $N(n,p)^{14}C$ (Fig. 2).

We can relate this gamma and high LET dose to known clinical experience. Assuming gamma and high LET dose ratios as given by Fairchild and Bond[2], one may first choose a clearly safe high LET whole brain dose and calculate the unavoidably resulting gamma dose.

To a first approximation 500 cGy of high LET dose results in 3,000 cGy gamma dose. One can speculate that this approximates the tolerance of whole brain to the 2 KeV beam with no contributing boron dose if the radiation is fractionated. It would clearly be

Tolerance

In a 2 KeV beam

- H(n,gamma)D
- $N(n,p)^{14}C$

relates to known experience

- if Bo concentration low in blood
- if Bo concentration low in skin

some skin sparing present

Fig. 2. Tolerance without Boron.

beyond tolerance in a single fraction where most therapists would be uncomfortable to deliver even one third of the above doses (Fig. 3).

Therefore, in this case, fractionated radiation therapy results in an increased boron dose by a factor of 2-3, since due to the high LET nature of the boron dose no repair is assumed between fractions in the tumor, whereas repair of the gamma dose will result in sparing of acute and late effects in normal tissues.

Very important questions remain unsolved in boron neutron capture therapy. We do not know with certainty if the periphery of the tumor may not be protected from any boron compound by the blood brain barrier. We have not demonstrated clearly that any compound is homogeneously distributed through the tumor and available to every cell in sufficient quantities. Therefore, we do not have conclusive evidence that any favorable results reported by Hatanaka are indeed only due to boron loading of all tumor cells. One cannot totally exclude the possibility that a single high dose of radiation to the tumor bed after debulking accounts for this result.

It may be appropriate to ask the question whether boron dose to tumor cells is the only useful parameter for therapeutic success. Since capture gamma and capture high LET dose cannot be avoided, their utilization in an optimum fractionation may add to the therapeutic success of the procedure (Fig. 4).

The incumbent ability to deliver a higher boron dose to the tumor will be advantageous in particular if one may speculate that fractionated delivery of one or several classes of boron compounds may yield higher and more homogeneous tumor uptake (Fig. 5).

It must, however, be clear that the epithermal dose may be reduced if ideal boron compounds become available and therefore lesser intensities of thermal neutron would be adequate. The epithermal dose must be reduced if the boron compound eventually chosen does not completely clear from blood, normal brain and skin. It is

Tolerance Dose of Epithermal Beams

relates to maximum tolerated

H(n,gamma)D and $N(n,p)^{14}C$

Estimate: 500 cGy $N(n,p)^{14}C$ dose
$>$ also results in 3000 cGy gamma - dose

Fig. 3. Tolerance estimate without Boron.

Limits of Effectiveness in BNCT

- Tumor periphery may be protected by BBB
- Inhomogeneous Bo uptake

? Is Bo-dose the only parameter

? Is gamma and p dose important for therapeutic success

Fig. 4. Critical issues in BNCT.

Conclusion

500 cGy High LET
+ 3000 cGy gamma

= beyond tolerance of single dose
= within tolerance fractionated

Fractionation results in

1) increased Boron dose (additive since no repair)

2) therapeutic effect to suboptimally Bo-loaded tumor

? May fractionated compound delivery also increase Bo-tumor uptake

Fig. 5. Advantage of fractionation.

further emphasized that tolerance doses depend on a given beam, a particular boron compound and its distribution, and have to be approached in a dose escalation study, first in animals and then in Phase I human studies.

Unless compounds are developed clearing from blood immediately, continued cell growth between compound delivery and irradiation limits the availability of boron to all cells. This strongly supports the use of fractionated radiation and utilization of maximum radiation cell kill to affect non-boron loaded cells for cell lethality and cell cycle effects.

REFERENCES

1. R. Gahbauer, J. Horton, F.Q. Ngo, W. Roberts, and J. Blue, Biological considerations for treating alternate fields vs all fields daily with high and low LET radiation, Strahlentherapie, 161:771 (1985).
2. R.G. Fairchild, and V.P. Bond, Current status of ^{10}B-neutron capture therapy: enhancement of tumor dose via beam filtration and dose rate, and the effects of these parameters on minimum boron contents: a theoretical evaluation, Int. J. Radiation Oncology Biol. Phys., 11:831 (1985).

DELAYED EFFECTS OF NEUTRON IRRADIATION ON CENTRAL NERVOUS SYSTEM MICROVASCULATURE IN THE RAT

J.H.Goodman, J.M.McGregor, N.R.Clendenon, W.A.Gordon, and
A.J.Yates, R.A.Gahbauer, R.F.Barth, R.G.Fairchild*

Ohio State University College of Medicine
Columbus, Ohio

*Brookhaven National Laboratories
Upton, New York

INTRODUCTION

Pathologic examination of a series of 14 patients with malignant gliomas treated with BNCT showed well demarcated zones of radiation damage characterized by coagulation necrosis. Beam attenuation was correlated with edema, loss of parenchymal elements, demyelination, leukocytosis, and peripheral gliosis. Vascular disturbances consisted of endothelial swelling, medial and adventitial proliferation, fibrin impregnation, frequent thrombosis, and perivascular inflammation. Radiation changes appeared to be acute and delayed. The outcome of the patients in this series was not significantly different from the natural course of the disease, even though two of the patients had no residual tumor detected at the time of autopsy. The intensity of the vascular changes raised a suspicion that boron may have sequestered in vessel walls, resulting in selectively high doses of radiation to these structures (Asbury et al., 1972), or that there may have been high blood concentrations of boron at the time of treatment. The potential limiting effects of a vascular ischemic reaction in Boron Neutron Capture Therapy (BNCT) prompted the following study to investigate the delayed response of microvascular structures in a rat model currently being used for pre-clinical investigations.

Table 1. BNCT Dosimetry of Animals Examined

Specimen	Neutron Fluence	Boron
1.	8X10(12) N/cm2	none
2.	2X10(13) N/cm2	none
3.	6X10(12) N/cm2	50 mg/kg
4.	8X10(12) N/cm2	50 mg/kg

MATERIAL AND METHODS

Thirty CD Fischer 334 adult male rats were studied following exposure to thermal neutron beam irradiation provided by the Brookhaven National Laboratory Medical Reactor. B10 enriched sodium mercaptoundecahydrododecaborate (NA2B12H11SH), 50 mg/kg IV (26.9mg B10/kg) was given to one half of the rats 17-18 hours before treatment. Rats were immobilized in a fixed head-holder, and right cerebral hemispheric irradiation was focused through a 1-cm diameter port centered 3mm to the right of midline, and 7mm anterior to the external meatal line. The rats were divided into groups based on the thermal neutron fluence received. Irradiation was performed in single fractions of various durations up to 8 minutes to obtain the desired fluences. Selected specimens were obtained for study of the late effects of BNCT (Table 1).

Nineteen months after treatment those rats selected for electron microscopy were anesthetized with ketamine (100mg/ml) in a ketamine/xylazine mixture of .12 ml/.1 mg given in the dose 0.1 ml/100 gm body weight by i.p. injection. They were killed by whole body perfusion fixation, using half-strength Karnovsky's solution, consisting of 2% Paraformaldehyde and 2.5% Glutaraldehyde in 0.12 molar Sorensen's phosphate buffer, pH 7.4, containing 60 mM sucrose and 0.5 mM calcium chloride. Fixation was performed via intra-aortic cannulation at a perfusion pressure of 140 cm. of water. This procedure provided adequate fixation of the CNS. The brains were removed and serial coronal sections 1mm thick were cut. Tissue blocks 1mm3 were obtained from the right caudate nucleus, corpus callosum and cerebral cortex.

Tissue blocks for electron microscopy were fixed for one hour at room temperature in the half-strength Karnovsky's solution. Samples were rinsed several times in a 0.1 molar phosphate buffer with 0.1 molar sucrose at 4 degrees centigrade and placed in 1% osmium tetroxide in buffer for 2 hours at 4 degrees centigrade. The tissues were rinsed in cold buffer and stored 24 hours at 4 degrees centigrade, then subsequently dehydrated in graded ethanol and two changes of propylene oxide. The tissues then were infiltrated with spurr resin (1:1 spurr/propylene oxide) for 1 hour, rinsing twice in spurr resin, 1 hour each, and embedding. The tissue was post-stained with lead citrate and uranyl acetate before analysis. Electron micrographs were obtained on Phillips EM 300 and EM 301 electron microscopes.

Whole mount coronal sections were processed for histological study and stained with hematoxylin and eosin, phosphotungstic acid-hematoxylin, Bodian and luxol fast blue.

Adult control rats, not matched for age, received neither irradation nor boron compound and were analyzed in the same manner.

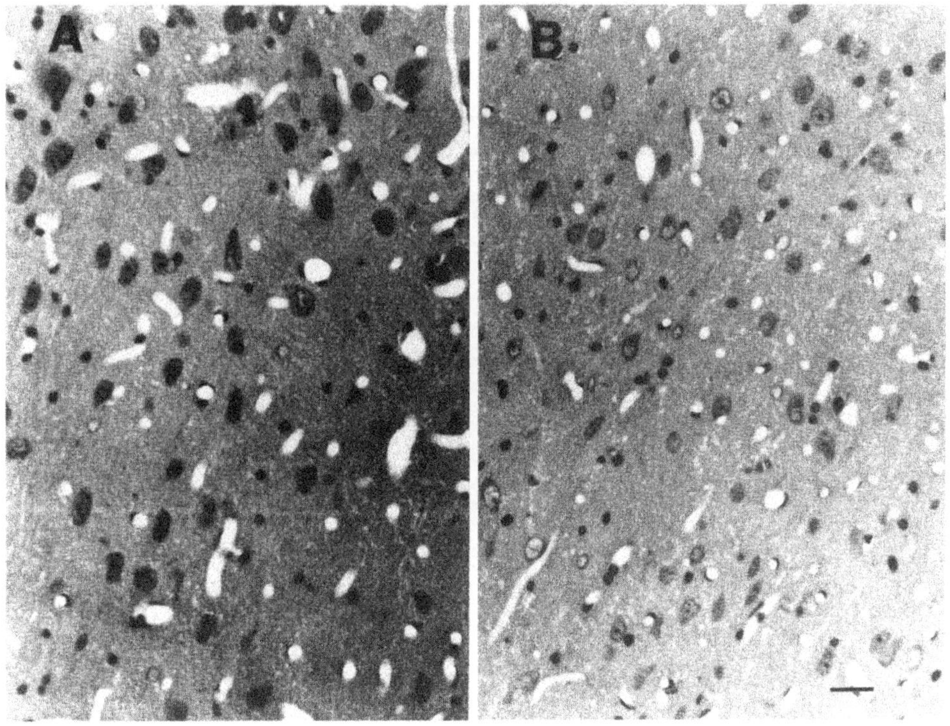

Fig. 1. Rat caudate nucleus. Photomicrographs taken of right caudate nucleus beneath the neutron radiation port. (A) normal control. (B) rat treated with BNCT (specimen 4). Similar vascular patterns are noted. Reactive changes including gliosis and perivascular infiltration are absent in irradiated tissue. Hematoxylin and eosin stain. Scale represents 0.1mm.

RESULTS

The observations reported focus solely on the microvascular architecture and perivascular structures in gray matter.

Light Microscopy

Coronal whole brain sections were used to correlate histopathology with samples taken for electron microscopy. Cortical gray matter and caudate nucleus beneath the beam port were examined following histochemical staining. Perfusion fixation resulted in distended vessels uniformly distributed throughout the tissues examined. Those animals undergoing neutron irradiation alone and neutron irradiation with boron showed similar vascular patterns as seen in the controls. Uniform thickness of capillary endothelium, lack of gliosis, and no evidence of tissue necrosis characterized all samples (Fig. 1). PTAH-stained sections did not show evidence

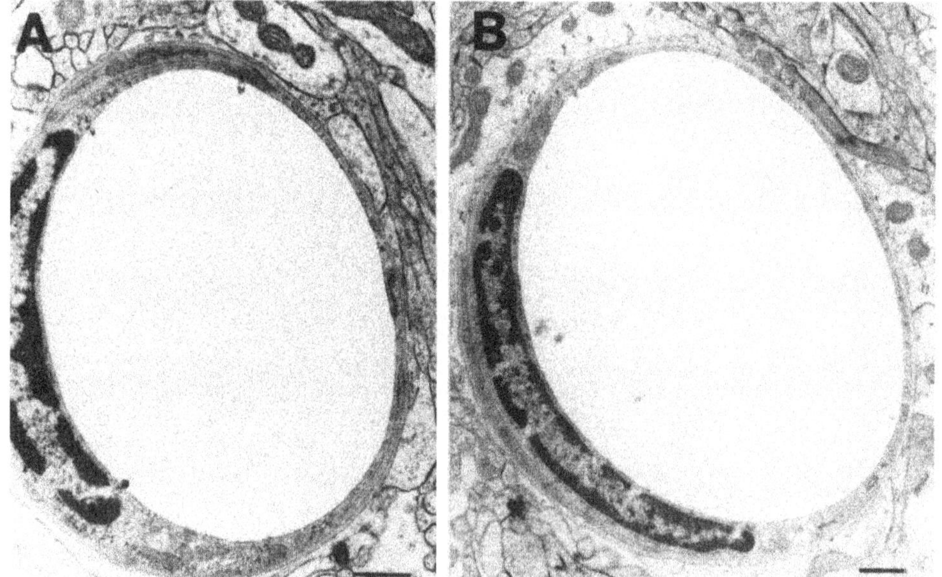

Fig. 2. Electron micrographs of capillaries from right caudate nucleus. (A) normal control. (B) rat treated with BNCT (specimen 4). Endothelial cytoplasm and basal laminae display uniform thickness and regular margins. Junctional complexes are noted. Intracytoplasmic organelles have a uniform appearence in both specimens. Pericyte processes maintain their perivascular relationships. Scale represents 1μ.

of gliosis that might have been related to direct tissue effects of radiation or secondary vascular ischemic changes.

Ultrastructural observations

The capillary endothelium appeared to have a uniform thickness with the usual number of intracytoplasmic organelles. Occasional pinocytotic pits and vesicles were encountered. Endothelial junctional complexes demonstrated sites of increased cytoplasmic density. The endothelial nuclei appeared morphologically normal (Fig. 2). The basal lamina was of uniform density and thickness, and completely encircled all vessels. Pericytes and pericyte processes were completely enclosed within the basal lamina. In larger vessels, collagen filaments were noted. Those larger vessels considered to be precapillary arterioles and postcapillary venules contained both collagen and smooth muscle cells. Pericytes

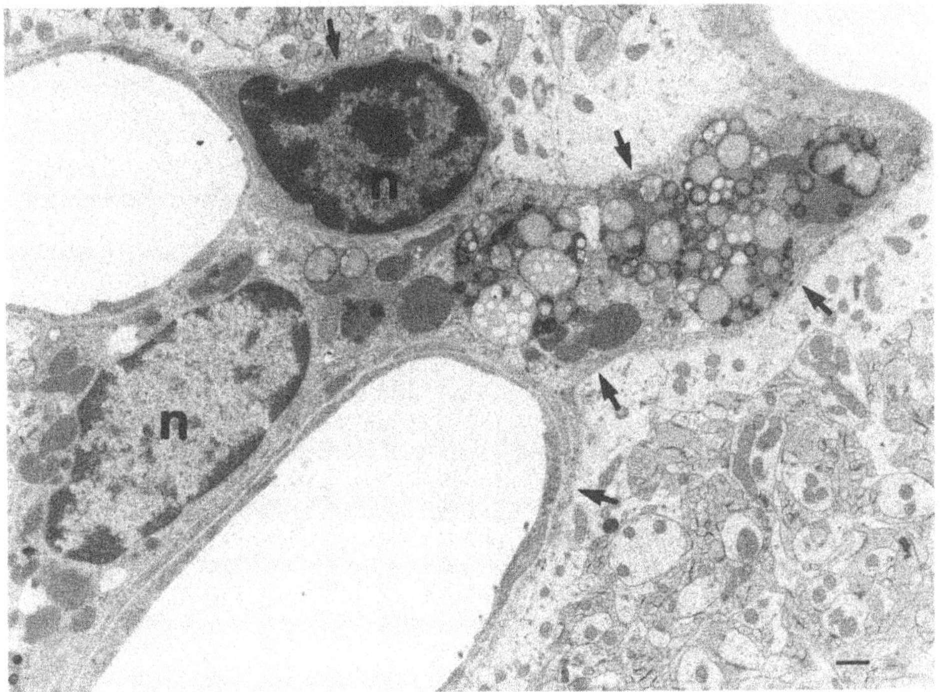

Fig. 3. Right caudate nucleus from a rat treated with BNCT (specimen 4). Two pericyte nuclei (n) are seen between the capillaries. The basal lamina completely encloses the cytoplasm of the pericyte (arrows). Note the numerous pleomorphic dense bodies within the cytoplasm, consistent with the phagocytic activity of these cells. Scale represents 1μ.

contained within the basal lamina of irradiated animals showed occasional accumulations of numerous dense bodies within the cytoplasm consisting of either lipid or condensed exogenous protein (Fig. 3). A glial investment consisting of clear and fibrous astrocytes surrounded the capillaries, arterioles, and venules.

There were no obvious differences between the control samples and radiated animals in the endothelium, basal lamina, or perivascular glia. Evidence of pathologic changes seen in pericytes consisted of vacuolization within membrane bound organelles in the radiated animals.

DISCUSSION

Radiation damage to the nervous system can be related to dose and latency, with damage appearing as late as 2 years after radiation to the spinal cord of the rat (Hubbard and Hopewell, 1978). Radiation of normal rat brain with 2000 cGy causes progressive vascular alterations over a period of two years, consisting of increased vascular density and telangiectasias (Reinhold and Hopewell, 1980). CNS vascular responses to varying doses and latencies are shown by antipyrine extraction studies to be progressive over several months to one year (Moustafa and Hopewell, 1979). Late focal vascular occlusions in the irradiated rat brain have been reported (Hopewell, 1974). Ultrastructural evidence of capillary tolerance to BNCT in the cerebral cortex of the dog was reported by Al-Samarrai et al. (1975).

Our current studies involve a group of animals treated with neutron fluences from 6X10(12) to 2X10(13) N/cm2. Animals receiving a higher radiation dose of 4X10(13) N/cm2 do not survive and typically die within two weeks. The dosages tested are being used to evaluate BNCT in a nitrosourea-induced glioma model, and this report indicates that late radiation vasculopathy at such doses is minimal. Pericyte phagocytic activity is a nonspecific reaction that occurs following pathologic conditions and has been observed 28 days after 1000 rad neon radiation in the mouse (Polak et al., 1982), and following 6000 rad alpha-particle irradiation to rat cerebral cortex (Maxwell and Kruger, 1965).

Vascular complications associated with BNCT clinically, and the known delayed CNS radiation effects justify further studies to establish normal tissue tolerances. The potentially devastating late vascular complications must be avoided. Cross-species testing to confirm tolerance limits in the dog and in primates will aid in planning clinical protocols. Further investigations will provide insights into the vascular mechanisms by which BNCT provides therapeutic effects, to determine the optimal parameters for future clinical trials.

REFERENCES

Al-Samarri, S.F., Takeuchi, A., and Hatanaka, H., 1975, Electron microscopic study on the response of the normal canine brain to boron-neutron capture therapy, Gann, 66:663.

Asbury, A.K., Ojemann, R.G., Nielsen, S.L., and Sweet, W.H., 1972, Neuropathologic study of fourteen cases of malignant brain tumor treated by Boron-10 slow neutron capture radiation, Neuropath and Exp Neurol., 31:278.

Hubbard, B.M., and Hopewell, J.W., 1978, The dose-latent relationship in the irradiated cervical spinal cord of the rat, Radiology, 128:779.

Hopewell, J.W., 1974, The late vascular effects of radiation, Br J Radiol., 47:157.

Maxwell, D.S., and Kruger, L., 1965, Small blood vessels and the origin of phagocytes in the rat cerebral cortex following heavy particle irradiation, Exp Neurol., 12:33.

Moustafa, H.F., and Hopewell, J.W., 1979, Late functional changes in the vasculature of the rat brain after local X-irradiation, Br J Radiol., 53:21.

Polak, M., D'Amelio, F., Johnson, J.E., and Haymaker, W., 1982, Microglial cells origins and reactions, in: "Histology And Histopathology Of The Nervous System," W. Haymaker and R.D. Adams, eds., Charles C. Thomas, Springfield, Illinois.

Reinhold, H.S., and Hopewell, J.W., 1980, Late changes in the architecture of blood vessels of the rat brain after irradiation, Br J Radiol., 53:693.

PRE-CLINICAL STUDIES ON BORON NEUTRON CAPTURE THERAPY

Rolf F. Barth, Albert H. Soloway, Fazlul Alam, Nancy R. Clendenon, Thomas E. Blue, Naoki Mafune, Joseph H. Goodman, Wanda Gordon, Bhaskar Bapat, Dianne M. Adams, Alfred E. Staubus, Melvin J. Moeschberger, Reinhard Gahbauer, Allan J. Yates, Carl P. Boesel, Timothy F. Mengers, James F. Curran, Chris K. Wang, George E. Makroglou, Jone-Jiun Tzeng and Ralph G. Fairchild

The Ohio State University, Columbus, Ohio 43210 and Brookhaven National Laboratory, Upton, New York 11973

INTRODUCTION

Boron neutron capture therapy (BNCT) is based on the nuclear reaction that occurs when boron-10 is irradiated with thermal neutrons to yield stripped down helium nuclei (alpha particles) and recoiling lithium-7 nuclei.[1]

$$^{10}B + {}^{1}n \rightarrow [^{11}B] \rightarrow {}^{7}Li + {}^{4}He\ (\alpha) + 2.79\ MeV$$

In order for BNCT to be therapeutically effective a sufficient fluence of thermal neutrons and a critical amount of ^{10}B must be delivered to individual tumor cells. Monoclonal antibodies (MoAbs) directed against tumor associated antigens potentially might provide a means for selectively delivering ^{10}B to tumors.[2] Another possibility is to use chemical compounds or drugs, which for one or another reason preferentially or selectively localize in tumor cells. One such compound is di-sodium mercaptundecahydro-closo-dodecaborate ($Na_2B_{12}H_{11}SH$), whose tumor localizing properties originally were described by Soloway et al.[3] Alternatively, boron containing chlorpromazine [4,5] or promazine derivatives[6] might be useful for the targeting of ^{10}B to melanomas. Animal models may be useful for assessing the therapeutic efficacy of boronated antibodies and drugs prior to their use in clinical trials. Quantitation of ^{10}B at the level of individual tumor cells would provide direct evidence for selective delivery, which is essential if BNCT is to succeed. At the present time thermal neutrons are derived as a product of the fission reaction that occurs in the core of a nuclear reactor. There would be significant advantages to a more compact source of neutrons, such as a particle accelerator, that could be used for BNCT. The purpose of the present report is to provide a brief overview of research activities in each of the above areas that currently is in progress at The Ohio State University.

Optimization of Methods for the Conjugation, Purification, and Characterization of Boronated Monoclonal Antibodies

Monoclonal antibodies (MoAbs) directed against tumor associated antigens may be useful for the selective targeting of boron-10. One of our major areas of research has been to optimize the conditions for linking a large number of boron atoms to antibody molecules, to develop methodology for the purification of the immunoconjugates, and to characterize them both *in vitro* and *in vivo*. MoAb 17-1A, directed against human colorectal cancer[7] and IB16-6, directed against the murine B16 melanoma[8], were boronated by means of the following procedure. A boron containing polymer was prepared by reacting an isocyanate polyhedral borane $Me_3NB_{10}H_8NCO^-$, with poly-DL-lysine to yield boronated poly-lysine.

$$Me_3NB_{10}H_8NCO^- + \text{Poly-Lys-}(NH_2)_x \rightarrow \text{Poly-Lys-}(NHCOHB_{10}H_8NME^-,)_x$$

This boronated macromolecule (BPL) contained 23% boron by weight and >1700 boron atoms. The attachment of BPL to the MoAbs was carried out by means of a three step procedure, shown in Figure 1. In the first, masked sulfhydryl groups were introduced into BPL by reacting it with the heterobifunctional reagent, N-succinimidyl 3-(2-pyridyldithio) propionate to yield Cpd 1.

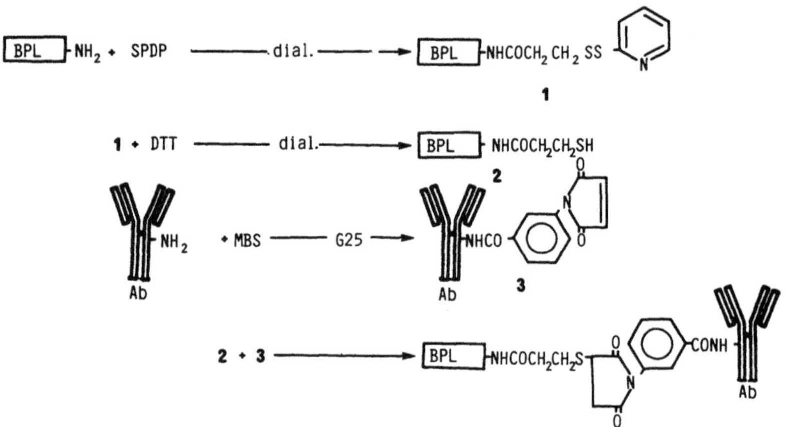

Figure 1. Conjugation of MoAbs with boronated poly-lysine (BPL).

After removal of unreacted SPDP, unmasking of the sulhydryl groups was accomplished by treatment with dithiothreitol to yield BPL-SH (Cpd 2). In the second, maleimido groups were introduced into antibody molecules by means of m-maleimidobenzoylsulfo-succinimide ester (sulfo MBS), to yield MoAb-MB (Cpd 3). Excess sulfo-MBS was removed by gel filtration on a Sephadex G25 column. In the third, sulfhydryl containing BPL (Cpd 2) was reacted with the maleimido groups on the antibody molecules (Cpd 3) to yield BPL-MoAb immunoconjugates. The conjugate was separated from the reaction mixture by gel filtration through a Sephacryl S-300 column. Immunoreactivity was determined by means of an enzyme-linked immunosorbent assay (ELISA) against semi-confluent cultures of SW 1116 colorectal cancer cells for 17-1A, and by membrane immunofluorescence against B16 cells for IB16-6. Boron concentrations of the purified immunoconjugates were determined by alpha track autoradiography using the polycarbonate resin CR-39 as a solid state nuclear track detector or by prompt gamma emission.

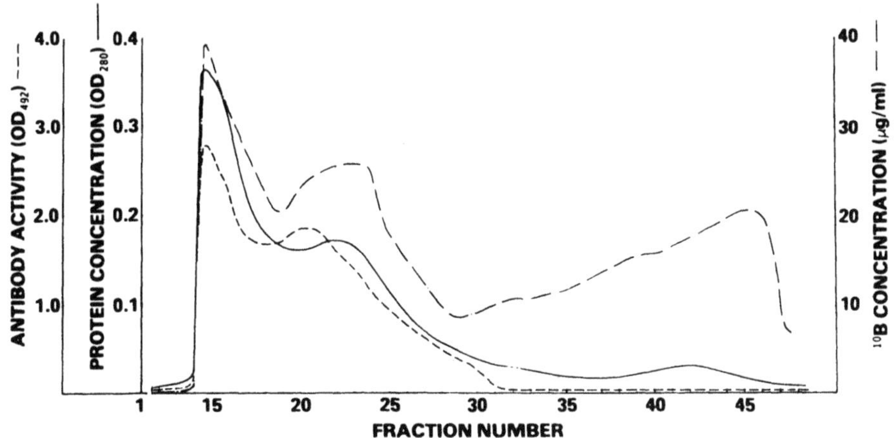

Figure 2. Elution pattern of boronated MoAb 17-1A on Sephacryl S-300 gel column chromatography. Purified immunoconjugates were characterized by three methods: (1) protein concentration, as determined by absorbance at 280 nm (2) antibody activity as determined by ELISA and (3) ^{10}B content, as determined by alpha track autoradiography. Fraction 15 had the highest protein concentration, antibody activity and boron content.

Immunoreactivity of boronated 17-1A ranged from 40 to 90% of that of the native MoAb, and was stable over 24 hours incubation at 37°C. Boron content was upto 10^4 atoms per molecule for 17-1A and 2.7×10^3 for IB16-6. Based on previous determinations of the K_A of 17-1A ($1.05 \times 10^8 M^{-1}$)and IB16-6 (1.5-6.0 x 10 M^{-1}) and the number of antigenic receptor sites per cell (10^6 and 2.5×10^5 respectively), these antibodies theoretically should be capable of delivering enough ^{10}B to sustain a lethal n, α reaction at the cellular level. Studies currently are in progress to define these antibodies activity following *in vitro* irradiation of tumor cells with thermal neutrons, and their *in vivo* tumor localizing properties.

Synthesis of Boronated Compounds for Neutron Capture Therapy

This section briefly describes the preparation of boron-containing compounds and macromolecules that potentially could be used as capture agents for BNCT. These are described in more detail elsewhere in this same volume. We have reported on the preparation of boronated polylysine (BPL) containing approximately 24% boron by weight and 1500 boron atoms per molecule, and the linkage of BPL to monoclonal antibodies.[2] To minimize the problems in purifying the conjugate and to increase yields, we have made three changes in methodology.

(1) The $Me_3N\underline{B}_{10}H_8NCO^-$ used to boronate polylysine was synthesized from $B_{10}H_{10}^{=}$ by a four step procedure. Changes in the first two steps involving amination of $B_{10}H_{10}^{=}$ and then methylation of the amino group has led to a doubling of the previously reported yield.[9] This is important because we have undertaken the synthesis of the 95% ^{10}B enriched compound for neutron irradiation studies.

(2) The poly-DL-lysine is now labeled with fluorescein isothiocyanate (FITC), either prior to or following boronation. This has permitted the rapid determination of BPL and, indirectly, boron in column fractions and in the immunoconjugates.

(3) The BPL is fractionated on a Sephadex G-150 column to obtain BPL of a narrower molecular weight range to minimize problems in purifying the conjugate. Utilizing these improvements, we have been able to incorporate 1500-9000 boron atoms into MoAbs with the retention of a high degree of immunoreactivity.

Phthalocyanines are known to localize in some tumors. We have synthesized boronated phthalocyanines containing an average of 15 boron atoms per molecule by chlorosulfonation of phthalocyanine with chlorosulfonyl chloride followed by reaction with p-aminophenylcarborane. The tumor localizing properties of p-boronophenylalanine (BPA) have stimulated us to synthesize carboranylalanine, which contains 10X more boron than BPA. Distribution studies of both of these compounds in tumor bearing mice should determine whether they can be used for the selective delivery of ^{10}B for BNCT.

Chlorpromazine is known to localize in melanomas and melanin containing cells.[4,5] Distribution studies in hamsters and mice bearing transplantable melanoma by Fairchild et al. indicate that boronated analogues of chlorpromazine potentially could be used to deliver a sufficient concentration of boron-10 for the BNCT. Five boronated promazine structures now have been synthesized by us. These contain 9-20 boron atoms per molecule as either 1,2-ortho-carborane or nidocarborane moieties linked to the phenyl moieties of the promazine structure. These compounds were tested for acute toxicity in C57Bl/6 mice and BALB/c mice. Single doses as high as 50 mg/kg body weight by iv administration in 25 μl DMSO was well tolerated by the mice. Significant sedation, similar to that observed with chlorpromazine, was observed with several of these compounds. Studies currently are in progress to define their tumor localizing properties in C57Bl/6 mice carrying the B16 melanoma and BALB/c mice carrying the Harding-Passey melanoma.

Boron Neutron Capture Therapy of Rat Glioma

The anaplastic glioma clone, F98, implanted stereotactically into caudate nuclei of syngeneic CD-Fischer rats, produces tumors with biologic characteristics similar to human glioblastomas.[10] These neoplasms kill at precisely defined time intervals that correlate positively with tumor mass. They do not metastasize and are highly resistant to all therapeutic modalities attempted to date. This is an established, highly reliable rat brain tumor model, that is well suited for experimental studies on the efficacy of BNCT.

Our *in vitro* studies with F98 cells demonstrated a 3-4 log reduction in surviving fraction using ^{10}B-enriched $Na_2B_{12}H_{11}SH$ at concentrations of 50 and 100 μg/ml at a thermal neutron fluence of 2×10^{13} n/cm^2. Pharmacokinetic studies revealed the compound injected i.v. at a dose of 50 mg/kg body wt behaved in a two compartment model fashion with a biological half-life of 6.17 hr.

In vivo survival studies utilized an animal holder, designed by D.N. Slatkin, Brookhaven National Laboratory to position the rat so that the tumor would be in the field of maximum neutron flux, and thus minimize irradiation to other areas. ^{10}B-enriched $Na_2B_{12}H_{11}SH$ was administered i.v. at a dose of 50 mg/kg body wt at different times prior to neutron irradiation at the BNL Medical Research Reactor. Neutron fluences also were varied. Fluences of 2, 4, or 6×10^{12} n/cm^2 showed no therapeutic effect, while 4×10^{13} n/cm^2 was uniformly lethal. The Kaplan-Meier plot of a representative survival study is shown in Figure 3. The mean survival time was 31.2 days for rats irradiated with a fluence of 10^{13} /cm^2 and 35.4 days with a fluence of 2×10^{13} n/cm^2 compared to 27.7 days for non-irradiated controls, significant at $p<0.05$ and $p<0.01$, respectively, compared to controls. When the capture agent was administered 16 hours prior to neutron irradiation, survival was significantly increased to 41.0 days ($p<0.005$) at the higher fluence. No therapeutic gain was noted at the lower fluence.

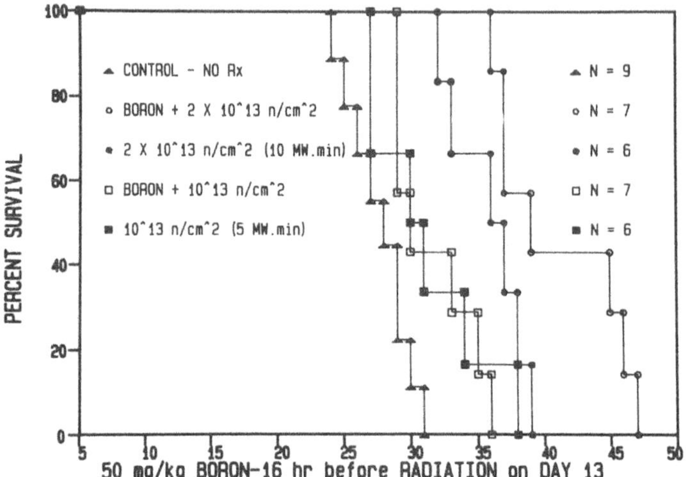

Figure 3. Kaplan-Meier survival curves for F98 tumor bearing rats following BNCT.

An attempt was made to increase the ^{10}B tumor concentration by varying the time between compound administration and irradiation. Figure 4 shows the percentage increase in life span for tumor bearing rats treated with a fluence of 2 x 10^{13} n/cm^2 and for animals given the capture agent at 3, 6, 13.5, 16, 18.5 or 23.5 hours prior to irradiation compared to non-irradiated controls. Significant therapeutic gains were observed at the 13.5, 16 and 23.5 hour intervals compared with neutron irradiated controls. Tumor size at the time of death for BNCT treated rats was similar to untreated and neutron irradiated controls.

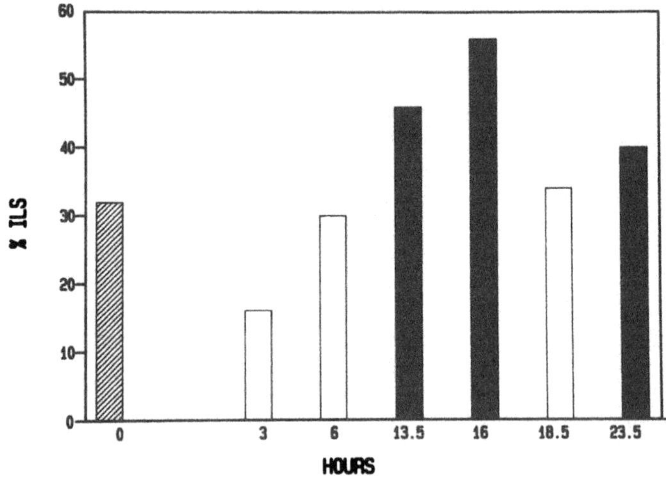

Figure 4. Relationship between time interval of administration of $Na_2B_{12}H_{11}SH$ and % ILS. ▨= irradiation only; □= no enhancement; ■= significant therapeutic gain.

Our in vivo survival studies suggest that a therapeutic gain has been achieved, as evidenced by regrowth delay of the tumor and increase of life span for BNCT treated rats compared to either irradiated or non-irradiated control animals. Studies currently in progress should tell us if tumor concentrations of ^{10}B can be increased by multiple dosing or sustained infusion by means of osmotic pumps.

An Accelerator-Based Neutron Irradiation Facility for BNCT

A design study of an accelerator-based neutron irradiation facility (ANIF) for BNCT was performed using three-dimensional Monte Carlo transport calculations. The major components of the ANIF are a radio frequency quadrupole (RFQ), a lithium target, and a moderating assembly. Neutrons were generated by bombarding the lithium target with 2.5 MeV protons. The neutrons emerging from the lithium target were too energetic to be used for BNCT, and therefore had to be moderated. Calculations showed that, among all materials for the ANIF, beryllia (BeO) and heavy water (D_2O) were the best moderators. Between them, beryllia provided better neutron spectra, but D_2O gave higher neutron intensities Adding alumina (Al_2O_3) to D_2O improved the neutron spectra, but it also increased gamma-ray contamination.

The overall performance of an ANIF was evaluated for a moderating assembly that was composed of a beryllia cylinder, which was 20.0 cm in height and 12.5 cm in radius, reflected by 30.0 cm of alumina (Figure 5).

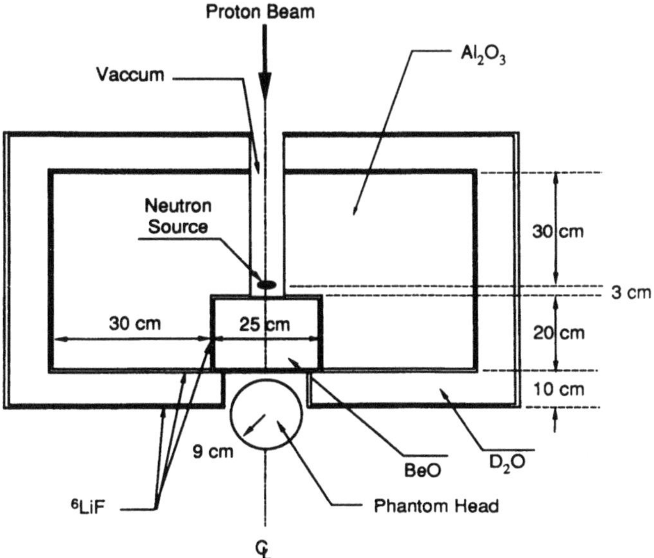

Figure 5. The configuration (side view) of the final design of ANIF.

Calculations showed that the addition of the alumina reflector doubled the epithermal neutron intensity at the irradiation port. A layer of ^{6}Li 0.025g/cm^{2} thick was placed between the beryllia moderator and the alumina reflector to reduce the number of thermal neutrons escaping from the beryllia, and therefore the capture gamma rays produced by aluminum in the reflector. Also, a layer of ^{6}Li 0.01g/cm^{2} thick was placed at the irradiation port of the moderating assembly to remove thermal neutrons from the irradiation field. Finally, a neutron shield of D_2O 10.0 cm thick wrapped with ^{6}LiF was placed around the moderating assembly except at the irradiation port. The maximum therapeutic gain for the neutrons from the moderating assembly was calculated to be 4.0 at 3.5 cm for 35 μg of ^{10}B/g-tumor and a 3.5 μg of ^{10}B /g-normal tissue. The treatment was 75-90 minutes for a 10-mA proton current. If the beryllia were replaced by heavy water in the moderating assembly, then the treatment time would be reduced to 20 minutes, at the price of a higher entrance dose to patients, and thus lower therapeutic gains.

Boron-10 Concentration Measurements Using the Solid State Nuclear Track Detector CR-39 and Automatic image Analysis

(1) Automatic Image Analysis

The alpha track autoradiographic technique for the determination of the boron concentration of blood requires the analysis of CR-39 Solid State Nuclear Track Detectors.

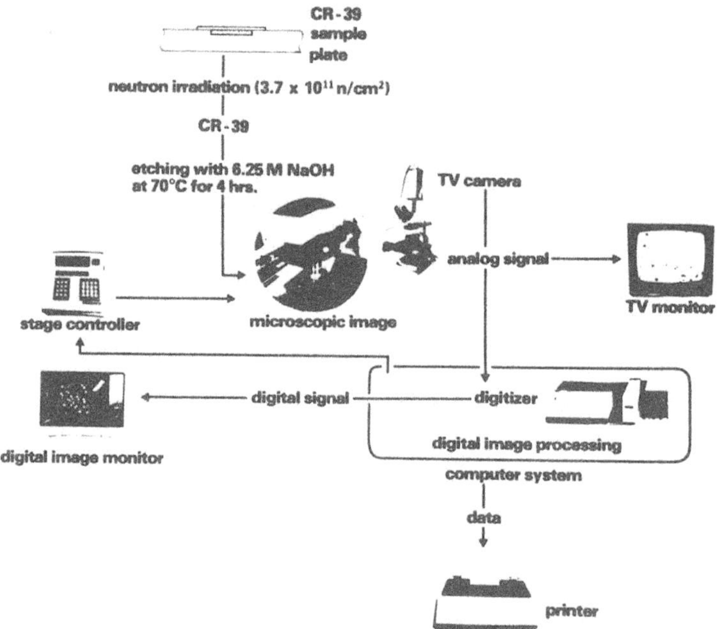

Figure 6. Boron-10 concentration measurements using CR-39.

The track detectors were analyzed using an image analysis system.[11] In order to reduce operator interaction with the image analysis system, an automatic focus system has been developed. In the focus system, the signal from the CCTV camera, which is the first stage of the image analysis system, is split and passed through an op-amp derivative circuit. An analog gate is combined with a synch-pulse stripping circuit to remove the video retrace pulses from the signal. The remaining signal is rectified and integrated to produce a focus dependent DC voltage. This signal is sent to an A/D converter attached to an IBM compatible personal computer. An iterative TURBO Pascal algorithm samples the signal and sends controlling logic pulses to a stepping motor driver. The attached motor turns the focus knob on the microscope. Measurements with constant focus indicates the resolution for alpha tracks is 2.49 $\pm$ 0.01%. With autofocus the resolution is 2.50 $\pm$ 0.01%. In addition, by completely automating the system, we have reduced operator time from thirty-five minutes per detector to less than five minutes per detector.

(2) Boron-10 Concentration Measurements

A method has been developed for determining the kinetics of boronated compounds in the blood of rats, by sampling many time points from individual rats, fitting the blood serum concentration measured at these time points to kinetic models, and averaging the kinetic model fitting parameters over a group of rats.

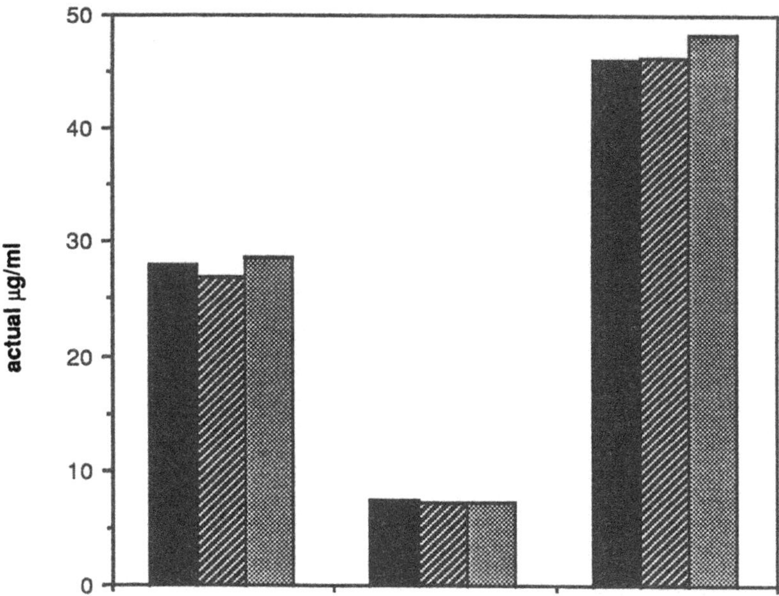

Figure 7. Comparison of different methods for the determination of boron concentrations in blood. ■= actual amount (µg/ml); ▨= prompt γ; ■= track etch.

Figure 7 is a comparison of the determination of the boron concentrations of unknown samples of blood by the prompt-gamma technique at BNL, and the track etch technique at OSU. The boron concentrations determined by the track etch method agreed well with those determined at BNL, and with the actual amount (μg/ml) placed in solution.

The steps in the development of the method for the determination of blood boron concentrations, which have been accomplished to date are:

(a) The development of an alpha track autoradiographic method for blood boron concentration measurement, that requires only 50 μl of blood per well.

(b) The development of a cannulation technique for removing blood samples of ~100 μl, and their replacement with equal volumes of saline by slow injection. The boron concentration measurement technique has been tested by determining the boron concentration of unknowns.

Studies are currently in progress to develop methodology to quantify ^{10}B at the cellular level by means of alpha track autoradiographic techniques.

SUMMARY

The present report provides an overview of the multidisciplinary research effort on BNCT that currently is in progress at The Ohio State University. Areas under investigation include the preparation of boron containing monoclonal antibodies, the synthesis of boron containing derivatives of promazines and phathalocyanines, the development of a rat model for the treatment of glioblastoma by means of BNCT, the design of an accelerator-based neutron irradiation facility, and ^{10}B concentration measurements using alpha track autoradiographic methods. Progress in each of these areas is described and the direction of future research is indicated.

ACKNOWLEDGMENTS

The work described in this report has been supported by grant 5 R01 CA41288 from the National Institutes of Health, contract DE-AC02-82ERG0040 from the Department of Energy and a grant from the Office of Research and Graduate Studies, The Ohio State University. We thank Dr. Zenon Steplewski, The Wistar Institute, Philadelphia, PA from providing us with MoAb 17-1A, Dr. Daniel Slatkin, Brookhaven National Laboratory, Upton, LI, NY for allowing us to use his rat holder for neutron irradiations, Ms. Peggy Micca and Brenda Laster for boron determinations, Ms. Joan Rotaru for technical assistance and Mrs. Ada Morgan for secretarial assistance.

REFERENCES

1. G. L. Locher, Biological effects of therapeutic possibilities of neutrons. Amer. J. Roentgenol. 36:1 (1936).

2. R. F. Barth, F. Alam, A. H. Soloway, D. M. Adams, and Z. Steplewski, Boronated monoclonal antibody 17-1A for potential neutron capture therapy of colorectal cancer. Hybridoma 5: Suppl. 1: S43 (1986).

3. A. H. Soloway, H. Hatanaka, and M. A. Davis, Penetration of brain and brain tumor. VII. Tumor-binding sulfhydryl boron compounds. J. Med. Chem. 10:714 (1967).

4. Y. Mishima and T. Shimakage, Thermal neutron capture treatment of malignant melanomas using ^{10}B-Dopa and $^{n}B_{12}$-chlorpromazine compounds. Pigment Cell 2:394 (1976).

5. R. G. Fairchild, D. Greenberg, K. P. Watts, S. Packer, H. L. Atkins, P. Som, S. J. Hannon, A. B. Brill, I. Fand, and W. P. McNally, Chlorpromazine distribution in hamsters and mice bearing transplantable melanoma. Cancer Res. 42:556 (1982).

6. A. H. Soloway, F. Alam, R. F. Barth, N. Mafune, B. Bapat and D. M. Adams, The development of boron compounds for use in neutron capture therapy. Proc. Imboron VI Meeting June 22-26, 1987, Rez, Czechoslovakia (1988, In Press).

7. M. Herlyn, Z. Steplewski, D. Herlyn and H. Koprowksi, CO 17-1A and related monoclonal antibodies: their production and characterization. Hybridoma 5: Suppl. 1: S3 (1986).

8. C. W. Johnson, R. F. Barth, D. Adams, B. Holman, J. E. Price and I. Sautins, Phenotypic diversity of murine B16 melanoma detected by anti-B16 monoclonal antibodies. Cancer Res. 47:1111 (1987).

9. F. Alam, A. H. Soloway, R. F. Barth and D. M. Adams, Chemoradiotherapy of cancer: boronated antibodies and boron containing derivatives of promazine for neutron capture therapy. in "Neutron Capture Therapy." Proc. Second Int'l Sympos. on Neutron Capture Therapy pp 8-16. H. Hatanaka, ed. Nishimura, Niigata, Japan (1986).

10. N. Kobayashi, N. Allen, N. R. Clendenon and L. Ko, An improved rat brain tumor model. J. Neurosurg. 53:808 (1980).

11. T. E. Blue, T. C. Roberts, R. F. Barth, J. W. Talnagi and F. Alam, Boron-10 concentration measurements using the solid-state nuclear track detector CR-39 and automatic image analysis. Nuclear Technology 77:220 (1987).

BORON COMPOUNDS FOR NEUTRON CAPTURE THERAPY

F. Alam, A.H. Soloway, B.V. Bapat, R.F. Barth, and
D.M. Adams

College of Pharmacy and Department of Pathology
The Ohio State University
Columbus, Ohio 43210

INTRODUCTION

There have been two main approaches to the development of boron compounds for neutron capture therapy (BNCT). One has involved the synthesis of boronated analogues of organic structures which possess a high degree of selectivity for neoplastic cells. These include amino acids, nucleic acid precusors, porphyrins and promazines. The second approach has emphasized the use and incorporation of boron compounds into monoclonal antibodies targeted against tumor associated antigens. There have been several important requirements in achieving the use of antibodies for BNCT. First, the conjugation of boron to monoclonal antibodies must occur with significant retention of the antibody's immunoreactivity. Second, sufficient numbers of boron atoms have to be incorporated and at least 10^3 boron atoms per protein molecule is necessary if a goal of 10^9 boron atoms per tumor cell is to be attained. Third, separation of the boron-containing antibody from the unconjugated species and from the boron entity used in the conjugation is essential. Finally, the boron-loaded antibody must have the ability for targeting all the tumor cells, under *in vivo* conditions with a high degree of selectivity. Research at The Ohio State University on the incorporation of boron-containing polymers into monoclonal antibodies has already been described[1]. The work presented herein outlines the synthesis of boronated analogues of promazines and phthalocyanines, structures which have a demonstrated proclivity for certain neoplasms. The tissue distribution data in tumor-bearing animals for certain of these compounds are presented.

BORON-CONTAINING PROMAZINES

Fairchild et al[2] had observed high concentrations of chlorpromazine (CPZ) in the tumors of melanoma-bearing animals. Concurrently, Mishima and his colleagues[3] had prepared boronated derivatives of CPZ in which a boron species was attached to the basic nitrogen functionality. These two studies prompted the synthesis of five carborane-containing promazines shown in Figure 1. The rational for this research was the desire to preserve the S-N-N axis of the promazine structure intact and unaltered so that the formation of the malanin-promazine complex would not be interfered with. Thus, the boron cages were attached to the aromatic rings. The attachment of the carborane moieties was the final step in the synthetic sequence and that situation offers a clear advantage of any of these structures were to be prepared with B-10 enriched material.

The synthesis of compounds I, III and IV have been described previously[4] and stem from the reaction of the appropriate promazine with lithiocarborane. Compound II was formed by the reaction of I with alcoholic KOH; this is a classical procedure for the degradation of the carborane cage to yield the corresponding *nido* structure. Compound V was prepared by reacting 7-aminochlorpromazine with 2-methylcarboran-1-ylcarboxylyl chloride. The requisite amino structure was obtained by nitration of CPZ followed by its catalytic hydrogenation. These compounds contain 9-20 boron atoms per molecule and if they behave comparable to CPZ from a biological standpoint, then the concentration of boron in tumor should be clearly adequate for use in BNCT.

In order to evaluate these compounds in animals, it was necessary to use organic solvents which were readily miscible with water and yet solubilized these carboranyl promazines to a significant extent. Dimethyl sulfoxide (DMSO) appeared to be the solvent of choice. However, at 100 μL injected volume, DMSO itself caused sedation and even death in C-57 black mice. The volume of DMSO that appeared to be well tolerated was 25 μL. Therefore, for toxicity studies and *in vivo* localization studies, the boronated promazines as well as CPZ were injected into mice in 25 μL DMSO.

Acute toxicity of these compounds was carried out in C-57 black mice. The basis for the selection of this rodent species was the fact that B-16 melanoma is carried in this species. With the exception the one *nido*-carborane, compound II, these compounds were well tolerated by the mice, at dosages of 62 mg/kg, and thus they are comparable with CPZ. Significant sedation was the major pharmacological effect which was observed. The *nido* compounds in other series[5] were significantly more toxic producing death at dosages of 50 mg/kg.

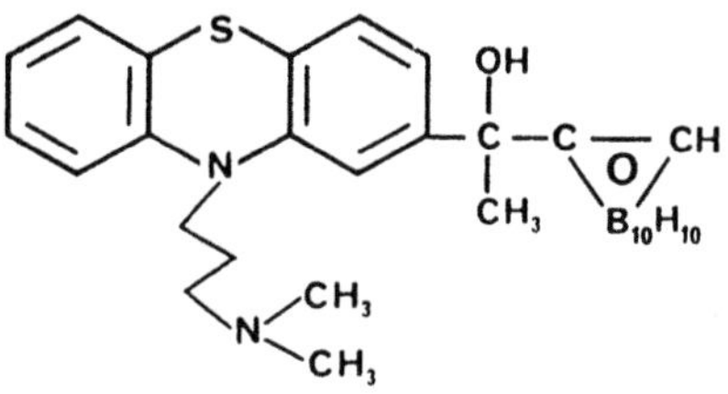

I

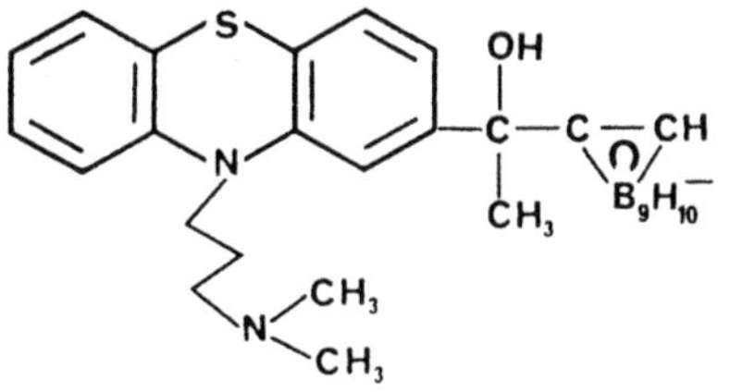

II

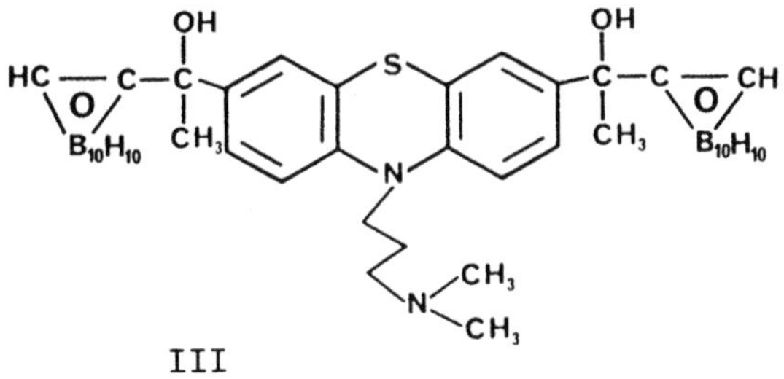

III

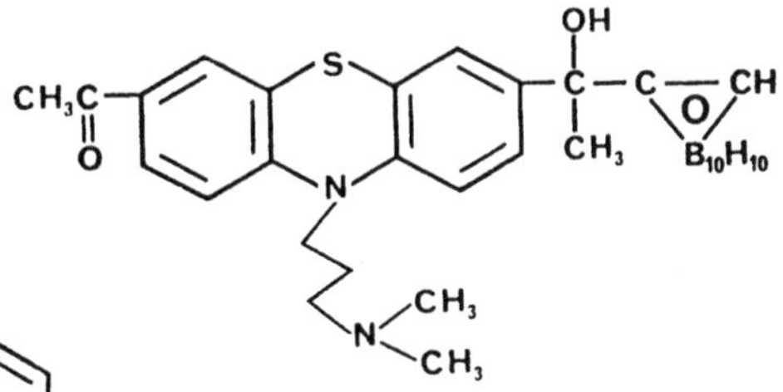

IV

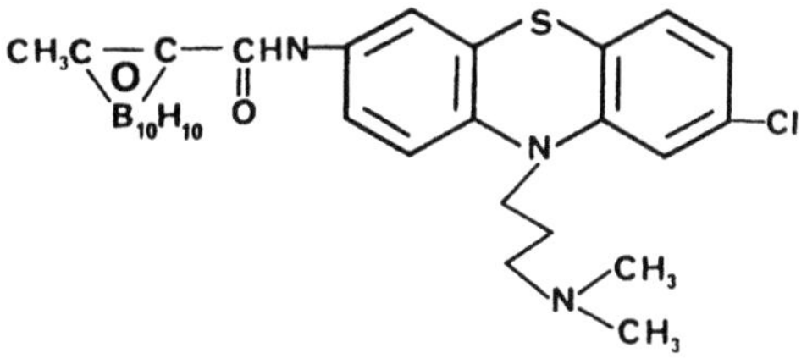

V

Figure 1. BORONATED PROMAZINES

These compounds are now being evaluated for tissue localization in B-16 melanoma-bearing C-57 black mice and in BALB/c mice with the Harding-Passey melanoma. Initial results with compound I have been disappointing since less than 2 μg B/g was obtained in the B16 melanoma with significantly higher concentrations in liver.

BORON-CONTAINING PHTHALOCYANINES

Phthalocyanines are very similar to porphyrins in their ability to localize in a variety of tumor. They have been used as radiodiagnostic agents[6] due to their ability to form highly stable metal chelates. Thus, the insertion of a radionuclide into the phthalocyanine nucleus has been the basis for their use diagnostically. This has been the basis for the synthesis of carborane-containing phthalocyanines.

As the first example in this new class of tumor-seeking boron compounds, we have succeeded in synthesizing the following phthalocyanine:

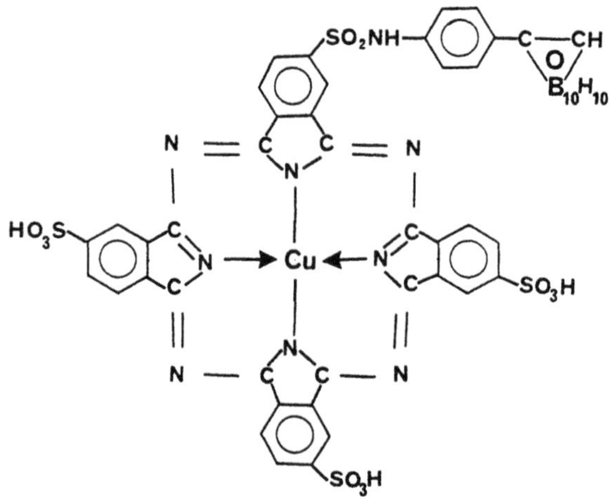

VI

The preparation of this compound involved first the synthesis of p-aminophenylcarborane by literature methods[7]. The phthalocyanine intermediate was prepared by the chlorosulfonation of copper phthalocyanine yielding copper phthalocyanine tetrasulfonylchloride. The reaction of this sulfochloride with p-aminophenylcarborane resulted in a mixture of boron-containing products with an average of 1.5 carborane cages per phthalocyanine nucleus. Work is now under way to separate the mixture and to isolate and fully characterize the precursor of compound VI. The unreacted sulfochloride groups can be readily hydrolyzed to the corresponding sulfonic acids. Such structures per se are water soluble or they may be converted to water-soluble alkali salts (e.g. SO_3Na). Their purification and full characterization will permit in vivo studies in tumor-bearing mice.

ACKNOWLEDGMENTS

The work described in this report has been supported by grant 5 R01 CA41288 from the National Institutes of Health, contract DE-AC02-82ERG0040 from the Department of Energy and a grant from the Office of Research and Graduate Studies, The Ohio State University.

REFERENCES

1. R. F. Barth, F. Alam, A. H. Soloway, D. M. Adams and Z. Steplewski, Boronated monoclonal antibody 17-1A for potential neutron capture therapy of colorectal cancer. Hybridoma 5:Suppl. 1:S43 (1986).

2. R. G. Fairchild, D. Greenberg, K. P. Watts, S. Packer, H. L. Atkins, P. Som, S. J. Hannon, A. B. Brill, I. Fand and W. P. McNally, Chlorpromazine distribution in hamsters and mice bearing transplantable melanoma. Cancer Res. 42:556 (1982).

3. Y. Mishima and T. Shimakage, Thermal neutron capture treatment of malignant melanomas using ^{10}B-Dopa and ^{10}B-chlorpromazine compounds. Pigment Cell 2:394 (1976).

4. F. Alam, A. H. Soloway, R. F. Barth, D. M. Adams and Z. Steplewski, Chemoradiotherapy of cancer: Boronated antibodies and boron-containing derivatives of promazine for neutron capture therapy, in: "Neutron Capture Therapy," H. Hatanaka, ed., Nishimura, Niigata, Japan (1986).

5. R. A. Spryshkova, L. I. Karaseva, V. A. Brattsev and N. G. Serebryakov, Toxicity of functional derivatives of polyhedral carboranes, Med. Radiol. 26:62 (1981).

6. W. H. Sweet, N. Shealey and A. H. Soloway, unpublished.

7. A. H. Soloway and D. N. Butler, Nitrogen Mustards, J. Med. Chem., 9:411 (1966).

FRACTIONATION CONSIDERATIONS FOR BORON NEUTRON CAPTURE THERAPY: THE PERSPECTIVE OF A CLINICIAN

Allen G. Meek

Department of Radiation Oncology
University Hospital at Stony Brook
Stony Brook, NY 11794-7028

Fractionation is the cornerstone of modern megavoltage photon therapy. The sparsely ionizing nature of x-ray therapy seems to necessitate fractionation for successful sterilization of malignant tumors. However, high-LET, densely ionizing radiations such as neutrons or alpha particles are less dependent on fractionation for their success. In this context, I will weigh the advantages and disadvantages of fractionation for boron neutron capture therapy for malignant gliomas.

The cell population effect of fractionation has been distilled into the "four R's" of Radiobiology; namely, Repair of sublethal injury, Reoxygenization of the tumor cell population, Redistribution of tumor cell ages, and Repopulation. For high-LET radiation, repair is of little significance, as most of the cell injury is irreparable. If there is a large gamma component in a neutron beam ($\geq$ approx. 90 cGy per fraction) then repair of the gamma component of cell injury between fractions may be important. Reoxygenation is less important for high-LET radiation as the OER is considerably less than for photon therapy. But again, if there is a large gamma contamination in the neutron beam, reoxygenation between fractions may be important. Redistribution also is less important for high-LET radiations compared to photons as there is less of a cycle dependence, but the same considerations hold as for reoxygenation. Repopulation of tumor cells is a disadvantage of fractionation, and thus minimizing fractions or the overall treatment time consistent with normal tissue tolerance is desirable. Time-dose data for tissue reactions from photon therapy are reasonably well understood for a limited range of fractionations, but this relationship is not nearly as well understood for high-LET radiations.

Based on these radiobiologic concepts and on clinical observations, the issue of fractionation is becoming better understood in photon therapy. The trend is toward increasing the number of fractions while keeping the overall treatment time the same (hyperfraction), or shortening it (accelerated fractionation). The concept then of treating a malignant glioma with a single fraction of radiation seems heretical. Though the radiobiologic basis of fractionation in high-LET radiations is not as strong as for low LET, there probably is some advantage (for the reasons given above), and this will be particularly true if there is a large gamma component to the neutron beam. Further argument potentially in favor of fractionation for high-LET radiation is that the RBE of densely ionizing radiations increases as the dose per fraction and the dose rate decrease. A greater RBE is probably desirable, though an unanswered question is: what are the relative effects on tumor-versus-normal tissue RBE; i.e., is there a therapeutic gain? The Boron "lens" should "focus" the beam selectively and provide the therapeutic gain.

Finally, another advantage of fractionation in boron neutron capture therapy is that multiple infusion of the boron compound could be given, increasing the probability of uptake by the tumor cells.

Looking at the other side, are there some clear disadvantages to fractionation? If anesthesia or craniotomy were necessary for each fraction, then this certainly would be a practical disadvantage. The epithermal beam should obviate this. If the boron were to be given as a monoclonal antibody, then it may not be possible to give multiple infusions due to the development of anti-antibodies, again arguing against fractionation. Thirdly, there may be some alteration of the blood-brain barrier by each fraction of radiation and this may effect the relative distribution of boron in the normal and tumor tissues--however, whether this is favorable or unfavorable is not obvious.

Overall, the arguments seem to favor some fractionation. Perhaps following the trend of the neutron trials, namely, a smaller number of fractions in a shorter period of time than used with photon therapy, is reasonable. A program of 7 to 8 fractions within a 3 to 4 week period, with treatment sessions lasting no more than 60 to, at most, 90 minutes, is a reasonable starting point. As a clinician, I would be comfortable recommending that to the patient under my care.

VASCULAR FACTORS AFFECTING DRUG DELIVERY TO BRAIN TUMORS

George Tyson, Joseph Fenstermacher, and Raphael Davis

Department of Neurological Surgery
Health Sciences Center
State University of New York at Stony Brook, Stony Brook, N.Y. 11794

A satisfactory agent for boron neutron capture therapy (BNCT) must bind tumor cells in preference to normal cellular elements of the brain. However, it must also be delivered in sufficient concentration to the tumor cells by the bloodstream. The latter depends upon the degree of uptake or binding of the agent by blood cells or plasma proteins, the blood flow within the tumor, the permeability of the tumor vasculature to the particular boronated agent, and the distribution volumes of the agent within the tumor and adjacent brain tissue[1,2].

This paper will briefly review the vascular factors that are important in selecting an agent for BNCT. In general, these particular factors -- tumor blood flow and microvascular permeability -- have not been considered critical limiting factors in BNCT . Although the normal cerebral capillary endothelium restricts the transfer of water-soluble drugs from blood to brain, the capillaries of malignant cerebral neoplasms are generally more permeable. Furthermore, blood flow in malignant brain tumors is generally normal or even increased, except in necrotic regions in which drug delivery is considerably less important.

Unfortunately, these generalizations may be inadequate for any form of drug therapy which is delivered by the bloodstream and which seeks to entirely eradicate a malignant brain tumor (or at least reduce the tumor burden to a level at which normal immunologic mechanisms can eliminate the residual tumor). Available multi-modality treatment programs fail to achieve a cure despite the fact that they can eliminate more than 99.99% of a tumor. Thus, novel forms of therapy are not needed for the vast majority of the tumor cells. Instead, all new forms of therapy -- including BNCT -- must concentrate on the .01% of tumor cells which are presumably "different" enough to escape destruction. In this perspective, general statements about tumor blood flow and microvascular permeability are of little value and the possibility of microregional heterogeneity becomes an important issue.

The rate of capillary blood flow may have a considerable effect on the quantity of a drug that is delivered to a brain tumor. Consider, for example, the effect of blood flow on the delivery of a chemotherapeutic agent such as chloroethyl-cyclohexyl-nitrosourea (CCNU) that crosses cerebral vascular endothelium relatively well.[3] If a particular region of a tumor had a blood flow of 100 ml/100 g/min, it would take only 6 seconds for the drug to achieve half-equilibration with the extracellular fluid of the brain. On the other hand, if another region of the same tumor had a blood flow of only 0.1 ml/100 g/min, the time required for the drug to achieve half-equilibration with the extracellular fluid would be 1.7 hours (and this assumes that the blood concentration of the drug does not decline during this period).

Does tumor capillary blood flow ever reach such a low level that it imposes a practical limitation on the delivery of a drug to tumor cells? Although physiologic imaging (e.g. PET scanning) of human brain tumors has demonstrated considerable heterogeneity in tissue blood flow rates, microregional flow has not been quantified because of the limited spatial resolution of *in vivo* imaging techniques. Therefore, most of the information on microregional blood flow in brain tumors has been derived from animal models.

Unfortunately, blood flow values and patterns of flow vary considerably among animal brain tumor models. In some models, there is an inverse relationship between the volume of the tumor and the rate of tumor blood flow. For example, in the Walker 256 metastatic carcinoma murine model,[4] the blood flow in small tumors (less than 1 mm in diameter) is approximately the same as in the surrounding white matter. In larger tumors, blood flow is reduced to as little as 10% of the white matter values. In fact, blood flow values below 10 ml/100g/min can be recorded from necrotic areas of larger tumors. A similar relationship between blood flow, tumor volume, and histological appearance can be discerned in certain other tumor models, such as the RT-9 transplanted tumor model.[5]

However, in still other models, such as the murine ethyl-nitroso-urea (ENU) induced glioma model,[6] blood flow is relatively normal and varies little from tumor to tumor, or from one region to another in an individual tumor. Conversely, blood flow is highly variable in rat brain tumors that are induced by the avian sarcoma virus.[7]

From animal data, as well as from the little human data that is available, it seems reasonable to conclude that tumor blood flow is potentially very heterogeneous, particularly in large tumors. Furthermore, the lowest levels of blood flow are often associated with tumor necrosis. The latter is not necessarily reassuring, since it is unclear whether histologically necrotic areas are completely devoid of viable cells (particularly on the periphery). It is also worth emphasizing that in some models, blood flow reductions are less circumscribed. For example, in the murine Walker 256 metastatic carcinoma model, even the "normal" white matter adjacent to large tumors had a blood flow that is only 50% of normal.[4] Although a 50% reduction is probably not significant enough to impose a practical limitation on the delivery of a chemotherapeutic agent, this finding is still important. The "normal" white matter adjacent to malignant human gliomas is infiltrated with neoplastic cells and this may represent an important reservoir of cells that survive present treatments. Since the blood-brain (and blood-tumor) barrier may be considerably less permeable in this region (see below), any degree of reduction in tissue blood flow takes on additional importance with regard to drug delivery.

Important as blood flow may be in limiting drug delivery to at least some portions of malignant brain tumors, the degree of capillary permeability is potentially more important. Most drugs that traverse the normal blood-brain barrier do so by dissolving in and diffusing through capillary endothelial cells. It is unlikely that any drug can pass through the tight junctions that join adjacent cerebral capillary endothelial cells. Furthermore, few drugs have any affinity for the highly-specific carrier mechanisms that mediate the transfer of solutes (such as glucose or leucine). Therefore, the rate of blood-to-brain transfer of a drug is directly related to its lipid solubility and inversely related to its molecular size (which influences its diffusivity). Clearly, drugs that have a relatively high water solubility and a large molecular size are at a disadvantage and many chemotherapeutic agents fit this description.

In general, the permeability of capillaries is increased in malignant cerebral neoplasms. However, this is not uniformly the case. Again, adequate data is lacking for human tumors and most of our information is based on animal models. In the Walker 256 carcinoma model,[3,8,9] permeability to amino-isobutyric acid (AIB, a small, neutral amino acid) is increased as much as 50-100 times in larger tumors. On the other hand, permeability is not increased at all in smaller tumors. Of potentially greater significance is the fact that permeability is only modestly increased (2-4 times the permeability of normal white matter) in the brain tissue immediately adjacent to larger tumors. Again, this is the region in which the tumor may infiltrate otherwise normal brain, at least in the case of malignant human gliomas.

It should also be noted that in some tumors, such as the astrocytomas that are induced by the avian sarcoma virus,[7] there is marked variation in permeability even within an individual tumor, and in other tumors (e.g. the ENU-induced gliomas) the increases in permeability are, for the most part, relatively small.[10,11]

In conclusion, it seems reasonable to state that capillary blood flow and permeability are not likely to limit the delivery of parenterally-administered chemotherapeutic agents to the vast majority of viable cells in a malignant brain tumor. However, a combination of low blood flow and relatively normal capillary permeability may limit drug delivery to a very small fraction of these cells (particularly those that infiltrate histologically normal brain tissue). Furthermore, it may be this fraction of cells that is partially responsible for the "recurrence" of tumors after present forms of multi-modality therapy have been administered.

Thus, the ideal boronated compound would have considerable lipid solubility (considering, of course, that any parenterally-administered compound must also be reasonably soluble in plasma) and would also be relatively diffusible. Nevertheless, any boronated compound would share the potential limitations of all therapeutic agents that must be delivered to a brain tumor by the bloodstream.

References

1. J.D. Fenstermacher, Drug transfer across the blood-brain barrier, in: "Topic in Pharmaceutical Sciences," D.D. Breimer and P. Speiser, eds., Elsevier, Amsterdam (1983)

2. J. Fenstermacher and J. Gazendam, Intra-arterial infusions of drugs and hyperosmotic solutions as ways of enhancing CNS chemotherapy. Cancer Treat. Rep. 65 (Suppl. 2): 27 (1981)

3. R.G. Blasberg, T. Kobayashi, C.S. Patlak, M. Shinohara, M. Miyoaka, J.M. Rice, and W.R. Shapiro, Regional blood flow, capillary permeability, and glucose utilization in two brain tumor models: Preliminary observations and pharmacokinetic implications. Cancer Treat. Rep. 65 (Suppl. 2): 3 (1981)

4. R.G. Blasberg, W.R. Shapiro, P. Molnar, C.S. Patlak, and J.D. Fenstermacher, Local blood flow in Walker 256 metastatic brain tumors. J. Neuro-Oncol. 2: 195 (1984)

5. R.G. Blasberg, P. Molnar, M. Horowitz, P. Kornblith, R. Pleasants, and J. Fenstermacher. Regional blood flow in RT-9 brain tumors. J. Neurosurg. 58: 863 (1983)

6. R.G. Blasberg, T. Kobayashi, M. Horowitz, J.M. Rice, D. Groothuis, P. Molnar and J.D. Fenstermacher. Regional blood flow in ethylnitrosourea-induced brain tumors. Ann. Neurol. 14: 189 (1983)

7. Molnar, R.G. Blasberg, and D. Goothuis. Regional blood-to-tissue transport in avian sarcoma virus (ASV)-induced brain tumors. Neurology 33: 702 (1983)

8. R.G. Blasberg, J. Gazendam, W.R. Shapiro, M. Shinohara, C.S. Patlak, and J.D. Fenstermacher. Clinical implications of quantitative autoradiographic measurements of regional blood flow, capillary permeability and glucose utilization in a metastatic brain tumor model, in: "Treatment of Neoplastic Lesions of the Nervous System," J. Holderbrand and D. Gangji, eds., Pergamon, New York (1982)

9. R.G. Blasberg, W.R. Shapiro, P. Molnar, C.S. Patlak, and J.D. Fenstermacher. Local blood-to-tissue transport in Walker 256 metastatic brain tumors. J. Neuro-Oncol. 2: 205 (1984)

10. R.G. Blasberg, T. Kobayashi, M. Horowitz, J.M. Rice, D. Groothuis, P. Molnar, and J.D. Fenstermacher. Regional blood-to-brain tissue transport in ethylnitrosourea-induced brain tumors. Ann. Neurol. 14: 202 (1983)

11. P. Molnar, R.G. Blasberg, M. Horowitz, B. Smith, and J. Fenstermacher. Regional blood-to-tissue transport in RT-9 brain tumors. J. Neurosurg. 58: 874 (1983)

CLINICAL CONSIDERATIONS IN THE USE OF THERMAL AND EPITHERMAL NEUTRON BEAMS FOR NEUTRON CAPTURE THERAPY

Robert G.A.Zamenhof*, Hywel Madoc-Jones*,
Otto K. Harling#, and John A.Bernard, Jr.#

*Department of Radiation Oncology
Tufts-New England Medical Center
Boston, Massachusetts 02111

#Nuclear Reactor Laboratory
Massachusetts Institute of Technology
Cambridge, Massachusetts 02139

INTRODUCTION

Two important developments in the field of neutron capture therapy (NCT) in recent years have been the ultra-wide thermal neutron beam[1] and the epithermal neutron beam.[2,3] Both these maneuvers improve the depth in tissue at which the therapeutic advantage falls to unity, often referred to as the "advantage depth".[3,4] Both neutron beams have contaminating dose components, i.e., those that are not tumor-cell specific. These include: incident gamma rays (those originating in the reactor core and those produced by neutron capture in the beam line's structural materials); induced gamma rays (produced mainly by thermal neutron capture by hydrogen within the target tissue itself); background thermal neutrons (which interact mainly with tissue nitrogen by neutron capture, producing proton emission); and incident epithermal and fast neutrons (producing mainly recoil protons by scattering with tissue hydrogen). Whereas incident gammas and epithermal and fast neutrons (above about 30 keV) can be reduced to acceptably low levels by judicious beam design, the induced gamma and background thermal neutron doses are largely irreducible, although higher concentrations of ^{10}B in tumor diminishes their magnitude on a relative basis. Incident epithermal neutrons of 0.5 eV-30 keV, however, are the desirable components of an epithermal neutron beam. Such neutrons thermalize at depth in tissue, thereby producing the desired ^{10}B reactions.

Very simplistically, an epithermal beam may be considered equivalent to a thermal beam "injected" at a couple of centimeters depth in tissue.

In this paper we shall review the capabilities of the existing thermal beam and anticipated epithermal beam at the MIT Research Reactor (MITR-II) Medical Therapy Facility (MTF), and discuss the comparative advantages and disadvantages of thermal and epithermal neutron beams for NCT. Although historically our team has concentrated on the applications of NCT to the treatment of high grade astrocytomas, we will not assume such a constraint in our analysis.

THERMAL BEAM FACILITY AT MITR-II

The MIT Research Reactor, located on the MIT campus in Cambridge, Massachusetts, first achieved criticality on July 21, 1958. The original design of the reactor incorporated a dedicated medical therapy facility in anticipation of future applications of this reactor for medical research, in particular neutron capture therapy. Between 1959 and 1961, sixteen grade III-IV astrocytoma patients were unsuccessfully treated by neutron capture therapy at the MIT reactor in collaborative trials with Massachusetts General Hospital. In retrospect the reasons for these and earlier failures of NCT are now identified and understood. Presently, the MIT reactor supports a large number of research and teaching programs at MIT and other surrounding universities, including nuclear engineering, physics, metallurgy and material science, earth and planetary sciences, nutrition and food science, and chemical engineering. The reactor also operates a neutron activation analysis facility. The reactor supports a number of medical research projects with various hospitals, including a newly developed program of radiation synovectomy using the isotopes dysprosium and holmnium in collaboration with Boston's Brigham and Womens' Hospital, the supply of radioactive gold seeds for interstitial cancer therapy to Boston's Deaconess Hospital, and in the past the supply of radioactive osmium/iridium generators to Boston's Childrens' Hospital for pediatric nuclear cardiological applications. Finally, since July, 1987 the reactor and its staff have been an integral component of the Tufts-New England Medical Center/MIT collaborative program in neutron capture therapy, funded by a $1,200,000 three-year grant from the U.S. Department of Energy.[5]

Fig. 1 is a cut-away view of MITR-II, and represents the current configuration which has existed since July, 1976 when a major upgrade of the reactor was completed. The MTF is seen at the bottom of the illustration. The MTF is tiled, has a sink with

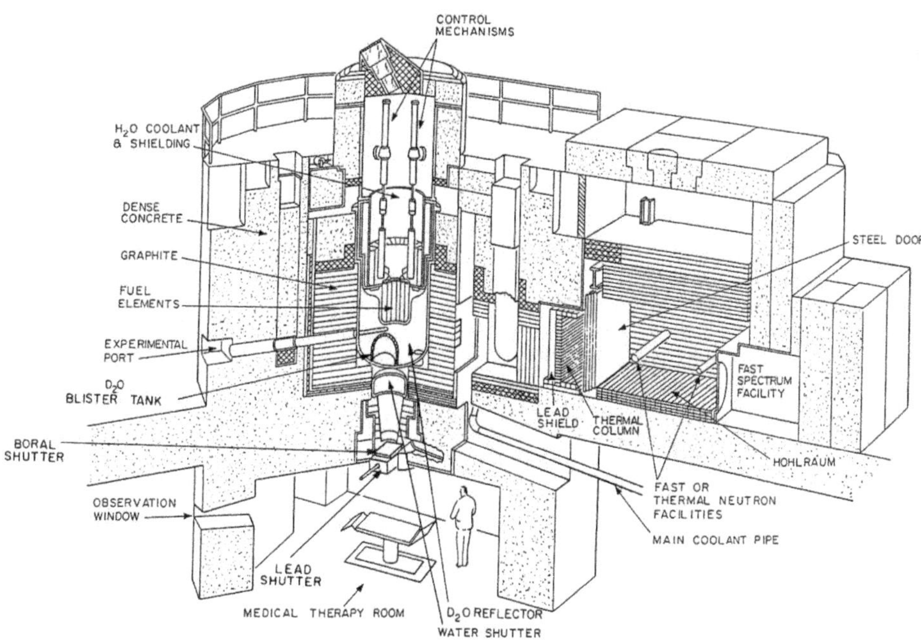

Fig. 1. Cut-away drawing of the Massachusetts Institute of Technology Research Reactor, MITR-II, showing the location of the medical therapy facility and medical therapy neutron beam line. A 6-foot tall person standing in the irradiation room indicates the scale of the drawing.

water supply, peripheral ultraviolet antibacterial lights, and contains a surgical couch on a hydraulic pedestal on which a patient can be raised up to the irradiation position near the ceiling. A water-filled observation window permits a direct view of the patient at all times while protecting personnel from radiation. A motorized shielded door separates the irradiation room from the surrounding area but allows fast access and egress when necessary for the safety of the patient. Beam control is achieved using three independent shutters. Starting with the topmost in Fig. 1, these are a light-water shutter, a lead shutter, and a boral shutter. When these shutters are all closed the dose rate within the irradiation room is at a completely safe level. The shutters are remotely controlled from outside the irradiation room and allow beam control independent of normal reactor operations. There is a large entrance door into the reactor building into which an ambulance can reverse to discharge a patient. Immediately next to this entrance inside is an elevator which can lower a patient on a stretcher to an area adjacent to the irradiation room. The MTF is a unique feature of the MIT Research Reactor.

As part of the reactor's upgrade during 1973-1976 the quality of the thermal beam in the MTF was greatly improved by reducing incident gammas and fast neutrons. Currently, at the patient irradiation position the thermal neutron flux is 4.10^9 $cm^{-2}s^{-1}$ (which can easily be increased 2-4 times) with a gold-cadmium ratio of 250:1, while the incident gamma and fast neutron dose rates are, respectively, 3 cGy/min and 0.3 cGy/min. A useful design aspect of MITR-II is a heavy-water tank (labelled "D_2O blister tank" in Fig. 1) which can be partially or completely emptied to provide a more intense epithermal and fast neutron component in the beam; this provides a desirable degree of flexibility for the development of an epithermal beam. The beam is shaped by collimators and has a maximum diameter of 20 cm at the patient position.

Fig. 2 depicts the tissue-surface dose rate components for the MITR-II thermal beam. The curved line shows the macroscopic ^{10}B dose rate as a function of ^{10}B concentration in tissue. A useful measure of the "purity" of a neutron beam for NCT is the equivalent ^{10}B concentration at which the "total background dose" and "^{10}B dose" lines cross. In the case of the MITR-II thermal beam this occurs at just over 10 microgram/g of ^{10}B. The lower this value the "purer" the beam and the greater the depth of therapeutic advantage.

The various dose components, as depicted in Fig. 2, can be grossly divided into two categories: those with linear energy transfers (LET) more than 100 keV/micron, and those with LET less than 100 keV/micron. With this partition, the ^{10}B dose falls into the first category while the other dose components fall into the second. It has been observed since the 1920's that fractionated irradiation of tissue with "low" LET radiation (such as X-rays or gamma rays) results in the ability to deliver substantially higher doses to achieve a given biological effect than with acute irradiation. In the upper limit, generally fractionation can approximately triple the low LET dose that can be delivered to achieve a given biological effect. With fractionated dose delivery a greater opportunity for the repair of sublethal radiation damage is believed to occur, the half-time for which is on the order of one hour. Also in Fig. 2 is a dotted horizontal line which is one half the value of the "total background dose", representing the amount of reduction in the effect of the lower LET background dose that might accrue under a maximally effective fractionation schedule. It is assumed that under the same fractionation schedule the effectiveness of the high LET ^{10}B dose would not be reduced. Under such illustrative conditions it can be seen that the purity of the MITR-II thermal beam would be improved to 3 microgram/g ^{10}B equivalent. Compared with other research reactor thermal beams potentially suitable for NCT, the present MITR-II thermal beam is sufficiently pure and very well suited for patient treatment.

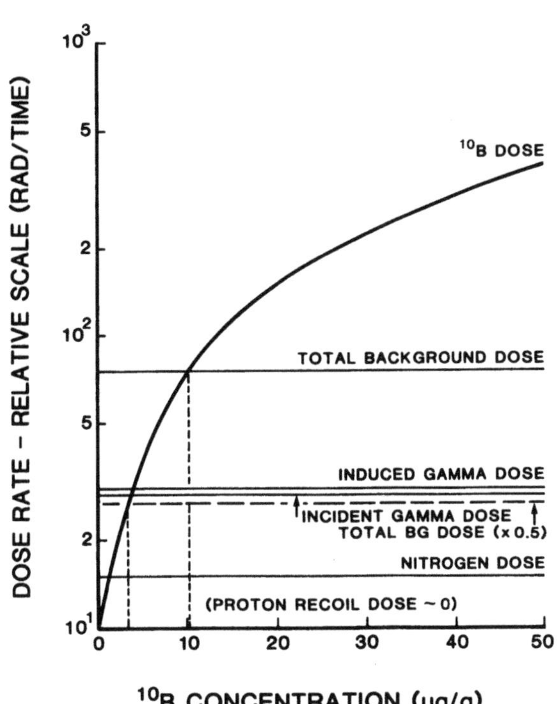

Fig. 2. Brain-tissue surface dose components for MITR-II thermal beam, illustrating the possible influence of dose fractionation or protraction on the effective purity of the beam. Time to deliver 2000 cGy total dose is approximately 1 hour.

Because of the relatively poor advantage depths typical of most thermal beams, the procedure for the NCT treatment of high-grade astrocytomas by Hatanaka in Japan was to initially surgically remove the bulk of the tumor, then to reflect the scalp and reopen the skull flap during NCT treatment, thus minimizing the tissue thickness overlying the deepest margin of the tumor.[6] By such means tumor margins lying 6 cm from the surface of the scalp--essentially beyond the advantage depth for a typical thermal beam under typical conditions--may after such surgical maneuvers be only 3 cm from the surgically modified and exposed surface of the brain, and thus within the advantage depth of the thermal beam. However, such an intraoperative NCT procedure, requiring surgery and remote general anesthesia at the reactor site, would not be conducive to fractionated irradiation; a protracted irradiation lasting up to 8-10 hours would not necessarily be out of the question, since patients treated by NCT in Japan have not infrequently been irradiated for over 6 hours.

Can the advantage depth of a thermal beam be substantially improved? Improving the purity of the beam and/or improving the depth-dose characteristic for the ^{10}B dose will increase the advantage depth. In the discussion above we already commented that the effective purity of a thermal beam can be improved both by protracted irradiation and judicious beam design, while recent data from Japan[1] showed that the ^{10}B depth-dose can be significantly improved by employing larger diameter beams.

Fig. 3 shows advantage depth curves based on dosimetric data for the MITR-II thermal beam. Assuming a tumor ^{10}B concentration of 30 microgram/g and a ^{10}B tumor:blood ratio of 4:1, Fig. 3 shows that with a diameter of 15 cm and no dose protraction an advantage depth of approximately 3 cm would be achieved. Analysis of the original depth-dose data from which Fig. 3 was constructed[3] reveals that protraction, as depicted in Fig. 2, might increase the advantage depth under the above ^{10}B distribution conditions to approximately 4 cm. Similarly, analysis of the 22-cm wide beam data from Japan[1] suggests that with no dose protraction an advantage depth of approximately 5 cm could be achieved, while with dose protraction this might further be increased to 6 cm. Advantage depths of 6-7 cm correspond to a patient's brain midline (from the lateral aspect) thus introducing the opportunity of treating midline tumors with a pair of parallel-opposed beams to approximately halve normal tissue dose near the surface. However, it is unlikely that with the current generation of blood-brain-barrier type boron compounds having comparatively poor tumor:blood ratios[6] that the unreflected scalp could tolerate the required high surface doses, even with parallel-opposed irradiation; but it might not be out of the question to consider a bilateral scalp reflection while leaving the skull intact. However, with improved tumor-seeking boron compounds exhibiting very high tumor:blood ratios even scalp reflection might not be necessary.

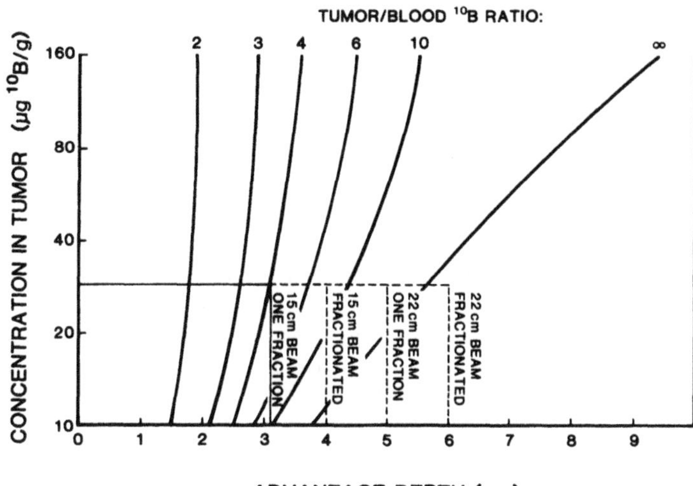

Fig. 3. Illustrative advantage depth curves based on the MITR-II thermal beam showing the anticipated advantage of ultra-wide beam and dose fractionation strategies. A ^{10}B tumor concentration of 30 microgram/g and tumor:blood ratio of 4:1 is assumed for illustrative purposes.

EPITHERMAL BEAM DEVELOPMENT AT MITR-II

As a part of the Department of Energy's funded NCT program, we are designing and constructing an epithermal beam at MITR-II. We previously argued that an optimal epithermal neutron beam for NCT should have an energy of approximately 40 eV[3]. There is no methodology at present for producing such monochromatic epithermal beams with adequate intensity for NCT, but it is possible to produce such beams having a broad spectrum in the eV and low keV region. Our approach is to design an epithermal beam having an energy range of approximately 0.5 eV-30 keV by employing s-wave resonance and potential scattering interference filters. We are presently using a Monte Carlo neutron/photon coupled transport code to optimize the thicknesses of aluminum, sulfur, heavy water, lithium-6, and bismuth filters to be placed in the medical therapy beam line. The goal is to design a broad spectrum epithermal beam with minimum incident gamma and fast neutron contamination while maintaining an incident neutron flux intensity of 10^8 $cm^{-2}s^{-1}$ or greater. This would permit a ^{10}B therapeutic dose to be delivered in approximately ten hourly fractions. A concommitant design goal is to construct these modification such that a switchover between thermal and epithermal beams, or vice versa, would be possible within approximately 24 hours. This would provide the flexibility of selecting the optimum beam or combination of beams for each patient, based on the tumor's size and location, geometry of the brain defect, and the ^{10}B distribution.

Epithermal beams potentially could provide greater advantage depths than thermal beams, while their ^{10}B depth-dose curves exhibit a characteristic build-up at 1.5-2.5 cm depth in tissue[2,3]. These two attributes make epithermal beams potentially suitable for NCT treatment through the intact skull and scalp. Although no epithermal beams suitable for treatment exist, one possible problem with such beams is that they may produce a relatively high background dose due to contamination with fast neutrons and incident gamma rays. Fig. 4 illustrates what might prove to be typical characteristics of filtered epithermal beams for NCT. Note that Figs. 2 and 4 were normalized to equal maximum thermal neutron flux (at the surface for the thermal beam and at 2 cm build-up depth for the epithermal beam). Consequently, the "nitrogen", "induced gamma", and "^{10}B" doses, which are dependent only on the thermal neutron flux level in tissue, are normalized to the same values for the two beams. For the epithermal beam the "proton recoil" dose, which is dependent on the incident epithermal and fast neutron flux levels, is seen to be significantly elevated compared to the thermal beam, while the "incident" gamma dose is seen to be slightly elevated. It should be reiterated that the parameters shown here for this generic epithermal beam are only illustrative and do not represent any specific design. As with the thermal beam, we may consider the "purity" of the epithermal beam as the ^{10}B equivalent concentration where the "^{10}B dose" and "total background dose" curves intersect; i.e., at 16-17 microgram/g--notably poorer than the 10 microgram/g for the thermal beam. Fig. 4 also shows an estimate of the reduced effective total background dose that might be obtained with fractionated or protracted irradiation. The effective purity of the beam under such circumstances improves to 8-9 microgram/g.

Fig. 5 shows advantage depth curves for the generic epithermal beam depicted in Fig 4. A few important features make these curves strikingly different from the ones for the thermal beam (Fig. 3). At very high tumor ^{10}B levels the epithermal beam roughly doubles the advantage depths of the thermal beam, but at low tumor ^{10}B levels it is not significantly superior. Also, in the typical tumor ^{10}B range of

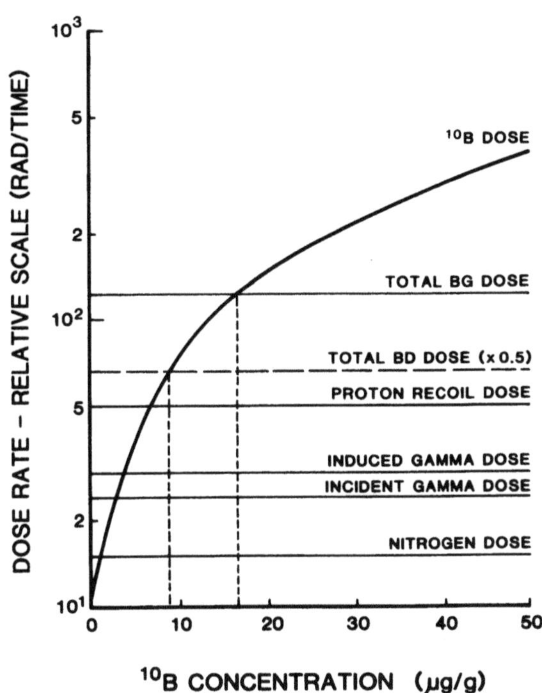

Fig. 4. Dose components at 2 cm depth in brain tissue for a "generic" filtered epithermal beam with relatively high background dose, illustrating the possible influence of dose fractionation on the effective purity of the beam.

10-30 microgram/g for available blood-brain-barrier type compounds (such as the monomer of the boron sulfhydryl compound used in Japan for brain tumor therapy) the advantage depths for the epithermal beam are much less sensitive to ^{10}B tumor:blood ratio than those for the thermal beam. This underscores an interesting difference between these beams. For a boron-carrying agent which exhibits comparatively low ^{10}B tumor levels but high tumor:blood ratios (e.g., 10 microgram/g and 10:1, respectively), a thermal beam might exhibit superior advantage depths to an epithermal beam, especially if the latter produces a comparatively high background dose. In contrast, if a boron carrying agent exhibits high ^{10}B tumor levels (e.g., >50 microgram/g), then an epithermal beam--even one of poor purity--would exhibit advantage depths greatly superior to a thermal beam. It is possible that a

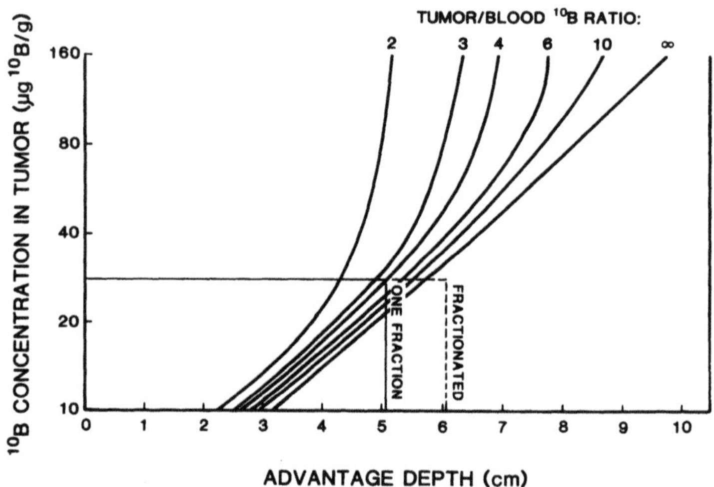

Fig. 5. Illustrative advantage depth curves for a "generic" filtered epithermal beam with relatively high background dose, illustrating the anticipated advantage of dose fractionation or protraction. A ^{10}B tumor concentration of 30 microgram/g and tumor:blood ratio of 4:1 is assumed for illustrative purposes.

monoclonal antibody agent might fall into the first category,[7] while an agent which is metabolically incorporated into tumor, such as p-borophenylalanine for the treatment of melanotic malignant melanoma, might fall into the second.[8] Fig. 5 also shows an estimate of the increase in advantage depth that might be incurred if the background dose component were "fractionated down" by a factor of 2. It is important to try and maximize the purity of epithermal beams unless high tumor ^{10}B levels are anticipated, in which case a reduction in the effect of the background dose would yield marginal benefit. We should like to underscore that there are many factors to be considered in the comparative evaluation of thermal and epithermal beams for NCT.

Figs. 2,3,4, and 5 do not include any relative biological effectiveness (RBE) weighting factors on the doses. While the RBE of the gamma dose components is close to unity, the RBE of the background neutron dose components probably lies somewhere between 1 and 2, while that for the alpha and ^{7}Li particles from the boron reaction lies somewhere between 2 and 4.[9,10] Whatever the true RBE values are it is highly likely that on a relative basis the ^{10}B dose is at least twice as biologically effective as the background neutron dose; Therefore, the purities of the thermal and epithermal beams and their respective advantage depths presented here are conservative estimates. In addition, Monte Carlo simulation[11] and analytic calculation[12] showed that the actual dose to endothelial cells from ^{10}B in the blood is 0.3-0.5 times the macroscopic dose. Such an effect can be represented on the advantage depth curves of Figs. 3 and 5 as a corresponding increase in effective ^{10}B tumor:blood ratio. For example, an actual tumor:blood ratio of 3:1 would translate to an effective ratio of 6:1 if the 0.5 factor above were assumed to apply. This would suggest that the advantage depth curves shown in Figs. 3 and 5 may be additionally conservative.

IRRADIATION STRATEGIES FOR THERMAL AND EPITHERMAL BEAMS

When treating a tumor by NCT, two fundamental criteria must be satisfied: (1) sufficient dose must be delivered to the most deeply located tumor cells; (2) a tolerance dose must be assured for normal tissue structures. Recognizing these criteria we developed the concept of "advantage depth"[3] which, despite its simplicity, is probably still the most useful criterion for treatment planning for NCT. In three dimensions we may think of advantage surfaces rather than advantage depths, with the goal of treatment planning being to ensure that the surface with the assumed limiting advantage ratio (usually assumed to be 1) is distal to all known regions of tumor or residual tumor bed.

Hatanaka's approach to brain tumor therapy by NCT involves thermal beam irradiation of a residual tumor bed with reflection of scalp and skull. Such a surgical maneuver protects the scalp from receiving an unacceptably high ^{10}B radiation dose (since the amount of blood/cc is much higher in the scalp than in the brain) and also eliminates 1-2 cm of overlying skull and scalp which would otherwise "eat into" the available advantage depth of the thermal beam. In contrast, the potential attractiveness of NCT using an epithermal beam is that it might possess sufficient advantage depth to alleviate the necessity of reopening the skull and possibly reflecting the scalp of the patient before irradiation. If the epithermal beam could be shown to have advantage depths at least 1-2 cm greater than a thermal beam, then there would be a clear advantage in using it. Fractionated or protracted irradiation should, as demonstrated earlier, further increase the advantage depths of both thermal and epithermal beams. However, if an ultra-wide thermal beam were used, such as proposed in Japan[1] Figs. 3 and 5 suggest that such a beam could match the advantage depth of an epithermal beam (at least a relatively impure one). In that case, failure to reflect scalp and skull when using the epithermal beam might render it actually less effective than an ultra-wide thermal beam delivered through a reflected scalp and skull. On the other hand, an epithermal beam could be delivered in a parallel-opposed geometry, thereby further increasing its advantage depth.

Could an ultra-wide thermal beam be used to advantage with a reflected bone window that is significantly smaller than the width of the beam? Would an ultra-wide epithermal beam demonstrate significant improvements in advantage depth? These are complex and relevant questions that we are attempting to answer through a combination of experimental measurements and Monte Carlo simulation.

We have mentioned these various treatment scenarios mainly to indicate why it would be useful to possess both a thermal and an epithermal beam capability at a reactor facility. Indeed, it might prove advantageous to perform irradiations using combinations of such beams. Treatment planning decisions would depend on the biological distribution characteristics of the ^{10}B agent employed, the location, size, and shape of the tumor or residual tumor bed, and on the condition of the patient--in particular the ability to tolerate extended general anesthesia in the case of a protracted intraoperative thermal beam irradiation. If an epithermal beam were to be used it would also need to be recognized that the integral dose characteristics of such beams would be quite different from those of thermal beams. Tolerance doses derived empirically for thermal beams may, therefore, need to be lowered when using epithermal beams.

CONCLUSION

Improved Federal support in the area of neutron capture therapy has produced a resurgence in neutron capture therapy research and interest in the United States. Encouraging clinical results from Japan in the treatment of glioblastoma multiforme and malignant melanoma brain metastases have spurred on a growing enthusiasm for neutron capture therapy among a wide range of scientific and medical disciplines. One area of intense debate and research is the issue of which types of neutron beams would be most suitable for starting new trials in the United States. In this paper we have reviewed some of the important issues regarding the relative merits of thermal and epithermal beams for neutron capture therapy. We are glad if we have prompted more questions than provided answers, since a rigorous treatment of the subject must include many more issues than we have addressed.

REFERENCES

1. T. Matsumoto and O. Aizawa, Depth-dose evaluation and optimization of the irradiation facility for boron neutron capture therapy of brain tumors, Phys. Med. Biol. 30:897 (1985)
2. R. G. Fairchild, Development and dosimetry of an epithermal neutron beam for possible use in neutron capture therapy. I. Epithermal neutron beam development, Phys. Med. Biol. 10:491 (1965)
3. R. G. Zamenhof, B.W. Murray, G.L. Brownell, G.R. Wellum, E.I. Tolpin, Boron neutron capture therapy for the treatment of cerebral gliomas. I. Theoretical evaluation of the efficacy of various neutron beams, Medical Physics 2:47 (1975)
4. G. L. Brownell, R.G. Zamenhof, B.W. Murray, G.R. Wellum, Boron neutron capture therapy, in: "Therapy in Nuclear Medicine," R.P. Spencer, ed., Grune and Stratton, New York (1978)
5. O. K. Harling, J.A. Bernard, R.G. Zamenhof, H. Madoc-Jones, A clinical trial of neutron capture therapy for brain cancer, in: Proc. of int. symp. on the utilization of multi-purpose research reactors and related international co-operation, I.A.E.A., Vienna (1988)
6. H. Hatanaka, S. Kamano, K. Amano, S. Hojo, K. Sano, E. Egawa, H. Yasukochi, Clinical experience of boron neutron capture therapy for gliomas--a comparison with conventional chemo-immuno radiotherapy, in: "Boron-Neutron Capture Therapy for Tumors," H. Hatanaka, ed., Nishimura, Niigata, Japan (1986)
7. G. R. Wellum, R.G. Zamenhof, E.I. Tolpin, Boron neutron capture therapy of cerebral gliomas. III. An analysis of the possible use of boron loaded tumor specific antibodies for the selective concentration of boron in gliomas, Int. J. Rad. Onc. Biol. Phys. 8:1339 (1982)
8. J. A. Coderre, J.D. Glass, R.G. Fairchild, U. Roy, S. Cohen, I. Fand, Selective targeting of boronophenylalanine to

melanoma in BALB/c mice for neutron capture therapy, Cancer Research 47:6377 (1987)

9. D. Gabel, R.G. Fairchild, B. Larsson, K. Drescher, W.R. Rowe, The biological effect of the $^{10}B(n,alpha)^{7}Li$ reaction and its simulation by Monte Carlo calculations, in: Proc. of 1 st. int. symp. on neutron capture therapy, Report #51730, Brookhaven National Laboratory, Upton, New York (1984)
10. M. A. Davis, J.B. Little, K.M.M.S. Ayyangar, A.R. Reddy, Relative biological effectiveness of the $^{10}B(n,alpha)^{7}Li$ reaction in HeLa cells, Radiat. Res. 43:534 (1972)
11. R. A. Rydin, O.L. Deutsch, B.W. Murray, The effect of geometry on capillary wall dose for boron neutron capture therapy, Phys. Med. Biol. 21:134 (1976)
12. K. Kitao, A method for calculating the absorbed dose near an interface from the $^{10}B(n,alpha)^{7}Li$ reaction, Radiat. Res. 61:304 (1975)

ACKNOWLEDGMENTS

We would like to acknowledge the contributions of S. Clement, N. Lizzo, R. Choi, and W. Fecych to this paper. This work is supported by Grant 87ER60600 from the U.S. Department of Energy.

A PROPOSED PROTOCOL FOR CLINICAL TRIALS OF BORON NEUTRON CAPTURE THERAPY IN GLIOBLASTOMA MULTIFORME

Ronald V. Dorn III, John H. Spickard, and
Merle L. Griebenow

Idaho National Engineering Laboratory
EG&G Idaho, Inc.
P.O. Box 1625
Idaho Falls, ID 83415-3519

and

Mountain States Tumor Institute
151 East Bannock
Boise, ID 83712

INTRODUCTION

Neutron Capture Therapy (NCT) was suggested in theory as a treatment for malignant tumors some 50 years ago. Since then, considerable data have accumulated on the mechanisms of action and possible application of this technique. This paper outlines a protocol for a controlled study of the use of Boron Neutron Capture Therapy (BNCT) for the treatment of Glioblastoma Multiforme (GM). The protocol is one component of a comprehensive national BNCT research program at the Idaho National Engineering Laboratory (INEL) directed towards validating (or invalidating) NCT as a treatment for human malignancies. This paper will address the following three points:

1. Provide a background of GM, as a tumor model, including current conventional treatment and research avenues.

2. Present an overview and framework of the clinical protocol.

3. Introduce questions on research that may well impact the protocol before it is used, including possible additional tumor systems to be studied.

BACKGROUND

We will study the use of BNCT in the treatment of GM. As shown in Fig. 1, a three-tiered classification of astrocytoma includes GM as the most malignant component of this tumor group. Histologically, the diagnosis of GM in this classification system relies on the presence of marked hypercellularity, pleomorphism, hyperchromatic nuclei, vascular proliferation, and necrosis. The presence of necrosis is a required criteria for the diagnosis of GM. Table 1 (Cancer: Principles and Practice of Oncology, 2nd Edition, 1985) shows the very poor survival associated with GM, represented on the table as Grade IV. This summary of many clinical studies shows that GM, or Grade IV astrocytoma, has a two-year survival of ten percent and almost no patients surviving at five years after both surgery and conventional radiation therapy (XRT). Median survival with this tumor is in the range of 45-50 weeks. Current conventional treatment of GM includes surgery for biopsy and documentation of the diagnosis, as well as sometimes removing as much tumor as possible without causing significant additional neurological deficit. Surgery then is followed with fractionated photon XRT, using multiple fields, to a total dose of 6000 to 6600 cGy over 42-56 days. This treatment is limited by the

I. Astrocytoma

II. Anaplastic astrocytoma

III. Glioblastoma Multiforme

3-tiered system after Brain Tumor Study Group (BTSG)

Fig. 1. A three-tiered classification of astrocytoma.

Table 1. Survival with Glioblastoma Multiforme

Grade	Surgery (±)	Radiation Therapy (±)	Survival (%)		
			1 Year	2 Years	5 Years
III	+	-	10 - 15	5 - 10	0
	+	+	40	30	15 - 20
IV	+	-	5	0	0
	+	+	25 - 50	10	0 - 3

normal brain's intolerance to XRT, with a rapidly increasing incidence of brain damage from radiation above these doses. A variety of experimental approaches have been and are being made in an effort to improve the dismal prognosis of this tumor. These experimental approaches include:

1. Argon laser activation of absorbed hematoporphoryn derivative,

2. Hyperbaric oxygen-enhanced XRT,

3. Combination of XRT with electron affinic sensitizers, such as metronidazole,

4. Combination of XRT with halogenated pyrimidines,

5. Hyperfractionated XRT,

6. Heavy particle XRT, including fast-neutron and negative pi-meson radiation,

7. Interstitial brachytherapy, and

8. Hyperthermia.

Unfortunately, no experimental treatment to date has resulted in a significantly increased survival from this highly malignant tumor. This clinical situation, therefore, lends itself to the study of any promising new treatment technique, such as BNCT.

PROPOSED PROTOCOL FOR CLINICAL TRIALS

The proposed protocol for the clinical trial of BNCT in GM is national in scope. It is hoped that the trial will involve the national resources of the Department of Energy (DOE), the National Cancer Institute (NCI), and the Radiation Therapy Oncology Group (RTOG). Gaining the support and cooperation of these national entities is important in the successful institution of the clinical protocol. It will be a Phase-I, -II study, investigating the safety and refinement of the technique and doses for the application. As the study progresses, effectiveness and control of GM would assume greater importance in the results. Patient recruitment for the clinical trials is anticipated to rely on the accrual of patients from the Idaho - northwest Rocky Mountain area, as well as nationally. (Hopefully, through the cooperation of an organization such as the RTOG).

Fig. 2 outlines the proposed protocol for the treatment of GM with BNCT. Eligible GM patients would fall in the Karnofsky performance status categories of 60-100 to allow their transportation to INEL for the treatment, and also adequate follow-up to permit assessment of endpoints. The patients then would undergo BNCT XRT in a nonrandomized fashion, and be followed for two years with assessment of a variety of endpoints, including treatment-related toxicity, evidence of local recurrence, and survival. Specific eligibility criteria for inclusion in the protocol would be:

1. Proof of GM from biopsy of the brain above the tentorium. To maintain a uniform population of patients, biopsy material would be reviewed by a single pathologist, who would ensure uniform diagnosis in the patients.

2. There should be reasonable expectation that the patients entering the study would complete the treatment and follow-up examinations.

3. Patients would begin therapy within four weeks of surgery.

4. Patients would be at least 18 but no older than 75.

5. Patients and their referring physicians would agree to the conditions of the pilot study.

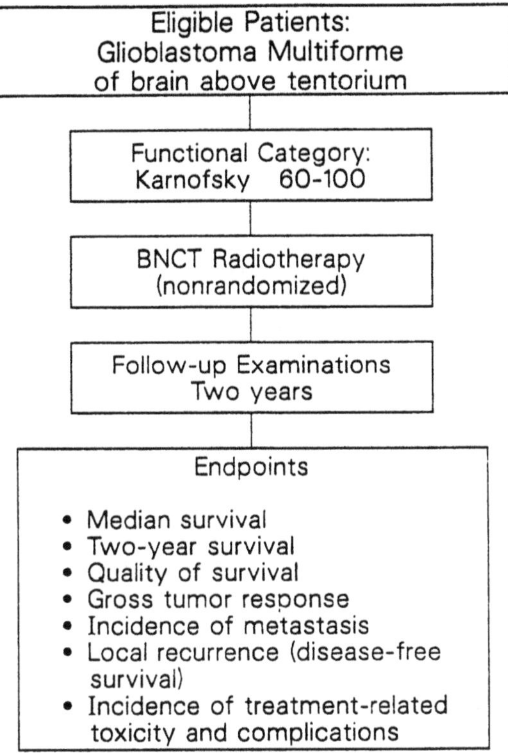

Fig. 2. The proposed protocol for the treatment of Glioblastoma Multiforme with BNCT.

6. Patients would complete all required consent forms.

Specific conditions for ineligibility would include:

1. Evidence of distant metastases.

2. Previous definitive therapy of the primary tumor, other than surgery.

3. Previous chemotherapy which might compromise the evaluation of the treatment.

4. Previous XRT to areas overlapping the projected treatment portals.

5. Active, uncontrollable infection in the intended vicinity of the radiation.

6. Medical, psychological, or other contraindications for the diagnostic or therapeutic measures.

7. Evidence of uncontrolled second malignancy.

8. Performance status of less than Karnofsky 60. The Karnofsky performance-status rating is shown in Fig. 3.

Upon entering the protocol, the patients would be stratified according to criteria that might affect the results of the treatment (Fig. 4). These criteria would be noted in the record, and reviewed at the time of data evaluation to determine what effect they might have on the patient's outcome from the treatment. Pretreatment evaluation would include a medical history and physical examination, standard laboratory tests listed in the protocol, imaging procedures to assess the tumor's volume (including computed tomography), magnetic resonance imaging, and possibly positron emission tomography. The imaging procedures used for a particular patient would be determined by the capability of the referring physician and treatment center, as well as by the particular needs determined by the study team. Following the pretreatment evaluation, standard study entrance forms and consent forms would be completed and the patient then would be assigned a code number and scheduled for nonrandomized treatment with BNCT XRT. The specific technique to be used (i.e., type and delivery technique of the boron compound, as well as the technique for exposure to epithermal neutrons) would be based on interim accrual of data from ongoing preclinical studies.

After the BNCT XRT, the patient would be followed closely, particularly with respect to:

1. Gross tumor response to treatment,

2. Long-term effects of BNCT XRT,

3. Time and site of local recurrence (if any),

4. Functional status during survival, and

5. Time of survival, in months or years.

Follow-up frequency would begin with monthly follow-ups for the first six months, then gradually lengthening to every three months for 18 months, every six

Able to carry on normal activity; no special care is needed	100	Normal; no complaints; no evidence of disease
	90	Able to carry on normal activity; minor signs or symptoms of disease
	80	Normal activity with effort; some signs or symptoms of disease
Unable to work; able to live at home and care for most personal needs; a varying amount of assistance is needed	70	Cares for self; unable to carry on normal activity or to do active work
	60	Requires occasional care for most needs
	50	Requires considerable assistance and frequent medical care
Unable to care for self; requires equivalent of institutional or hospital care; disease may be progressing rapidly	40	Disabled; requires special care and assistance
	30	Severely disabled; hospitalization is indicated, although death is not imminent
	20	Very sick; hospitalization necessary; active supportive treatment is necessary
	10	Moribund; fatal processes progressing rapidly
	0	Dead

Fig. 3. Criteria Used in the Karnofsky performance status rating.

months for the next year, and then continued follow-up at six-month intervals during the survival of the patient. Information would be gathered with the appropriate history and physical and standard laboratory tests (as well as repeat imaging studies such as CT, MRI, and PET) as appropriate to compare with the patient's imaging studies obtained at time of entry into treatment. Additional information would be gained by neurologic examination, evaluation of functional status, opthalmologic examination, and psychological testing. Because of the need to accurately determine the toxicity of this new treatment, it is proposed that all patients would agree to the performance of an autopsy in the event of death to document the toxic effects of treatment as well as tumor effects. The entire spectrum of data from the patient's follow-up and autopsy would be recorded on standard forms.

- Karnofsky performance status
  - 90-100
  - 70-90
  - 60-70
- Age
  - < 55
  - ≥ 55
- Extent of tumor removal
  - Needle or open biopsy
  - Subtotal removal

Figure 4. Stratification criteria.

RESEARCH QUESTIONS

Before the proposed clinical protocol starts, several questions will be investigated within the scope of this and other research programs in the United States and elsewhere. The findings will then be integrated into, and perhaps used to modify the details of, the proposed clinical protocol. The areas of investigation include:

1. Single dose tolerance,

2. Boron distribution and dosimetry,

3. Relative biologic effectiveness (RBE) of BNCT,

4. Appropriate use of single dose versus fractionated or protracted treatment,

5. Potential dose-rate effects,

6. Changes in the blood-brain-barrier (BBB) related to the ionizing components,

7. Potential BBB effects of corticosteroid administration which may affect the timing of the application of the boron compound,

8. Potential development of new boron compounds, and

9. Potential application of the BNCT technique to other tumors.

Perhaps the most intriguing question involves the development of new boron compounds and, therefore, the potential application of the BNCT technique to other tumors. The study team involved in the INEL research project will watch these developments closely. The proposed clinical protocol will likely include use of multiple different boron compounds, as well as addressing using the treatment technique in other tumor areas such as metastatic brain tumors, lower grade gliomas, other brain tumors, malignant melanoma, and other systemic malignancies.

REFERENCE

Kornbulith, P. L., et al., 1985, Neoplasms of the Central Nervous System, *in* Cancer: Principles and Practice of Oncology, DeVita, V. T., Hellman, S., Rosenberg, S. A., editors, 1985, Lippincott, Philadelphia.

ACKNOWLEDGEMENT

Work performed under the auspices of the U.S. Department of Energy, DOE Contract No. DE-AC07-76ID01570.

THE EFFECT OF IONIZING RADIATION ON THE BLOOD-BRAIN-BARRIER (BBB): CONSIDERATIONS FOR THE APPLICATION OF BORON NEUTRON CAPTURE THERAPY (BNCT) OF BRAIN TUMORS

Ronald V. Dorn III, John H. Spickard, and
Merle L. Griebenow

Idaho National Engineering Laboratory
EG&G Idaho, Inc.
P.O. Box 1625
Idaho Falls, ID 83415-3519

and

Mountain States Tumor Institute
151 East Bannock
Boise, ID 83712

INTRODUCTION

All methods of Boron Neutron Capture Therapy (BNCT) in use or envisioned for treatment of brain tumors have, as an inseparable component, an element of ionizing radiation (incident and induced). This paper reviews data on the effects of ionizing radiation on the blood-brain-barrier (BBB) and the blood-tumor-barrier (BTB) and the potential impact of the effects on the delivery techniques of BNCT. This paper has the following objectives:

1. Review the available technique for BNCT of brain tumors,
2. Review the literature on experimental and human studies regarding the effects of ionizing radiation on the BBB,

3. Discuss the impact of these effects on the fractionization question for BNCT, and

4. Draw conclusions from that information.

A CURRENT METHODOLOGY FOR BNCT OF BRAIN TUMORS

Most currently proposed techniques for the use of BNCT of brain tumors involve the application of a boron salt, $Na_2B_{12}H_{11}SH$. That compound appears to be very strongly bound to albumin once it is introduced into the bloodstream, although this remains to be more fully characterized. Localization of the boron compound into the brain tumor relies on breakdown of the BBB around the area of the tumor, resulting in a high concentration of the boron compound within the tumor, as compared to the surrounding normal brain. Once appropriate concentration of the boron compound is obtained in the tumor, the area is exposed to epiermal or thermal neutrons. An n,α reaction occurs, which results in activation of the boron. Important elements of the technique include a significant induced ionizing component as well as an incident ionizing comnent of the neutron beam. These components may result in significant ionizing radiation to the surrounding normal brain. It is the ionizing components of the treatment that we analyze in this paper, their effect on the normal BBB, and what effect this may have on the question as to the fractionization versus nonfractionization of BNCT using this technique. To that end, an extensive literature review was undertaken to evaluate data on the effects on the BBB of ionizing radiation. That data was divided into two parts: (1) experimental animal data, and (2) the data in the human clinical experience.

ANIMAL EXPERIMENTAL RESULTS

The effect of ionizing radiation on the BBB in experimental animal models has been evaluated by a number of researchers. Animal models that were studied include the rat, the dog, and the cat. These studies reveal that the radiation doses employed have ranged from 500 to 30,000 cGy in single doses, and 200 to 2500 cGy in fractionated techniques. Following delivery of the radiation, changes in the BBB were evaluated in times ranging from one hour to one month and beyond.

Table 1. Detection Techniques

131 RISA	Penicillin EEG
^{35}S sulfate	Contrast CT
Trypan blue	$^{99}Tc^{m}$
^{203}Hg	^{3}H-VM-26
Methotrexate	Bleomycin
^{14}C-Urea	Evans blue dye
^{3}H-Galactitol	Bicuculline EEG

A variety of detection techniques were used over the years (Table 1) including radionuclide-based techniques, physiologic dye uptake, and physiologic studies based on irritation of the brain produced by crossing of certain materials through the BBB. The techniques range in their sensitivity and involve study of both the cerebral spinal fluid (CSF) and brain tissue concentrations of these materials. The data published over the years generally shows an increase in the BBB permeability as a result of ionizing radiation throughout a wide range of doses and over a significant span of time. Exceptions include lack of evidence for permeability to ^{14}C-Urea, ^{3}H-VM-26 and bleomyocin (Levin et al., 1979)). Further, increasingly sensitive techniques have allowed better detection and accumulation of evidence of breakdown in the BBB. An example of typical experimental results can be found in the study by Storm et al. (1985). Rats were exposed to a single 2000 cGy dose of radiation. Methotrexate (MTX) concentration in brain tissue was investigated using ^{125}I RIA at 1 through 15 days post-radiation exposure. The results show an increase in the MTX concentration in the brain tumor by as much as a factor of four following the ionizing radiation exposure. Additional results from experimental animal models come from the references listed in Table 2.

CLINICAL STUDIES

A variety of data has been published over the years on the effect of radiation exposure on the BBB in the human clinical situation. A review of the literature in this area shows that radiation doses ranging from 0 to 24 cGy in a fractionated setting and 2500 to 3000 cGy

Table 2. References for Experimental Animal Models

Clemente and Richardson, 1962
Brownson et al., 1963
Nair and Roth, 1964
Schetter and Shealy, 1970
Olsson et al., 1975
Griffin et al., 1977
Levin et al., 1979
Remler and Marcusser, 1986
Fike et al., 1982
Lundquist et al., 1982
Storm et al., 1982
Remler et al., 1986

single dose have been investigated. Again, a wide post-radiation time frame has been evaluated, ranging from under 24 hours to a number of months. The detection techniques used in the clinical setting, of necessity, have primarily involved evaluating changing concentrations of material in the CSF. The CSF concentrations evaluated in the studies are listed in Table3. Those clinical studies again show, with one exception, an increase in BBB permeability following fractionated and single dose radiation therapy. An example of that type of study is illustrated in the paper by Livrea (1985). Children with leukemia were treated with CNS prophylaxis with MTX and radiation therapy (XRT) and the CFS concentrations of albumin, IgG, and alpha-II macroglobulin were studied. It was found that the concentration of these proteins were increased independently by both MTX and XRT, and that, the permeability secondary to the ionizing radiation increased in a stepwise fashion with each additional dose fraction of the XRT. Table 4 lists the clinical studies reviewed for this paper.

Table 3. Detection Techniques for CSF

Methotrexate
"Protein"
Albumin
IgG
α, macroglobulin
"Bromides, chlorides, sugar"

Table 4. References used to Review Clinical Studies

Hsu et al., 1936
Clemente and Richardson, 1962
Price and Jamison, 1975
Seshadri et al., 1979
Siemes et al., 1980
Stephani et al., 1982
Livrea et al., 1985

IMPACT OF THESE FINDINGS ON THE BNCT OF BRAIN TUMORS

Both experimental animal models, and clinical studies in general, suggest increased BBB permeability secondary to ionizing radiation. This BBB permeability can be detected both with large single doses and smaller fractionated doses of XRT. There is, therefore, a real concern that the induced and incident ionizing components of BNCT acutely increase BBB permeability in the normal brain might jeopardize subsequent preferential uptake of boron compound into the tumor over the normal brain. This would suggest a potential disadvantage to fractionating BNCT when the therapeutic advantage is based on differential BBB uptake of the boron compound.

CONCLUSIONS

1. The BNCT of brain tumors, which relies on the increased BBB permeability to the $Na_2B_{12}H_{11}SH$ compound, may best be applied as a single dose. Changes in the normal BBB from the initial ionizing dose may unfavorably alter the therapeutic ratio of the uptake of the boron compound.

2. At the very least, we feel that it is important to experimentally confirm changes in the BBB permeability to the boron compound.

3. These concerns underline the importance of developing new boron compounds that rely on other mechanisms for tumor uptake besides changes in BBB permeability (compounds that rely on active uptake of the boron compound into the tumor tissue).

4. For these reasons, emphasis needs to be placed on obtaining an epithermal or thermal neutron source with the lowest possible amount of incident ionizing component.

5. Confirmation of these results, as well as optimization of treatment techniques for BNCT, strongly support the use of facilities providing high-intensity, epithermal neutrons that will allow investigation of both single dose and fractionated treatment techniques.

REFERENCES

Brownson, R. H., Suter, D. B., and Diller D. A., 1963, Acute brain damage induced by low dosage radiation, Neurol., 13:181.

Clemente, C. D. and Richardson, H. E., 1962, Some observations on ex-irradiation effects on the blood brain barrier and cerebral blood vessels, in: "Response of the Nervous System to Ionizing Radiation", T. J. Haley and R. S. Schneider, Academic Press, New York and London eds.

Edwards, M. S., et al., 1979, Quantitative Observations of the Subacute Effects of Ex-Irradiation on Brain Capillary Permeability: Part II, International Journal of Radiation Oncology Biology Physics, 5:1633.

Fike, J. R., Cann, C. E., Davis, R. L., Phillips, T. L., 1982, Radiation Effects in the Canine Brain Evaluated by Quantitative Computed Tomography, Radiol., 144:603.

Griffin, T. W., Rasey, J. S., Bleyers, W. A., 1977, The Effect of Photon Irradiation on Blood Brain Barrier Permeability to Methotrexate in Mice, Cancer, 40:1109.

Groothuis, D. R. and Mikhael, M. A., 1986, Focal Cerebral Vasculitis Associated with Circulating Immune Complexes and Brain Irradiation, Ann. of Neurol., 19:590.

Groothuis, D. R., Vriesendorp, F., Mikhael, M. A., Blasberg, R. G., Patlak, C., 1984, Quantitative Measurement of Brain Tumor Capillary Permeability by CT: Application in Canine Gliomas and Implications for Use in Patients (Abstract), Neurol., Supp. 1-34:185.

Hsu, Y. K., Chang, C. P., Hsieh, C. K., Lyman, R. S., 1936, Effect of Roentgen Rays on the Permeability of the Barrier Between Blood and Cerebral Spinal Fluid, Chin. J. of Physiol., 10:379.

Levin, V. A., Edwards, M. S., Byrd, A., 1979, Quantitative Observations of the Acute Effects of Ex-Irradiation on Brain Capillary Permeability: Part I, Int. J. Radiat. Oncol. Bio. Phys., 5:1627.

Livrea, P., Trojano, M., Simone, I. L., Zimatore, G. B., Logroscino, G. C., Pisicchio, L., Lojacono, G., Colella, R., Ceci, A., 1985, Acute Changes in Blood-CFS Barrier Permselectivity to Serum Proteins After Intrathecal Methotrexate and CNS Irradiation, J. of Neurol., 231:336.

Lundquist, H., Rosander K., Lomanov, M., Lukjashin, V., Shimchuk, G., Zolotov, V., Minkkova, E., 1982, Permeability of the Blood Brain Barrier in the Rat After Local Proton Irradiation, Acta Radiol. Oncol., FASC.4, 21:267.

Nair, V. and Roth, L. J., 1964, Effect of Ex-Irradiation and Certain Other Treatments on Blood Brain Barrier Permeability, Radiat. Res., 23:249.

Olsson, Y., Klatzo, I., Carsten, A., 1975, The Effect of Acute Radiation Injury on the Permeability and Ultrastructure of Intracerebral Capillaries, Neuropath. Appl. Neurobiol., 1:59.

Price, R. A. and Jamieson, P. A., 1975, The Central Nervous System in Childhood Leukemia II: Subacute Leukoencephalopathy, Cancer, 35:306.

Remler, M. P. and Marcussen, W. H., 1981, Time Course of Early Delayed Blood Brain Barrier Changes in Individual Cats After Ionizing Radiation, Exper. Neurol., 73:310.

Remler, M. P., Marcussen, W. H., Tiller-Borsich, J., 1986, Delayed Effects of Radiation on the Blood Brain Barrier, Int. J. Radiat. Oncol. Biol. Phys., 12:1965.

Schettler, T. and Shealy, C. N., 1970, Experimental Selective Alteration of Blood Brain Barrier by Ex-Irradiation, Journal of Neurosurgery, 32:89.

Seshadri, R. S., Ryall, R.G., Rice, M. S., Leahy, M., Ellis, R., 1979, The Effect of Cranial Irradiation on Blood Brain Barrier Permeability to Methotrexate, Aust. Paediat. J., 15:184.

Siemes, H., Rating, D., Sieger, M., Hanefeld, F., Muller, St., Gadner, H., Riehm, H., 1980, Changes of CSF Protein Pattern in Children with Acute Lymphoblastic Leukemia During Prophylactic CNS Therapy (Berlin Protocol), Med. Paediatr. Oncol., 8:25.

Spence, A. M., Graham, M. M., O'Gorman, L. A., Siemes, H., Riehm, H., Hanefeld, F., 1987, Regional Blood to Tissue Transport in an Irradiated Rat Glioma Model, Radiat. Res., 111:225.

Stephani, U., Rating, D., Korinthenberg, R., Siemes, H., Riehm H., Hanefeld, F., 1983, Radiation Related Disturbance of Blood Brain Barrier During Therapy of Acute Lymphoblastic Leukemia, The Lancet, October 29, 1983, page 1036 (letter).

Storm, A. J., Van Der Kogel, A. J., Nooter, K., 1985, Effect of Ex-Irradiation on the Pharmacokinetics of Methotrexate in Rats: Alteration of the Blood Brain Barrier, Eur. J. Cancer Clin. Oncol., 21:759.

ACKNOWLEDGEMENT

Work performed under the auspices of the U.S. Department of Energy, DOE Contract No. DE-AC07-76ID01570.

COMPUTERIZED AXIAL TOMOGRAPHIC AND MAGNETIC RESONANCE IMAGING SCAN FOLLOW-UP OF TWO PATIENTS AFTER BORON NEUTRON CAPTURE THERAPY FOR GLIOBLASTOMA MULTIFORME

Stephen R. Marano, John H. Spickard, and Merle L. Griebenow

Idaho National Engineering Laboratory
EG&G Idaho, Inc.
P.O. Box 1625
Idaho Falls, ID 83415-3519

INTRODUCTION

Using computed tomography (CT) and magnetic resonance imaging (MRI), we are following a 30-year old, white female and a 64-year old, white male, both with biopsy-proven Glioblastoma Multiforme, from their preoperative through post-operative stages and pre- and post-BNCT treatment. The images visually demonstrate the evolving changes in the tumor and surrounding cortex. These patients were treated by Hiroshi Hatanaka of Teikyo University, at the Musashi Institute of Technology (MIT) reactor in Kawasaki, Japan. The MIT reactor is a 100 kW Triga-II facility that has been used by Hatanaka for many years for BNCT therapy.

The 30-year old female patient presented in June 1987, with a right parietal ring enhancing lesion that was subsequently excised subtotally (Figs. 1a and 1b). In August 1987, she traveled to Teikyo University for BNCT. A pre-treatment CT scan demonstrates effacement of the right lateral ventricle, shift of midline structure, and some increase in areas of contrast enhancement (Fig. 2). The pre-treatment MRI image (Fig. 3) showed large areas within the right cerebral hemisphere that are consistent with cerebral edema secondary to the presence of the tumor.

The patient's contrast enhancement CT image taken after the treatment (Fig. 4) demonstrated a remarkable decrease in ventricular effacement and midline shift. This image was obtained before the patient's departure from Japan and within the first two weeks after treatment. Four months subsequently, CT again demonstrated continued absence of ventricular effacement and midline shift with a small area of contrast enhancement that was interpreted by Hatanaka to represent the tumor undergoing necrosis (Fig. 5). The patient is near normal in her neurologic examination with only minimal left-sided paresis, is having no headaches, and is not presently on corticosteroids.

The 64-year old male, presented in July 1987, with left-sided hemiparesis, headaches, and some decline in mental status. The prebiopsy-enhanced CT (Fig. 6) demonstrated a large ring-enhancing right parietal lesion with significant mass effect, midline shift, and ventricular effacement. The lesion was a Glioblastoma Multiforme, and very little tumor was removed. He received BNCT in September, 1987. Follow-up contrast enhanced CT taken three months later (Fig. 7) demonstrated a persistent ring-enhancing lesion with mass effect and significant peritumoral edema. The lesion caused a "fullness" in the craniotomy site in contrast to the "sunken" craniotomy site of patient #1. The second patient had several months of dramatic improvements followed by a decline and is now in a long-term care facility.

Several significant differences in the treatment of the two patients may contribute to the vastly different outcomes: age, the quantity of tumor removed at the initial operation, and the initial size of tumor. Neither patient had conventional photon therapy. The follow-up will continue, and the data presented at appropriate intervals.

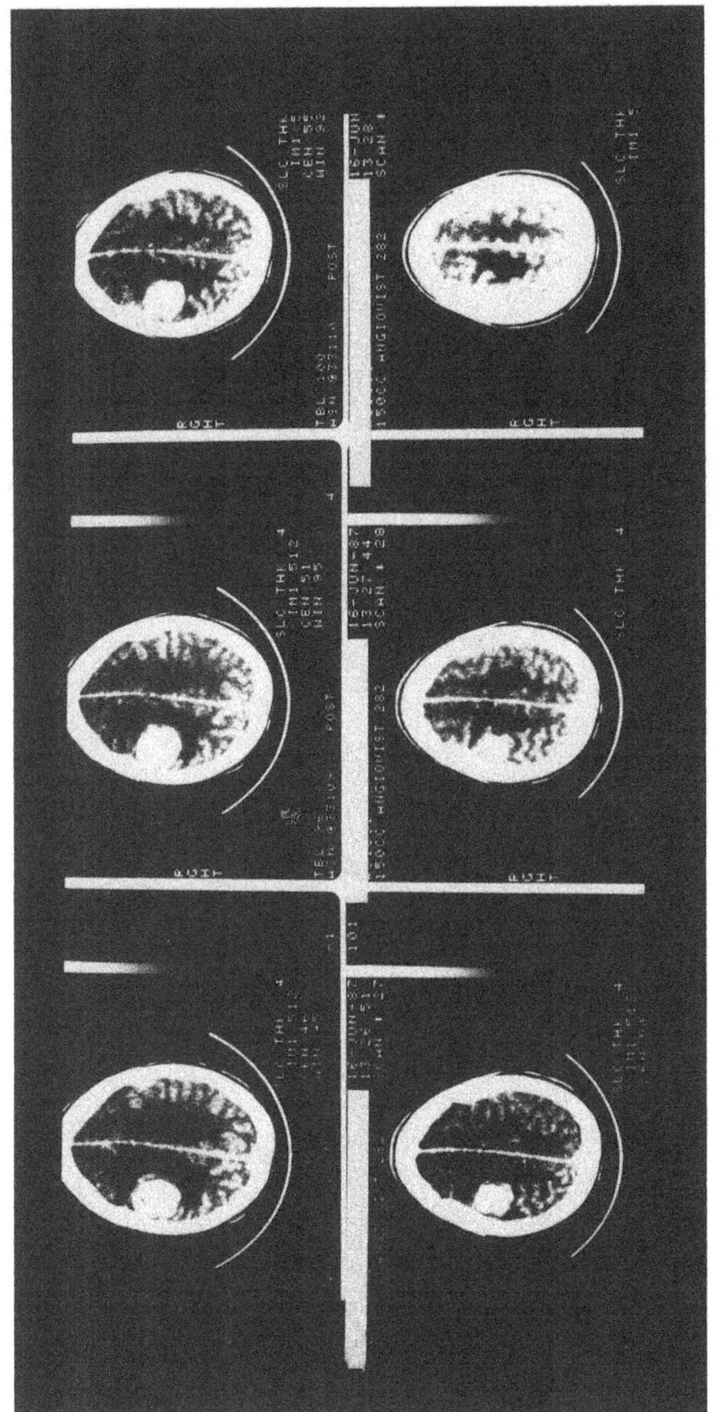

Figure 1a. Patient #1 - Right parietal ring-enhancing lesion that was subsequently excised subtotally.

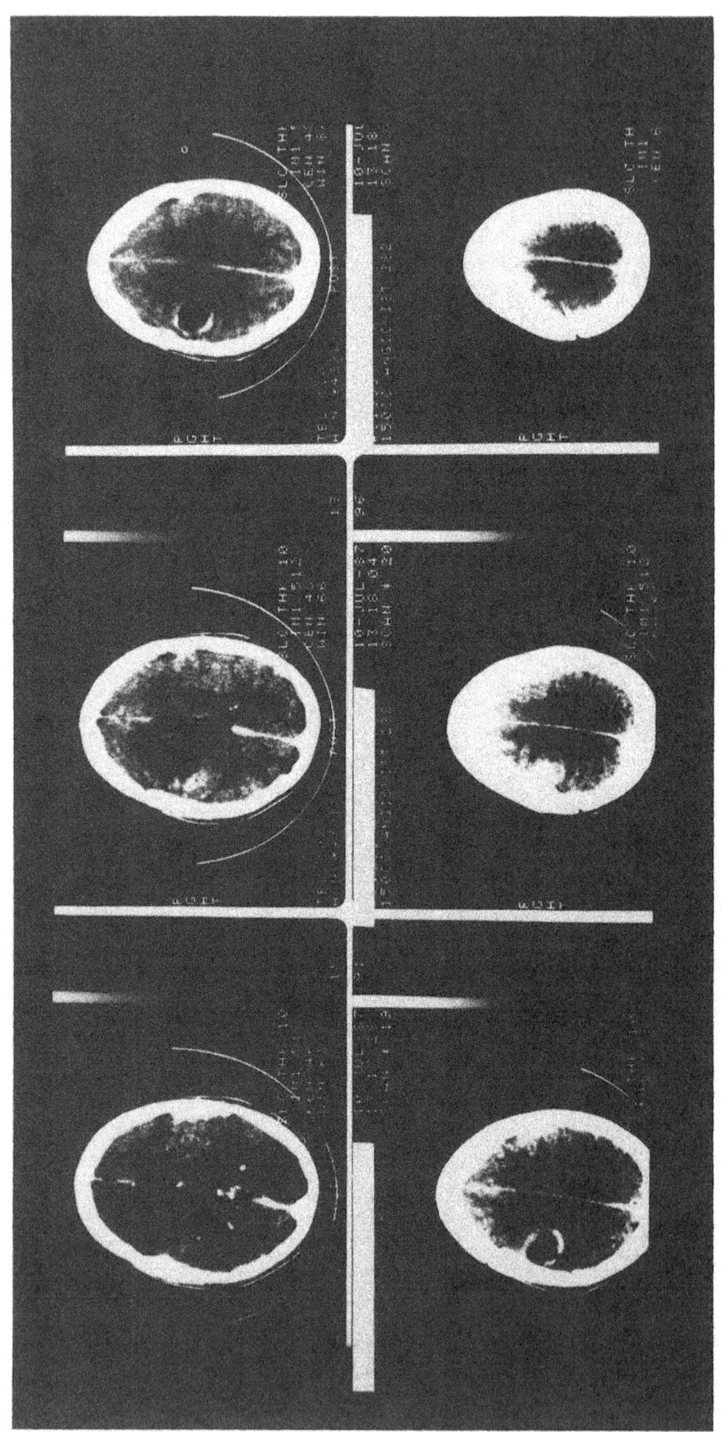

Figure 1b. Patient #1 - Right parietal ring-enhancing lesion.

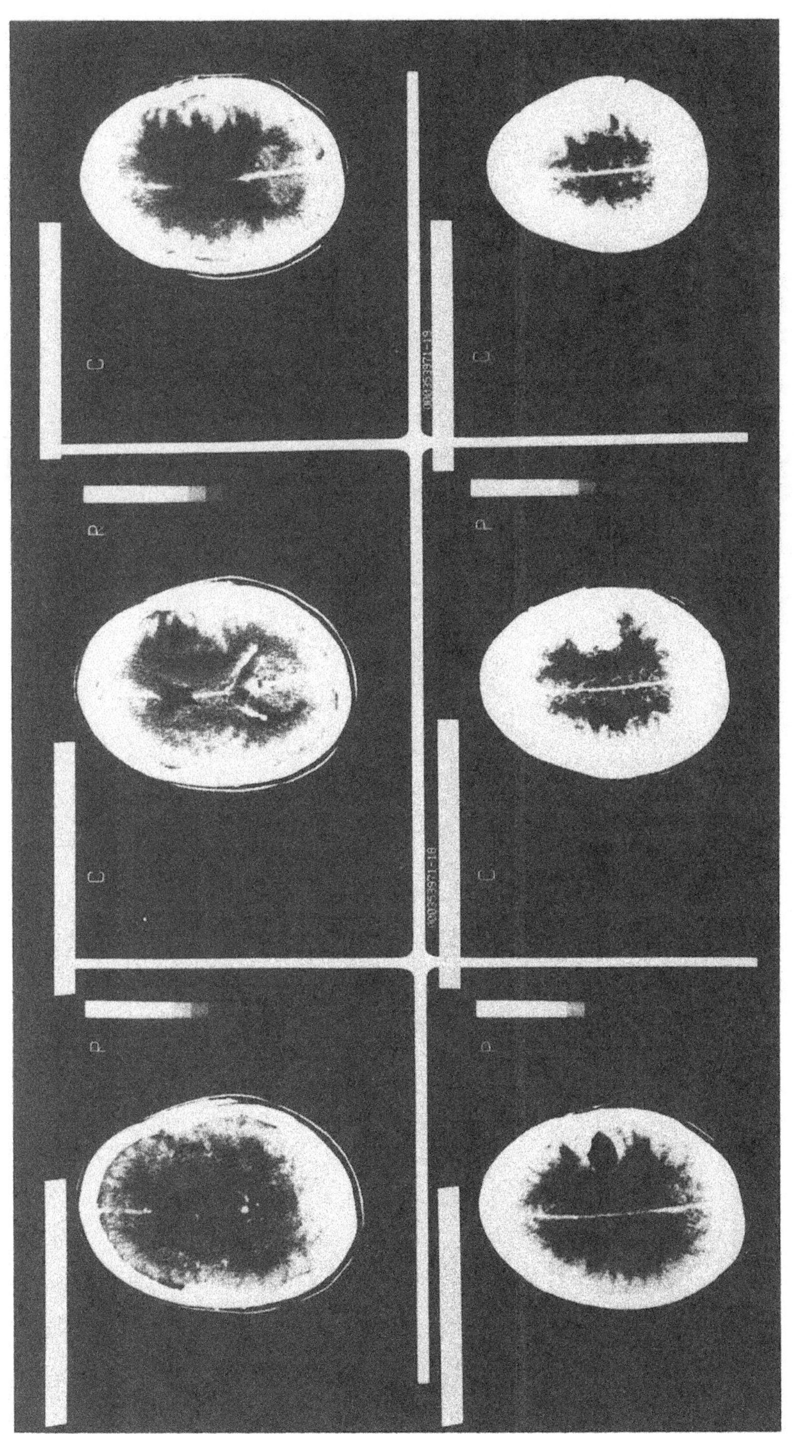

Figure 2. Patient #1 - Pretreatment CT scan.

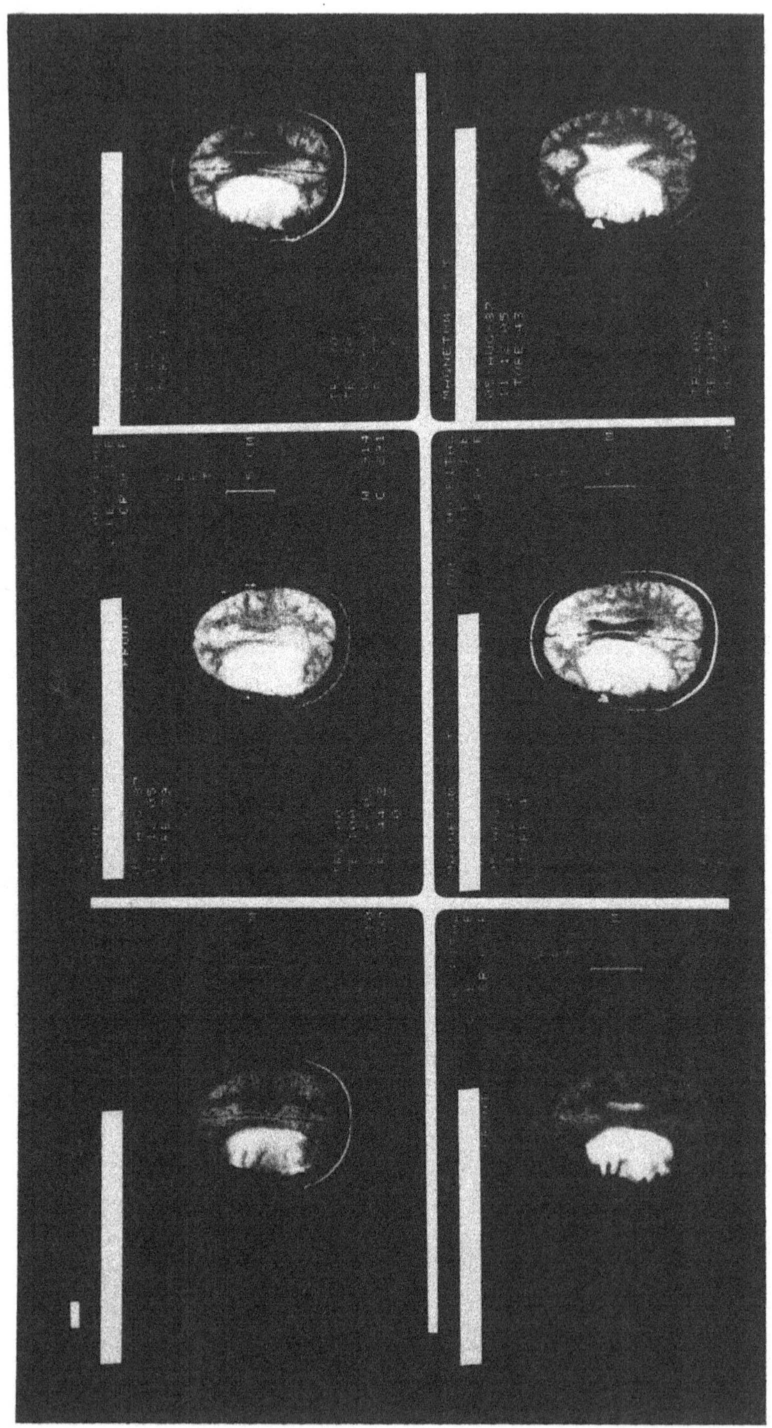

Figure 3. Patient #1 - Pretreatment MRI image.

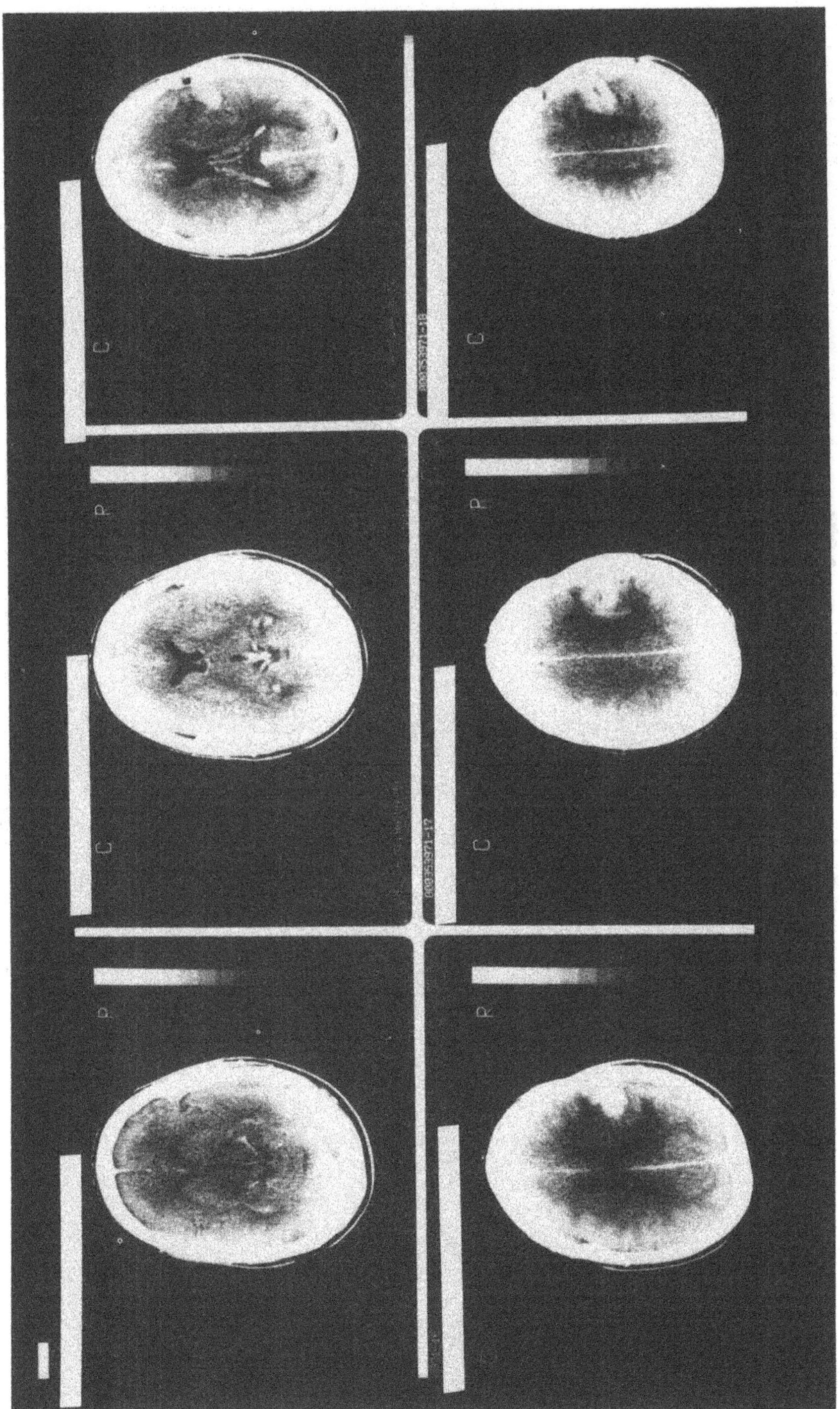

Figure 4. Patient #1 - Post-treatment contrast enhancement CT image.

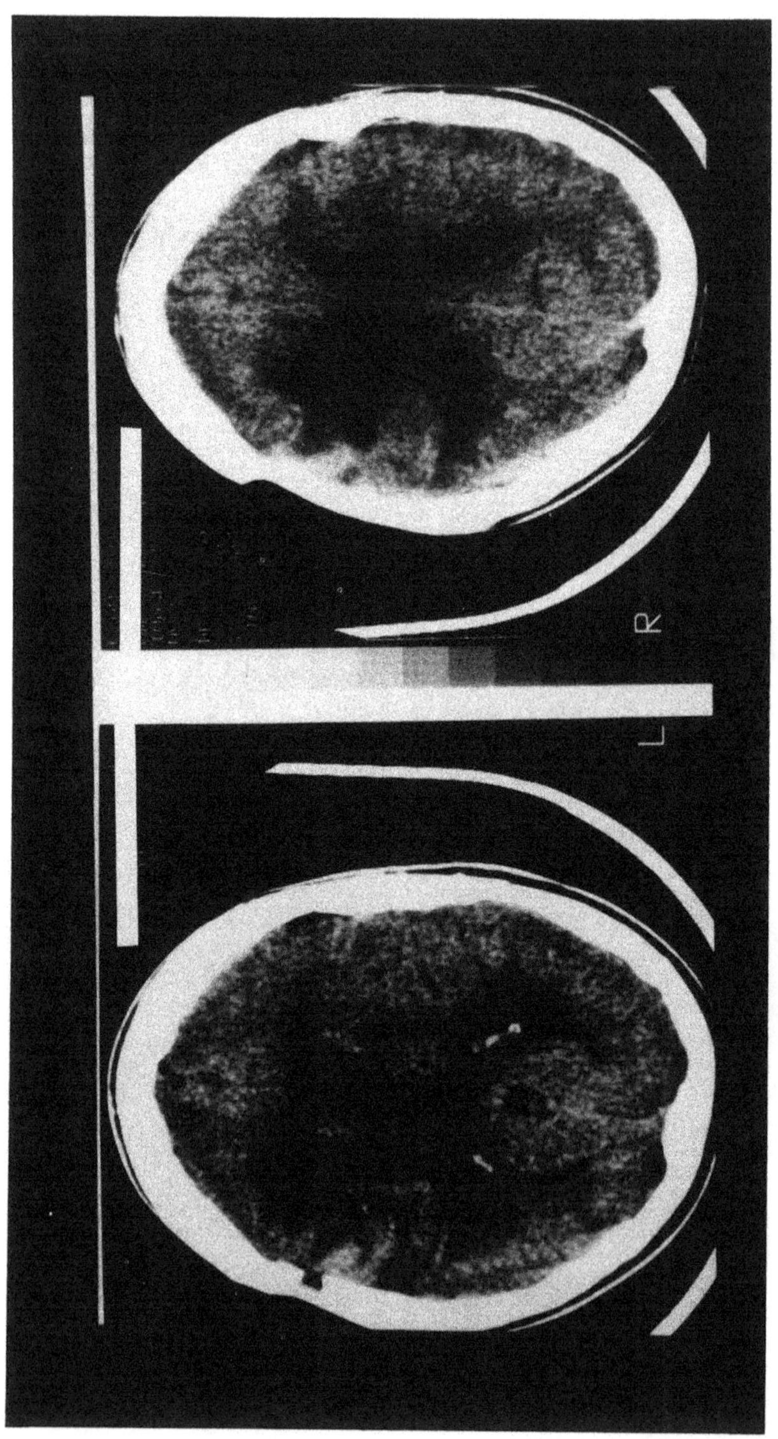

Figure 5. Patient #1 - Four months post-treatment CT scan.

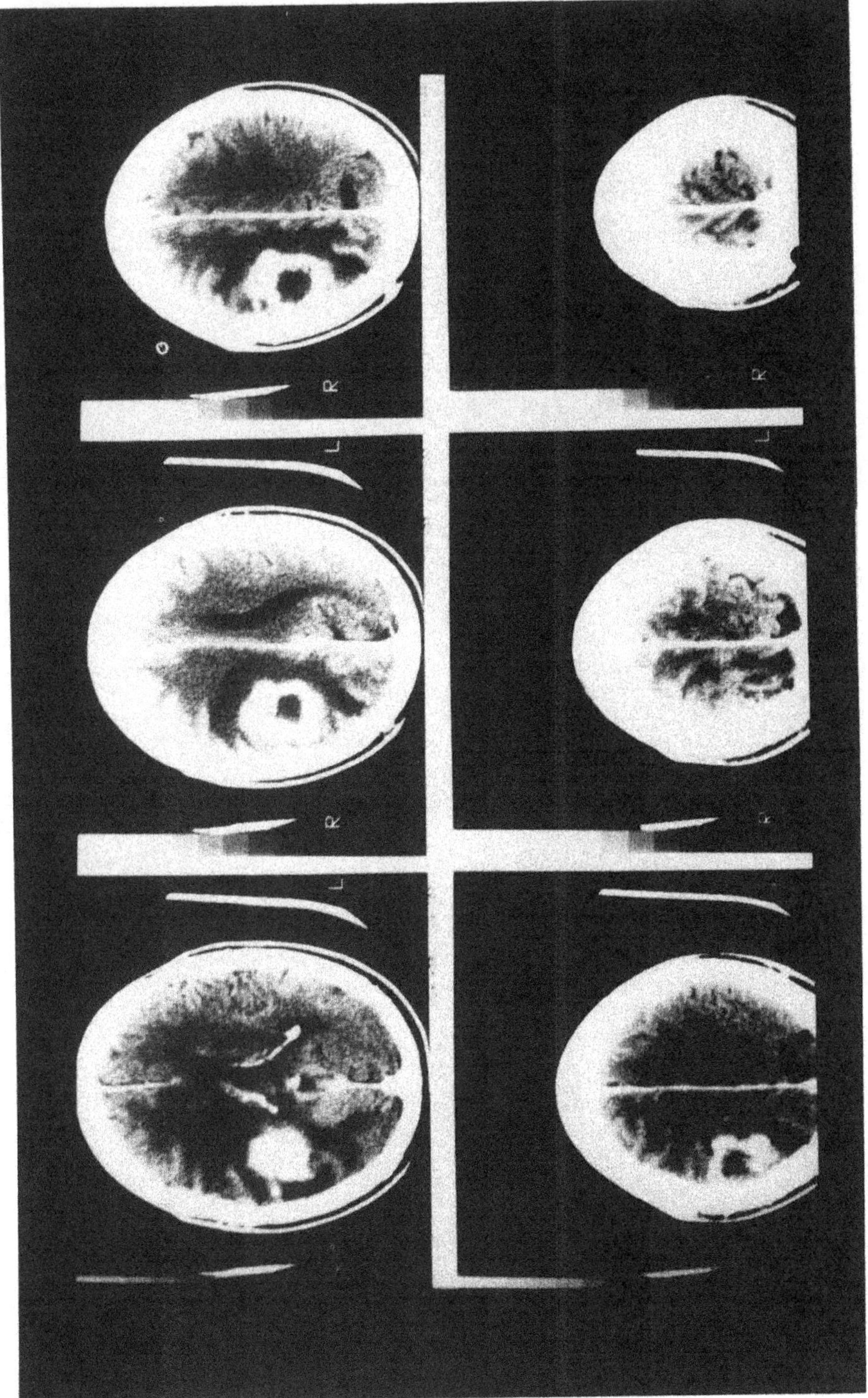

Figure 6. Patient #2 - Prebiopsy-enhanced CT scan.

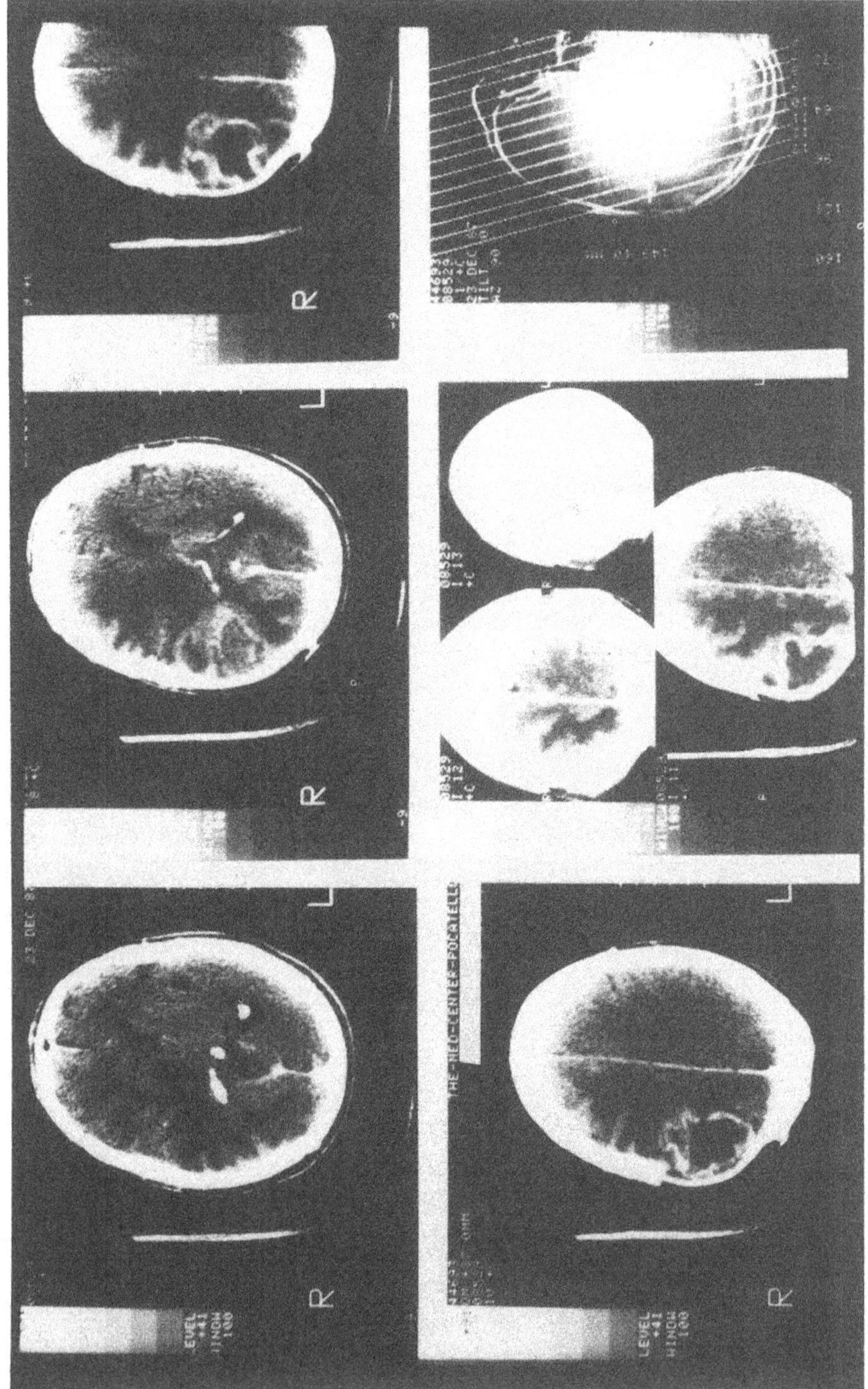

Figure 7. Patient #2 - Three-month followup contrast-enhanced CT.

ACKNOWLEGEMENT

Work performed under the auspices of the U.S. Department of Energy, DOE Contract No. DE-AC07-76ID01570.

A STOCHASTIC MODEL FOR HIGH-LET RESPONSE FOR BORON NEUTRON CAPTURE THERAPY (BNCT)

Floyd J. Wheeler, Merle L. Griebenow, Daniel E. Wessol, David W. Nigg, and Robert A. Anderl

Idaho National Engineering Laboratory
EG&G Idaho, Inc.
P.O. Box 1625
Idaho Falls, ID 83415-3519

INTRODUCTION

There is evidence showing that there is a significant variation in tumor-boron and blood-boron concentrations for individual patients. There also is a wide variation in the size and location of the tumor. This diversity creates a situation in which treatment must be carefully tailored to the specific needs of each patient. Patient treatment planning will require computer modeling of the various radiation transport and interaction processes expected to occur, coupled with a display of the results in easily interpretable form. Such an analytical evaluation will allow the radiation oncologist to select the beam configuration, specify the irradiation field and positions of local thermal neutron shields, establish the optimum time after boron administration to begin irradiation, and specify the duration of irradiation.

The computational model will be implemented on a high-performance graphics computer of the workstation type. The basic calculations will provide distributions of neutron, gamma, and secondary-charged particle interaction rates, energy deposition rates, and estimated cell-survivor fractions in the scalp, skull, normal brain tissue, endothelial tissue, and tumor tissue. State-of-the-art computerized displays will be employed to present the results. Data describing each individual patient (for example, head dimensions, tumor size and location, and boron distribution) will be input by several alternative methods. These include (1) manual input based on information from the diagnostic procedures, (2) "standard man" type models, and (3) direct reading of medical imaging data (CAT, MRI).

The analytical determination of the gross neutron and gamma fields and the corresponding dose contours will be a challenge insofar as representing geometry and beam characteristics and displaying the desired results rapidly and conveniently. The transport codes and data available are such that, with development, it is anticipated that the radiation fields can be determined with precision.

Radiation effects due to the $^{10}B(n,\alpha)^7Li$ reaction for tumor and healthy tissue depend upon microscopic distributions. The basic concepts of microdosimetry have been developed extensively (Kellerer and Rossi, 1972), but the quantitative application is difficult because of the biological response relationships. It is becoming accepted that the simple concepts of absorbed dose and RBE are not adequate to describe tissue effects.

A stochastic model is required for the $^{10}B(n,\alpha)^7Li$ effect. The application of such a model requires a microscopic biological-response function. Research and experience will be required before the models and response functions can be precisely quantified, but useful qualitative information on basic trends can be determined from simple models and trial response functions. This paper describes a proposed model based on the lineal response, which is very applicable to BNCT. The model is not limited to single-event response, but only requires the applicability of a response function which is independent of other events. Experiments support such a model for the $^{10}B(n,\alpha)^7Li$ reaction. This paper describes the model, provides details for basic charged-particle information and simulation methods, and provides a simple demonstration of the model's importance by evaluating the endothelium tolerance to BNCT.

Simulation studies previously were performed for the microvascular system (Deutsch and Murray, 1975; Rydin, et al., 1975; Kitao, 1975). Those studies have determined the absorbed dose to the capillary wall and zero-event distributions to the endothelial nucleus. They suggest a high tolerance by the endothelium to the $^{10}B(n,\alpha)^7Li$ reaction. The results of this study agree with those conclusions as long as the endothelium is relatively free from boron.

Canine experiments (Takeuchi, et al., 1985) were conducted where a thermal neutron field was applied to the brain vasculature with high blood-boron content to produce high $^{10}B(n,\alpha)^7Li$ doses generated within the blood. Takeuchi's results show a high tolerance of the endothelium to BNCT.

MODEL

The $^{10}B(n,\alpha)^7Li$ reaction is a relatively rare event during BNCT and, accordingly, requires a stochastic approach. The average number of $^{10}B(n,\alpha)^7Li$ fragment interactions with a 3.8 μm-radius spherical cell nucleus is about 2 ± 1.4 for an absorbed dose of 1 Gy from this reaction. In contrast, the same nucleus would experience about 1000 ± 31 events (electron tracks) for 1 Gy absorbed dose from ^{60}Co radiation. Thus, the variation in the dose, or the specific energy (z), for the $^{10}B(n,\alpha)^7Li$ reaction contains much more information than the specific energy for low-LET high-dose radiation.

Even more information is contained in the individual components (events) of specific energy, $f_y(z)$. The hit-size effectiveness function (Bond et al., (1985)) is a response based on lineal energy density (y). The distribution of y, f(y), corresponds to single-event components of lineal energy. For response to a spherical volume, y is proportional to the geometric cross-section times z, and thus is an effective measure of biological response.

For analytical modeling where analog tracking is performed by stochastic methods, it is not always possible to deal with specific energy and lineal energy density for single events because volumes and average chord lengths are not available to the computer code nor are they easily obtainable by the user for generalized geometry. The energy, E_s, deposited in a region by a single track is available in the computer model; and the distribution of this quantity is the subject of this paper. For this paper, the quantity,

E, or impulse energy, is defined. E is the energy deposited by one alpha track, one lithium ion track, or the sum of the alpha and lithium ion track in the case of capture within the volume of interest.

The frequency distribution of E within a region of interest is designed W(E), and the conditional probability of biological response, given an event of magnitude E, is designated K(E). Thus, in this model, all the biological response information is contained in the response function K(E), which is obtained from biological research, and all the physical information is contained in the frequency distribution W(E), which is obtained by the analytical model. Information for biological response as a function of dose, specific energy, or lineal energy can be used to construct (incompletely or ideally, completely) the K(E) used for this analytical model.

For the case with reproductive death as the biological response function, assuming the response function is independent, the fractional survivors (FS) of the population is given by (see Appendix A):

$$FS = e^{-N\int W(E)\ K(E)\,dE}$$

where N is the average number of events in the radiosensitive volume. Given the biological response function, simulation studies using Monte Carlo methods, chord length distributions, or other methods, can provide the N and W(E) which correlates with FS, or other response, of the population. Figure 1 shows a hypothetical biological response function. Similar functions were proposed by others (for example, Bond, et al., 1985). The biological response to an energy deposition event is zero for zero energy, increases with energy, and approaches unity for high values of deposited energy.

CHARGED-PARTICLE DATABASE

Stopping powers for the ions shown in Table 1 were derived from first principle considerations of charged-particle transport (Ziegler et al., 1985) using the TRIM-88* ion transport code. The TRIM code allows

*Ziegler, J. F., Cuomo, G., and Biersack, J. P. (1984, 1985, 1986, 1987, 1988).[c]

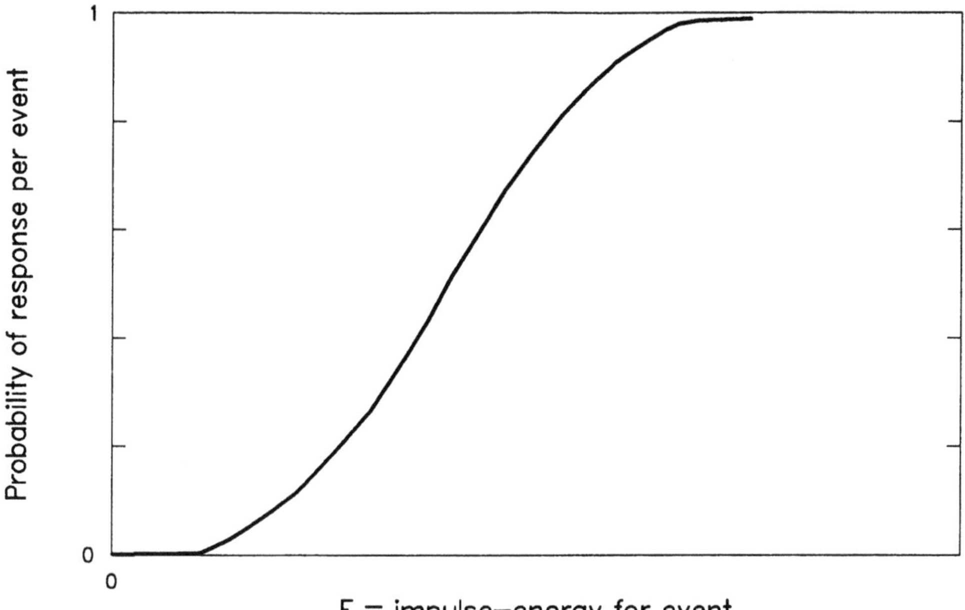

Fig. 1. Hypothetical biological response function (K(E)).

Table 1. Target Database for Initial ^{4}He and ^{7}Li Ion Energy of 1.5 MeV

Target	Target Composition (atom %)	ρ(g/cc)
Water	H(66.7%) - O(33.3%)	1.00
Brain	H(63%) - O(28%) - C(8%) - N(1%)	1.04
Blood	H(64%) - O(30%) - C(5.5%) - F(0.5%)	1.06

for a maximum of four constituent elements in a single target composition. For brain tissue and blood we explicitly represented the three most prevalent elements and charge-weighted the residual. Figures 2 and 3 show the stopping powers (expressed as keV/μm) for energetic helium and lithium ions as they slow down in water. Comparisons between TRIM-derived data and the Northcliffe and Schilling (1970) data are presented.

Gabel et al. (1987) fit the Northcliffe and Schilling data for a 1.49 MeV-He ion and a 0.85 MeV-Li ion slowing down in water with Equations 1 and 2, respectively. R is the penetration distance (microns) into the target and dE/dR is the stopping power expressed as keV/μm. Over the appropriate range limits, Equation 1 integrates to 1.5 MeV (1.49 MeV exact) and Equation 2 integrates to 0.8 MeV (0.85 MeV exact). Table 2 gives the range information.

$$dE_{He}/dR = -4.05(R-1.36)^2 + 234.0 \qquad (1)$$

$$dE_{Li}/dR = 92.232R - 7.1009R^2 \qquad (2)$$

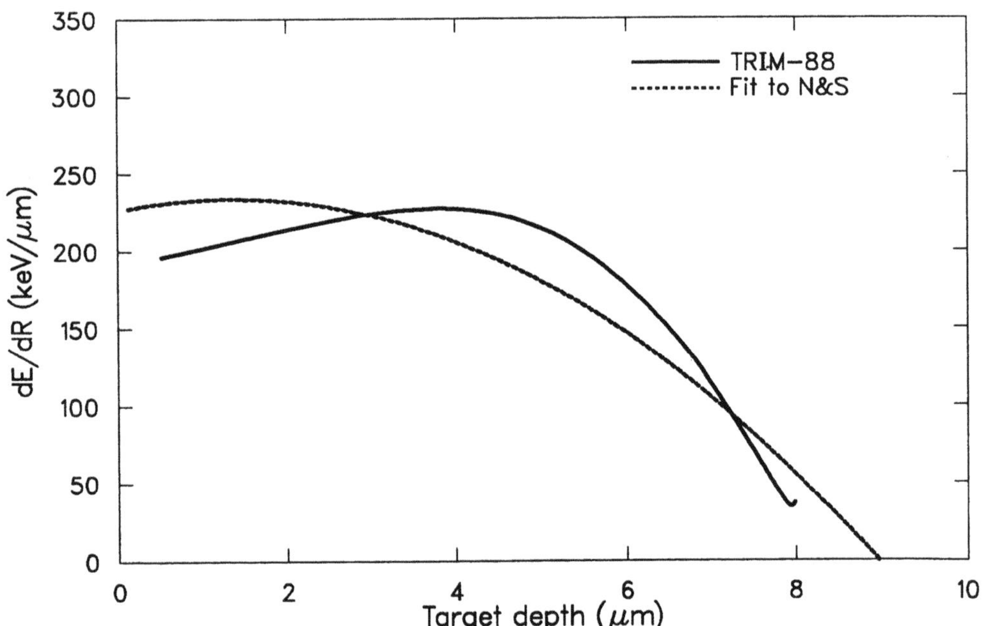

Fig. 2. Stopping power of He ions in water. TRIM vs Gabel fit to Northcliff and Schilling data.

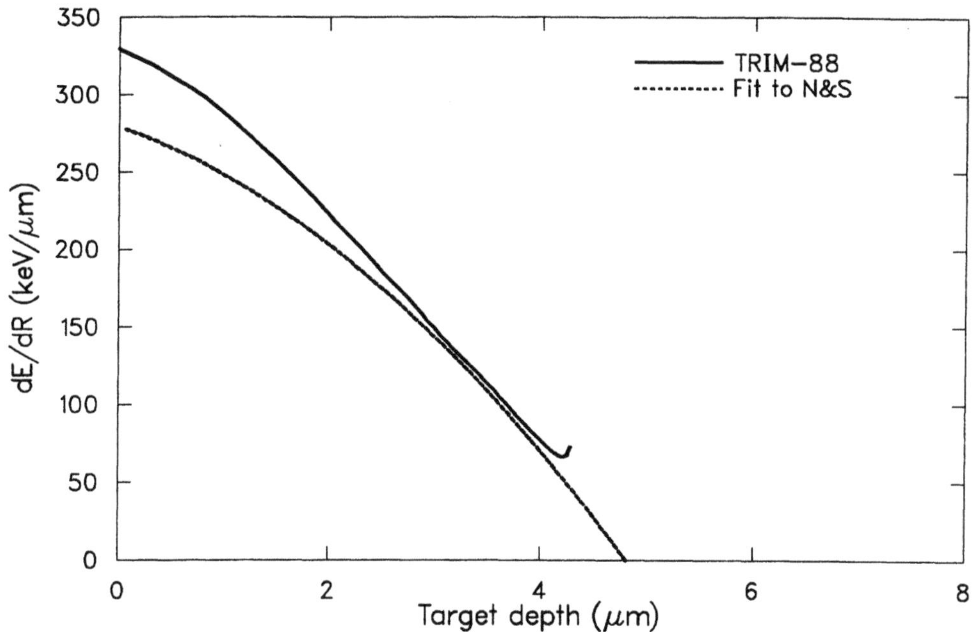

Fig. 3. Stopping power of ^{7}Li ions in water. TRIM vs Gabel fit to Northcliff and Schilling data.

Table 2. Range Data

Ion	Initial Energy (MeV)	Target	Range (m) TRIM/N&S
He	1.5	Water	8.01/8.96
He	1.5	Brain Tissue	7.68/----
He	1.5	Blood	7.60/----
Li	0.85	Water	4.13/4.81
Li	0.85	Brain Tissue	3.92/----
Li	0.85	Blood	3.89/----

The shape of stopping power curves for brain tissue and blood are similar to that for H_2O except for the relatively small deviation in range (Figs. 2 and 3).

There is a cusp in the curves at the end of the range. At this point, the forward component of the ion direction is no longer dominate when the ion begins to straggle. As the ions slow down, larger fractions of the energy losses will be attributable to inelastic (nuclear recoil) collisions, vacancy production (for example, free radical formation), and phonon vibrations (heat). Inevitably, this energy dependence should be factored in any model that accurately treats tissue lethality at the molecular level. There are noticeable differences in the stopping values among the various charged-particle data bases (TRIM vs Northcliffe and Schilling). For a given database, the differences in the stopping powers in targets composed of water, blood, or brain tissue are much smaller.

APPLICATION TO THE CAPILLARY RESPONSE

Monte Carlo simulations of alpha particles and ^{7}Li ions were performed for cells with uniform ^{10}B distributions and for endothelial cells with ^{10}B only in the lumen. For the case of uniform ^{10}B, the nucleus was assumed to be 3.8 microns. The model for the endothelial cells is shown in Fig. 4. The capillary was assumed to have an internal diameter of 10 microns and 1 micron of tissue separates the lumen from the endothelial cell nucleus. This Monte Carlo simulation determined the W(E) for each cell type. The K(E) can be determined only by experiment. For a trial exercise, we can use the experiments of Gabel (1983) for V79 Chinese hamster cells. The investigators determined a $D_o$value of 0.66 Gy for the ^{10}B reaction for these cells. They also observed no rate effects; the slope of the fractional survival relationship was constant with ^{10}B content and with fluence. The observation of no rate effect supports the model's assumption of an independent response function.

The shape of the response function cannot be determined by the results of the measurements, but the trial function shown in Fig. 5 reproduces the measured D_o value when employed in the model with the calculated W(E) for the cells with uniform ^{10}B. The trial response function also was used for the endothelial model and a comparison of the calculated fractional survival relationships is shown in Fig. 6. This figure shows the fractional survival relationships for tumor cells with 25 ppm ^{10}B. The tumor cells are assumed to be at a 6-cm depth and the neutron fluence is that

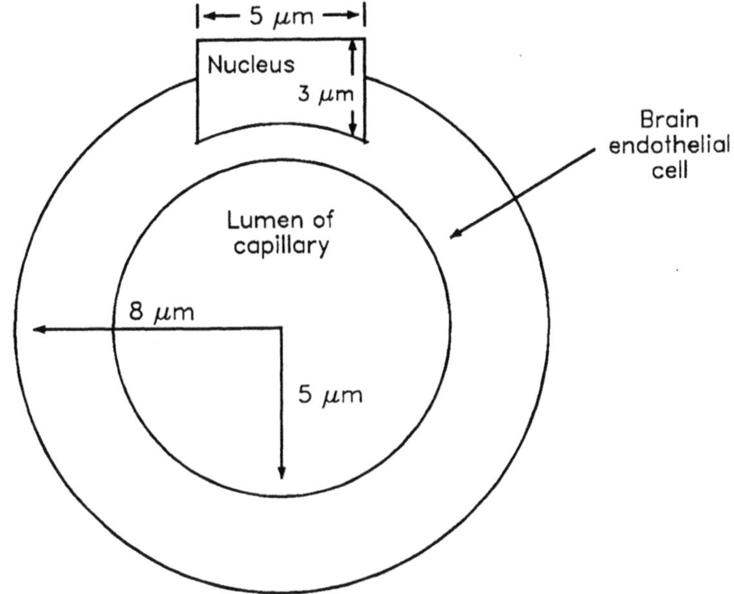

Fig. 4. Monte Carlo model of brain capillary with one micron of cytoplasm separating the lumen and the endothelial nucleus.

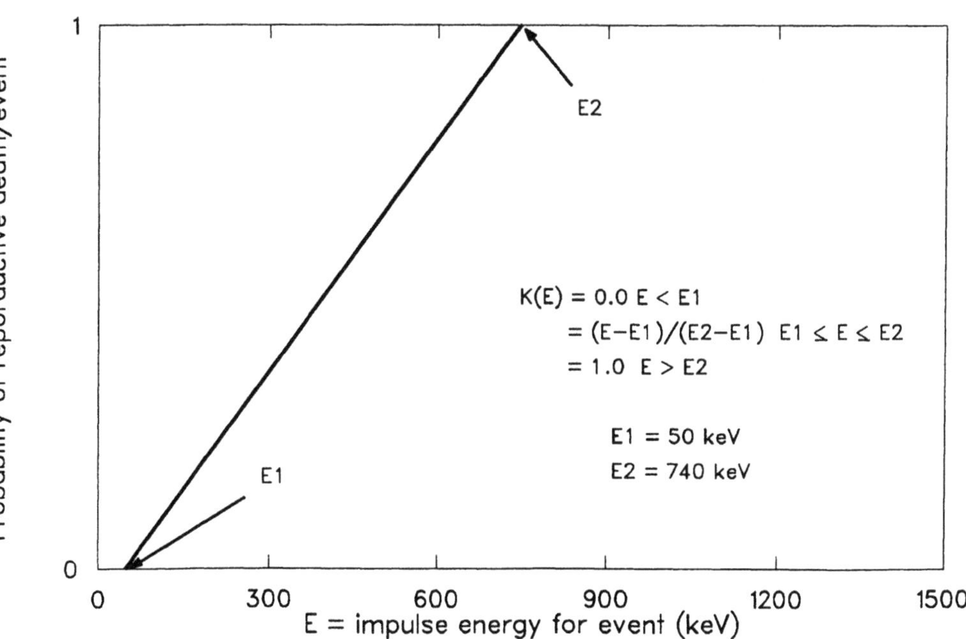

Fig. 5. Trial response function.

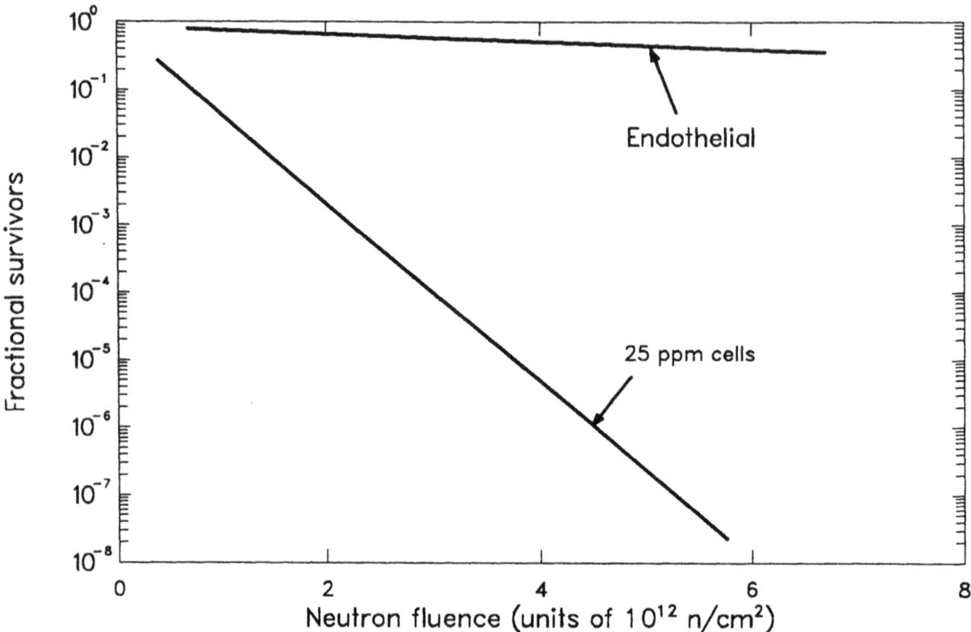

Fig. 6. Results of trial for ^{10}B response vs neutron fluence at 6-cm control depth in tissue. The endothelial response is at the thermal flux peak where the fluence is 1.7 times that at the control depth.

occurring at this depth. The endothelial cells are assumed to be at the peak thermal flux, where the fluence is 1.7 times the 6-cm fluence. The blood-boron content also is assumed to be 25 ppm. The comparison shows a tremendous advantage for killing tumor cells with the ^{10}B reaction and the high tolerance of the endothelium. These results are only qualitative since the actual biological response is not known, but the results would not change significantly for a different response function. The results are consistent with the analytical studies cited and with the canine experiments. It is felt that our model will be very useful for designing and interpreting experiments, and also will lead to an increased understanding for tissue response during radiation therapy.

APPENDIX A

An energy deposition event from a charged-particle track in a region is a random event and the frequency of occurrence is given by the familiar Poisson distribution:

$$W(m) = \frac{N^m}{m!} e^{-N}$$

where W(m) is the frequency of m events in a region that sees an average N events.

Suppose an individual event in a cell causes a biological response with probability K. Assume this conditional probability is independent of other events in the cell. Then, for a cell that experiences exactly m events, the probability experiencing no effect, or the survival probability for that cell is:

$$(1-K)^m.$$

The density of surviving cells, S(m), then can be defined as the fraction of the total cells in an irradiated population that experiences exactly m events and subsequently survives. This is given by the probability that a cell will experience m events when the population average is N events per cell, multiplied by the probability that a cell, having experienced m events, does indeed survive. Given the statistical assumptions shown above, this may be stated as:

$$S(m) = \frac{N^m}{m!} e^{-N} \cdot (1-K)^m$$

$$= \frac{(N(1-K))^m e^{-N}}{m!}.$$

The fractional survival for the entire population is given by:

$$FS = \sum_{m=o}^{\infty} S(m)$$

$$= e^{-N}[1+N(1-K) + \frac{[N(1-K)]^2}{2!} + \ldots] = e^{-N}e^{N(1-K)}$$

$$FS = e^{-NK}$$

Finally, define K(E) as the energy-dependent response function for impulse-energy E, where impulse energy is the energy deposited by either one charged-particle track or the sum of energy deposited by two charged-particle tracks from one capture in the region. Then, defining W(E) as the density of E in the region of interest, the effective response probability is equal to:

$$K = \int W(E)K(E)dE,$$

where W(E) can be obtained from analytical expressions or from simulation studies with Monte Carlo techniques, or other transport models.

These concepts are essentially in agreement with single-event theory developed in detail by earlier investigators (Kellerer and Rossi, 1972).

REFERENCES

Bond, V. P., Varma, M. N., Son Dnaus, C. A., and Feinendegen, L. E., 1985, An alternative to absorbed dose, quality, and RBE at low exposures, Radiat. Res., Suppl. 8, 104, S-52-S-57.

Deutsch, O. L. and Murray, B. W., 1975, Monte Carlo dosimetry calculation for boron neutron capture therapy in the treatment of brain tumors, Nucl. Technol., 26:320.

Gabel, D., Fairchild, R.G., Larsson, B., Drescher, K., Rowe, W. R., 1983, The biological effect of the $^{10}B(n,\alpha)^{7}Li$ reaction and its simulation by Monte Carlo calculation, in: Proc. of the First International Symposium on Neutron Capture Therapy, Cambridge, MA, USA (R. G. Fairchild and G. L. Brownell, eds), BNL-51730, 128.

Gabel, D., Foster, S., and Fairchild, R. G., 1987, The Monte Carlo simulation of the biological effect of the $^{10}B(n,\alpha)^{7}Li$ reaction in cells and tissue and its implication for boron neutron capture therapy, Radiat. Res. 111, 14.

Kellerer, A. M. and Rossi, H. H., 1972, The theory of dual radiation action, Current Topics in: Radiat. Res. Quarterly, 8:85.

Kitao, K., 1975, A method for calculating the absorbed dose near interface from $^{10}B(n,\alpha)^{7}Li$ reaction, Radiat. Res., 61:304.

Northcliffe, L. C. and Schilling, R. F., 1970, Range and stopping power tables for heavy ions, Nucl. Data Tables, A7:233.

Rydin, R. A., Deutsch, O. L., and Murray, B. W., 1975, The effect of geometry on capillary wall dose for boron neutron capture therapy, Phys. Med. Biol., 21:134.

Takeuchi, A., Nagata, T., Ohashi, F., Sasaki, N., Ushio, Y., and Hatanaka, H., 1985, Tolerance of canine brain to boron neutron capture therapy, Jpn. J. Vet. Sci., 47: 859.

Ziegler, J. F., Biersack, J. P., and Littmark, U., 1985, "The Stopping and Range of Ions in Solids", Pergammon Press, New York.

ACKNOWLEDGEMENT

Work performed under the auspices of the U.S. Department of Energy, DOE Contract No. DE-AC07-76ID01570.

DISTRIBUTIONS OF SULFHYDRYL BORANE MONOMER AND DIMER IN RODENTS AND MONOMER IN HUMANS: BORON NEUTRON CAPTURE THERAPY OF MELANOMA AND GLIOMA IN BORONATED RODENTS

D.N. Slatkin, D.D. Joel, R.G. Fairchild,
P.L. Micca, M.M. Nawrocky, B.H. Laster,
J.A. Coderre, G.C. Finkel, C.E. Poletti*,
and W.H. Sweet*

Medical Department
Brookhaven National Laboratory
Upton, New York 11973

*Department of Neurological Surgery
Massachusetts General Hospital
Boston, Massachusetts

INTRODUCTION

Boron neutron capture therapy (BNCT), a form of radiation therapy based on the $^{10}B(n,\alpha)^{7}Li$ nuclear reaction,[1,2] has been used in Japan for radiation therapy of human malignant gliomas after total or partial neurosurgical excision of visible tumor.[3] Japanese data for ^{10}B distribution in the blood and tumor of 30 patients with malignant glioma have been summarized.[4] The stable isotope ^{10}B was introduced into the tumor during a 1-2 hour intra-arterial infusion of a ^{10}B-enriched preparation of the sulfhydryl borane monomer $Na_2B_{12}H_{11}SH$ to a total dose in the range 30-80 mg ^{10}B per kg total body weight. The tumor bed was irradiated for 5-7 hours at a 100-kW nuclear reactor, 11 to 16 hours after the infusion. The average tumor ^{10}B concentration just before irradiation was 22 μg $^{10}B/g$, while the average blood ^{10}B concentration was 18 μg $^{10}B/g$.[4] Despite low tumor:blood ^{10}B concentration ratios just before irradiation (average ratio = 1.2:1.0), post-operative survival after BNCT was unexpectedly prolonged for some patients--indeed astonishingly so for a 66-year-old Japanese man who is neurologically and neuroradiologically stable nearly sixteen years after visibly incomplete removal of a malignant glioma.[4]

Boron is taken up more avidly by mouse melanoma and by mouse liver after slow infusion of the sulfhydryl borane dimer $Na_4B_{24}H_{22}S_2$ than of its parent monomer $Na_2B_{12}H_{11}SH$.[5] After slow infusion of the dimer into a rat, concentrations of boron in an intracerebral transplanted glioma are about the same as in blood.[6,7]

In this paper, boron distributions after infusion of monomer into two patients with malignant glioma are summarized. Preliminary studies are described of the effects of BNCT on intracerebral transplanted gliomas in rats infused with ^{10}B-enriched dimer and on subcutaneous transplanted mouse melanoma in mice infused with ^{10}B-enriched dimer or monomer. Distributions of ^{10}B in rats after prolonged intraperitoneal and intravenous infusions of the sulfhydryl boranes are also presented.

METHODS AND RESULTS

Distribution of Sulfhydryl Borane Monomer $Na_2B_{12}H_{11}SH$ in Humans

The first patient was terminally ill with a malignant astrocytoma in the left frontal lobe, which had been diagnosed by open biopsy 15 weeks previously. With the informed consent of next-of-kin and the approval of the Massachusetts General Hospital Committee for ethical clinical investigation, a 25-hour continuous intravenous infusion of 95 atom% ^{10}B-enriched $Na_2B_{12}H_{11}SH$ was carried out to give a total dose equivalent to 13.5 mg ^{10}B/kg body weight. The patient's condition continued to deteriorate as it did before the infusion, and death ensued 19 hours after infusion was stopped. Postmortem examination showed tumor in the left frontal lobe and in the pia mater of the sacral spinal cord and cauda equina. Neutron-induced alpha radiographs of air-dried cryostat sections of the unfixed cerebrum (Fig. 1) and of the sacral spinal cord showed ^{10}B in every zone of tumor that was examined, in zones of peritumor cerebral edema and in the tunica media of small arteries. Concentrations of ^{10}B in microscopic zones of tumor were in the 2-6 μg/g range and prompt gamma (478 keV) neutron activation analysis of several ~0.5 g portions of unfixed cerebral tumor indicated ^{10}B concentrations in the 1-3 μg/g range. Little or no ^{10}B was seen in the parenchyma of normal cerebrum or in the parenchyma of the sacral spinal cord.

The second patient was a middle-aged man who underwent partial resection of a large malignant astrocytoma of the right temporal lobe about 26 hours after a 20-hour intravenous infusion of 95 atom% ^{10}B-enriched $Na_2B_{12}H_{11}SH$ to a total dose equivalent to 15 mg ^{10}B/kg body weight. During the operation, several small and large portions of edematous, tumor-bearing temporal lobe tissue, cystic tumor fluid, spinal fluid, and

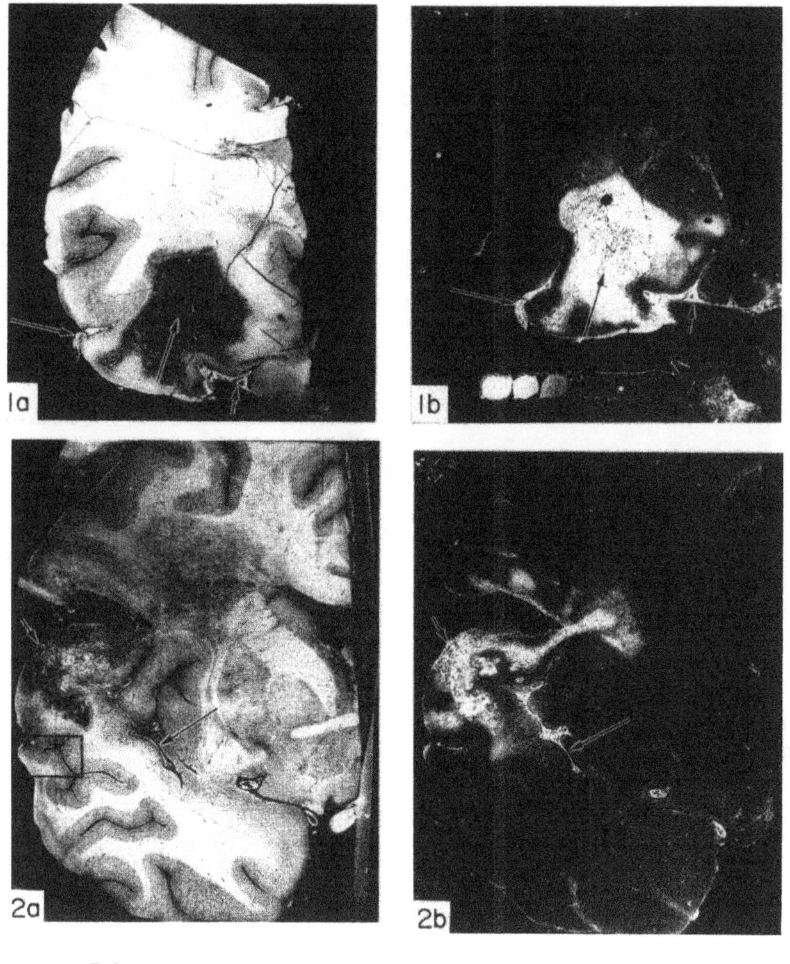

Fig. 1. Air-dried, unstained 50 μm cryomicrotome sections (upper and lower left frames) of an unfixed frozen coronal slice of glioma-bearing cerebrum (mainly postero-inferior left frontal lobe) with corresponding alpha-track-etched cellulose nitrate plastic films (Kodak-Pathe, Paris, France; type LR-115). The whitest areas of the films indicate ^{10}B-bearing zones of the matching brain sections.

blood were removed for ^{10}B analysis. Measurements of a 50 μm-thick cryomicrotome section of the largest temporal lobe specimen by an alpha-track-etch radiography technique showed ^{10}B concentrations in the 2.1-5.2 μg/g range. Analyses of small portions of edematous brain tissue containing macroscopically visible tumor by the 478 keV prompt gamma technique indicated ^{10}B concentrations in the 1.8-3.6 μg/g range. Fluid from a tumor cyst was centrifuged promptly and separated into an amber-colored supernate and a hemorrhagic sediment, which contained 5.3 and 2.7 μg ^{10}B/g, respectively. A lumbar sample of cerebrospinal fluid taken during the operation contained no measurable ^{10}B. In this patient, the effective average half-time for clearance of ^{10}B from blood plasma after infusion of the sulfhydryl borane monomer, 9.8 hours, was practically identical to that of ^{10}B from trichloroacetic acid-precipitable plasma proteins, 9.7 hours. This was in accord with observations that about 90% of ^{10}B in the patient's blood was in the blood plasma.

Distribution of the Sulfhydryl Borane Dimer $Na_4B_{24}H_{22}S_2$ in Rats

The distribution of boron from dimer has been reported[6,7] in eight male CDF rats (Charles River, Wilmington, MA), in four of which ~5 x 10^5 syngeneic glioma cells[8] had been injected stereotactically into the right frontal lobe. Osmotic pumps (Alza Corp., Palo Alto, CA; Model 2ML1), containing sufficient 95 atom% ^{10}B-enriched dimer to deliver a total dose equivalent to 147-240 mg ^{10}B/kg body weight, were inserted surgically into the peritoneum. After ~9 days of intraperitoneal infusion, when ^{10}B concentrations in macroscopic glioma tumor tissue averaged 20.1 μg/g, ^{10}B concentrations in whole blood averaged 21.2 μg/g; in blood plasma, 31.6 μg/g; in blood cells, 4.8 μg/g; in cerebrum, 2.7 μg/g.[6,7] Concentrations of ^{10}B in the tissues of similarly infused rats euthanized on days 12, 15 or 17 after implanting the pumps are shown in Table 1.

Average half-times for clearance of ^{10}B from the blood and from most tissues of the rat after pumping had ceased were in the range of 31-91 hours. These dimer-^{10}B clearance rates are an order of magnitude slower than the clearance of ^{10}B from blood and from intracerebral glioma in similar rats after prompt injection of ^{10}B-enriched monomer (1.7 and 2.6 hours, respectively; D.N. Slatkin and P.L. Micca, unpublished.). After slow infusion of the dimer into rats, concentrations of ^{10}B are about five times greater in blood plasma than in blood cells. It was found by thin-layer chromotography that the monomer, not the dimer, is excreted in the urine of dimer-infused rats (P.L. Micca, unpublished). Since the net rate of ^{10}B clearance from the kidneys of a dimer-infused rat is exceptionally slow (Table 1), we suggest that some dimer may be reduced to monomer in the kidneys.

Studies on 3- and 4-day intraperitoneal infusions of sulfhydryl boranes via external catheter into tethered, glioma-bearing rats show that dose rates of 50-60 mg ^{10}B per kg body weight per day result in roughly 50 μg ^{10}B per gram of tumor or blood from 95 atom% ^{10}B-enriched dimer and roughly 20 μg ^{10}B per gram of tumor or blood from 95 atom% ^{10}B-enriched monomer. Moreover, the rate of clearance of ^{10}B from the tumor is slower after infusion of the dimer than of the monomer (Fig. 2).

Experimental BNCT of Rat Gliomas and Mouse Melanomas

We attempted to treat the transplantable rat gliomas of Yoshida and Cravioto[8] and of Clendenon et al.,[9] using ^{10}B-enriched dimer delivered in ~9-day infusions from intraperitoneally implanted osmotic pumps. Anesthetized rats were held supine in a Li_2CO_3-TFE Teflon slow-neutron shield with the tumor-bearing zone of the head exposed to neutron-rich reactor radiations through a 1.5-cm diameter aperture at the apex of a conical slow-neutron collimator. The collimator walls are inclined 45° to the normal direction through the 27-mm thickness of a 10" x 10" square, 50% epoxy plastic/50% ^{6}LiF slow-neutron shield in which the collimator had been molded. Irradiations resulted in no more prolongation of life with the dimer than without it (Table 2). Irradiated, glioma-bearing rats lost much more weight than unirradiated, glioma-bearing rats (Fig. 3). Marked perinasal edema and a precipitous post-irradiation decrease in the number of circulating lymphocytes indicate that whole-body gamma and fast-neutron irradiation, irradiation of normal brain endothelium by alpha and ^{7}Li particles from ^{10}B in plasma,[10] and dehydration from the inanition caused by nasopharyngeal irradiation contributed to death.

We have also attempted BNCT of subcutaneously transplanted Harding-Passey melanoma[11] in mice without success using monomer (Fig. 4) and with only marginal success using dimer (Fig. 5). Each borane was infused in its 95 atom% ^{10}B-enriched form via intraperitoneal osmotic pump.[5]

CONCLUSION

Slow infusion of the sulfhydryl borane monomer into two patients with malignant glioma yielded roughly similar boron concentrations in tumor, peritumor edematous brain and blood plasma, with little boron in normal brain. Slow infusion of the monomer $(B_{12}H_{11}SH)^{2-}$ and dimer $(B_{24}H_{22}S_2)^{4-}$ forms of sulfhydryl borane in melanoma-bearing mice and in glioma-bearing

Table 1. Concentrations of ^{10}B (μg/g) in Blood and Other Tissues of Rats Euthanized after Cessation of ~9 Days of Intraperitoneal Infusion of $Na_4B_{24}H_{22}S_2$ to a Total Body ^{10}B Dose of ~200 mg/kg.

Tissue	Rat No.	Days after ~9 days of infusion				Average ^{10}B Clearance Half-Time (Hours)
		0	3	6	8	
Whole blood	1	35.1	10.5	--	--	41
	2	40.2	14.1	3.8	--	43
	3	34.5	11.4	3.2	1.2	43
Cerebrum	1	[5.6]	0	--	--	--
	2	[6.1]	--	--	--	--
	3	[5.2]	--	--	0	--
Cerebellum	1	[3.6]	0	--	--	--
	2	[4.0]	--	0	--	--
	3	[3.4]	--	--	0	--
Liver	1	[154.8]	31.6	--	--	31
	2	[168.6]	--	37.6	--	67
	3	[144.8]	--	--	19.1	65
Spleen	1	[88.8]	19.5	--	--	34
	2	[96.8]	--	19.0	--	62
	3	[83.0]	--	--	12.6	70
Kidney	1	[392.1]	209.4	--	--	79
	2	[427.2]	--	217.8	--	149
	3	[366.7]	--	--	153.1	154
Heart	1	[22.1]	5.4	--	--	36
	2	[24.1]	--	4.9	--	62
	3	[20.7]	--	--	3.4	74
Skeletal Muscle	1	[10.3]	3.6	--	--	48
	2	[11.2]	--	3.8	--	91
	3	[9.6]	--	--	0	--

Each bracketed concentration [day 0] is the average extrapolated tissue ^{10}B concentration from similar infusions into eight rats[6,7] after multiplication by a correction factor which normalized the blood ^{10}B concentration in rat 1, 2 or 3 on day 0 to 21.2 μg/g, the average blood ^{10}B concentration in the eight rats after such infusions.[6,7]

rats yield twice as much boron in tumor from dimer than from monomer. Similarly, plasma and liver concentrations are higher after infusion of dimer than of monomer.

Mixed field nuclear reactor irradiation of a rat cerebral glioma, mainly by thermal neutrons, tended to prolong the life of a tumor-bearing rat whether or not it had received ^{10}B-enriched dimer beforehand. Our failure to achieve better radiotherapeutic results with than without dimer may be attributed to low ^{10}B concentrations in the gliomas and to excessive whole-body radiation. Similar reactor irradiations of melanoma-bearing mice resulted in no better results with than without monomer, and in somewhat better results with than without dimer. The dimer may prove to be more useful than the monomer for BNCT of human gliomas if its hepatotoxicity can be tolerated by patients and if the high plasma boron concentration that follows infusion of dimer can be lowered by a procedure such as plasmapheresis[5,7] before slow-neutron irradiation of the tumor.

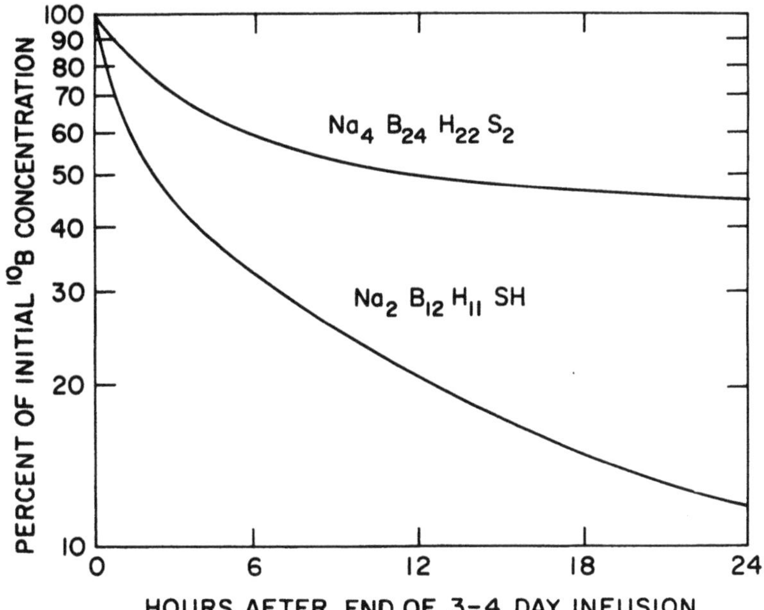

Fig. 2. Average ^{10}B concentrations in subcutaneously transplanted gliomas in the rat after the cessation of 3- or 4-day intraperitoneal infusions of monomer (lower curve) or dimer (upper curve), expressed as percent of average concentration at cessation of the infusions. Dose rate was 50-60 μg ^{10}B per gram body weight per day.

Table 2. Conditions of Irradiation and Post-irradiation Survival for BNCT of Rats with Intracerebrally Implanted Glioma of Either the Yoshida-Cravioto Type[8] (Experiments A and C) or the Clendenon et al. Type[9] (Experiment B).

Experiment, Rat No., Condition	Dose of Dimer (μg ^{10}B/gbw)	Rat Body Weight at Pump Insertion (tumor day), g	Percent of Rat Body Weight on (tumor day) at Irradiation	Death
A, 1, IB	238	(1) 150	(11) 93	(23) 77
2, IB	263	(1) 146	(11) 95	(180) 205^{s}
3, IB	243	(1) 150	(11) 93	(20) 95
4, IB	252	(1) 150	(11) 93	(44) 71
5, IB	250	(1) 143	(11) 102	(29) 78
1, IC	--	(1) 147	(11) 120	(22) 84
2, IC	--	(1) 153	(11) 110	(45) 137
3, IC	--	(1) 135	(11) 117	(41) 70
4, IC	--	(1) 135	(11) 120	(33) 73
5, IC	--	(1) 141	(11) 109	(29) 104
1, C	--	(1) 132	(11) 125	(36) 80
2, C	--	(1) 156	(11) 112	(23) 73

Supercript s indicates four rats that were euthanized after showing no neurological signs of brain tumor. Only in these rats was there no brain tumor found at necropsy. Superscript a indicates rats that received dimer unenriched in ^{10}B. Condition IB indicates rats that received 95 atom% ^{10}B-enriched dimer delivered slowly from intraperitoneally implanted osmotic pump for about 7-10 days after pump implantation, then irradiated under anesthesia at the BNL Medical Research Reactor operated at 1.25 MW power for 6.4 minutes (experiment A) or 8.0 minutes (experiments B and C). Rats were held supine in a tetrafluoroethylene Teflon-Li_2CO_3 slow-neutron body shield with their tumors centered at the apex of a 1.5-cm diameter aperture in a slow-neutron collimator. Condition IC indicates rats that received the same radiation but no dimer. Condition BC indicates rats that received dimer but no radiation. Condition C indicates rats that received neither dimer nor radiation. Data of experiment B are shown graphically in Figure 3. In each experiment, the flux of slow neutrons at the scalp was approximately 1.9×10^{10} cm^{-2} sec^{-1}.

Table 2. (cont'd)

A, 3, C	--	(1) 143	(11) 119	(18) 101
4, C	--	(1) 145	(11) 130	(13) 118
B, 1, IB	253	(2) 217	(14) 98	(33) 86
2, IB	261	(2) 232	(14) 96	(39) 68
3, IB	257	(2) 239	(14) 81	(36) 63
4, IB	241	(2) 238	(14) 89	(32) 66
5, IB	249	(2) 229	(14) 91	(39) 72
1, IC	--	(2) 264	(14) 101	(32) 50
2, IC	--	(2) 219	(14) 108	(34) 95
3, IC	--	(2) 255	(14) 102	(34) 56
4, IC	--	(2) 253	(14) 101	(36) 57
5, IC	--	(2) 236	(14) 102	(42) 67
6, IC	--	(2) 226	(14) 111	(35) 63
1, C	--	(2) 265	(14) 87	(17) 75
2, C	--	(2) 255	(14) 106	(24) 59
3, C	--	(2) 250	(14) 99	(19) 98
4, C	--	(2) 218	(14) 109	(18) 100
5, C	--	(2) 188	(14) 104	(20) 106
C, 1, IB	269	(1) 130		(7) 64
2, IB	295	(1) 140	(8) 68	(9) 65
3, IB	300	(1) 120	(8) 79	(15) 70
4, IB	292	(1) 140	(8) 64	(8) 64
5, IB	291	(1) 140	(8) 75	(15) 59
6, IB	295	(1) 131	(8) 81	(63) 81
1, BC	49[a]	(1) 132	(8) 78	(64) 217[s]
2, BC	54[a]	(1) 130	(8) 72	(36) 94
3, BC	48[a]	(1) 135	(8) 82	(64) 202[s]
4, BC	48[a]	(1) 120		(7) 68
5, BC	44[a]	(1) 140	(8) 81	(33) 66
1, IC	--	(1) 140	(8) 64	(8) 64
2, IC	--	(1) 130	(8) 100	(51) 108
3, IC	--	(1) 135	(8) 99	(16) 76
4, IC	--	(1) 140	(8) 104	(54) 96
5, IC	--	(1) 140	(8) 99	(28) 103
6, IC	--	(1) 125	(8) 100	(47) 95
1, C	--	(1) 115	(8) 83	(36) 83
2, C	--	(1) 133		(7) 67
3, C	--	(1) 135	(8) 75	(36) 69
4, C	--	(1) 136	(8) 104	(7) 74
5, C	--	(1) 129	(8) 94	(30) 88
6, C	--	(1) 120	(8) 85	(64) 223[s]

Other compounds, such as boronated porphyrins,[12] may also be useful for BNCT of gliomas. Whatever ^{10}B transport agent is used, BNCT of gliomas should take into account the influence of irradiation on the functions of effector and suppressor lymphocytes during the growth and regression of tumors.[13]

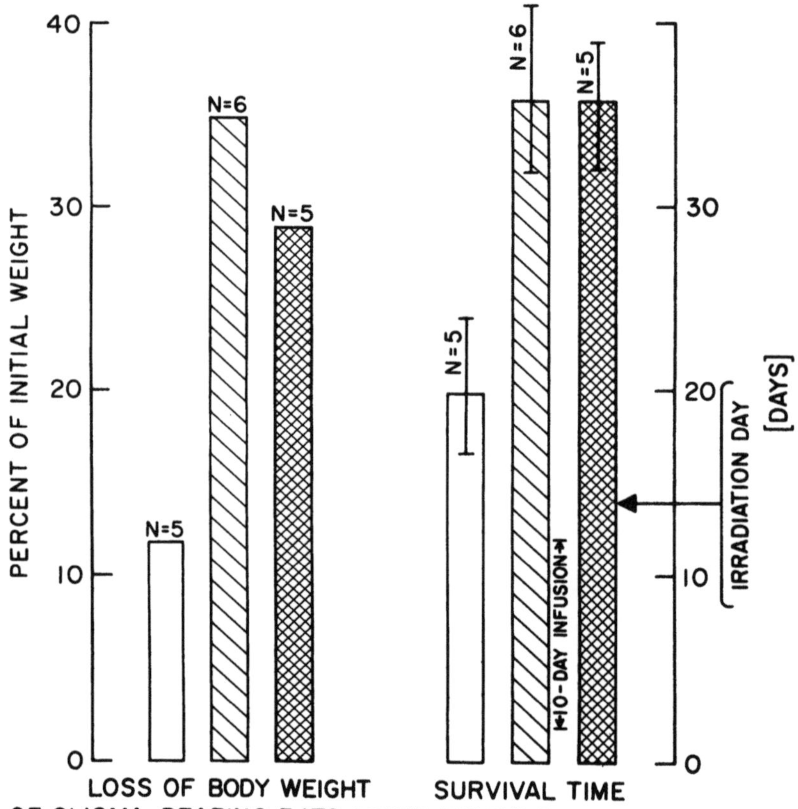

Fig. 3. Summary of body weight losses and survival times after intracerebral transplantation of gliomas[9] in rats (Table 2, experiment B). Each of the two groups of three vertical bars shows the results from same group of rats after treatment conditions C, IC and IB, respectively (see caption, Table 2). Glioma-bearing rats were provided by N. Clendenon et al., of the Ohio State University.

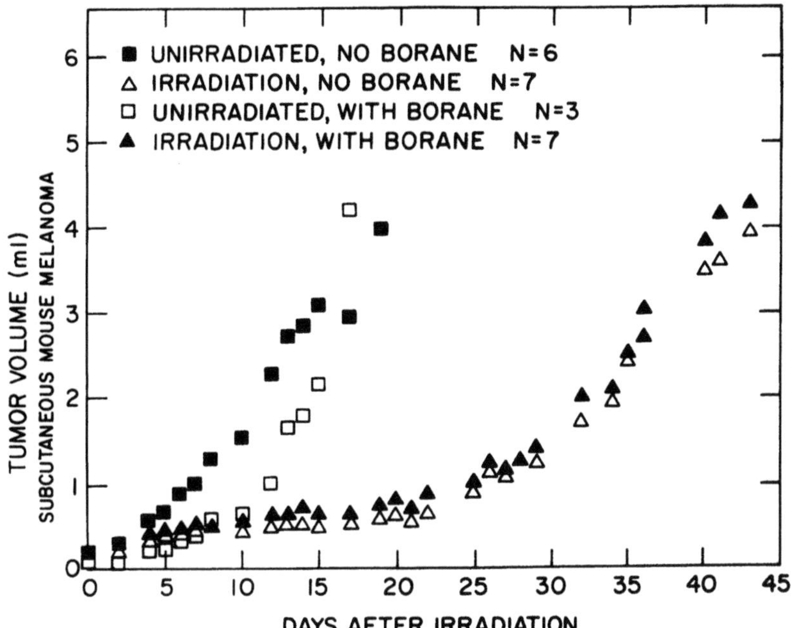

Fig. 4. Progression of growth of Harding-Passey melanomas implanted subcutaneously in thighs of BALB/cJ mice six days before start of ~9.3-day intraperitoneal infusions (average dose, 205 [range:199-282] μg ^{10}B/gram of body weight) of 95 atom% ^{10}B-enriched monomer.[5] BNCT with a slow neutron flux at the surface of the thigh of about 1.5 x 10^{10} cm^{-2} sec^{-1} was carried out at the end of infusion. The BNL Medical Research Reactor was operated at 1.25 MW. Irradiations lasted 6.4 minutes.

ACKNOWLEDGEMENTS

We are grateful to H. Cravioto and N. Clendenon for providing glioma-bearing rats and to F. Drnovski, J. Heinrichs, D. Greenberg, S. Stajnacki, H. Hauptman, G. Jackson, B. Armstrong, E. Jackle and T. Holmquist for technical assistance. Work was performed under Contract No. DE-AC02-76CH000016 with the U.S. Department of Energy.

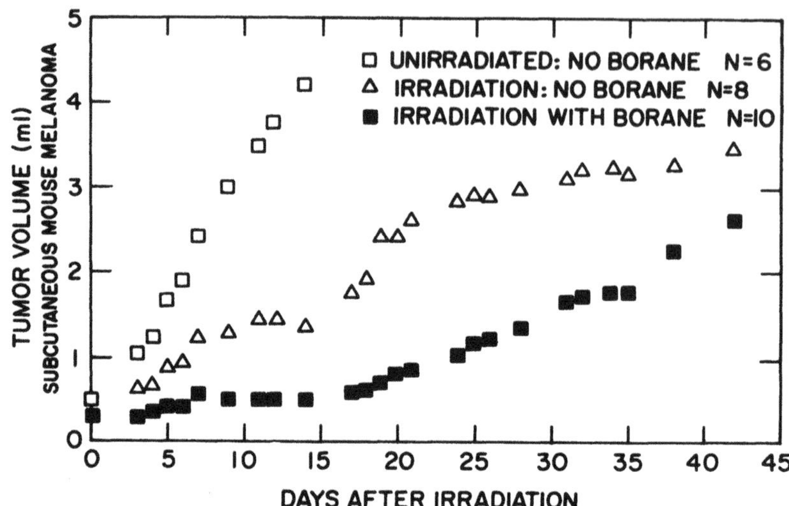

Fig. 5. Progression of growth of Harding-Passey melanomas implanted subcutaneously in thighs of BALB/cJ mice 12 days before start of ~9.7-day intraperitoneal infusions (average dose ~240 μg ^{10}B/gbw) of 95 atom% ^{10}B-enriched dimer.[5] BNCT with a slow neutron flux at the surface of the thigh of about 1.5×10^{10} cm^{-2} sec^{-1} was carried out at the end of infusion. The BNL Medical Research Reactor was operated at 1.25 MW. Irradiations lasted 6.4 minutes.

REFERENCES

1. M. Goldhaber, Introductory Remarks, in: "Workshop on Neutron Capture Therapy," R. G. Fairchild and V. P. Bond, ed., Brookhaven National Laboratory, Upton (1986).
2. D. E. Lea, "Actions of Radiations on Living Cells," 2nd Ed., University Press, Cambridge (1956).
3. H. Hatanaka, "Neutron Capture Therapy for Tumors," Nishimura and Co., Niigata (1986).
4. W. H. Sweet, Medical aspects of boron-slow neutron capture therapy, in: "Workshop on Neutron Capture Therapy," R. G. Fairchild and V.P. Bond, ed., Brookhaven National Laboratory, Upton (1986).
5. D. Slatkin, P. Micca, A. Forman, D. Gabel, L. Wielopolski, and R. Fairchild, Boron uptake in melanoma, cerebrum and blood from $Na_2B_{12}H_{11}SH$ and $Na_4B_{24}H_{22}S_2$ administered to mice, Biochem. Pharmacol. 35:1771 (1986).

6. D. N. Slatkin, P. L. Micca, and R. G. Fairchild, Distribution of boron in brain-tumor-bearing rats after infusion of $Na_4B_{24}H_{22}S_2$: Implications for neutron capture therapy, Radiology 157(P):311 (1985). Abstract.
7. D. N. Slatkin, P. L. Micca, B. H. Laster, and R. G. Fairchild, Distribution of sulfhydryl boranes in mice and rats, in: "Workshop on Neutron Capture Therapy," R. G. Fairchild and V. P. Bond, ed., Brookhaven National Laboratory, Upton (1986).
8. J. Yoshida and H. Cravioto, Nitrosourea-induced brain tumors: an in vivo and in vitro tumor model system, J. Nat. Cancer Inst. 61:365 (1978).
9. N. R. Clendenon, J. H. Goodman, R. F. Barth, F. Alam, A. H. Soloway, A. E. Staubus, W. A. Gordon, R. Gahbauer, J. R. Girvin, A. J. Yates, and M. L. Moeschberger, The use of an experimental rat brain tumor for boron neutron capture therapy, in: "Neutron Capture Therapy," H. Hatanaka, ed., Nishimura, Niigata (1986).
10. D. N. Slatkin, R. D. Stoner, K. M. Rosander, J. A. Kalef-Ezra, and J. A. Laissue, Central nervous system radiation syndrome in mice from preferential $^{10}B(n,\alpha)^7Li$ irradiation of brain vasculature, Proc. Natl. Acad. Sci. USA 85:4020 (1988).
11. H. L. Stewart, K. C. Snell, L. J. Dunham, and S. M. Schlyen, "Transplantable and Transmissible Tumors of Animals," Armed Forces Institute of Pathology, Washington, D.C. (1959).
12. S. B. Kahl, D. D. Joel, G. C. Finkel, P. L. Micca, M. M. Nawrocky, J. A. Coderre, and D. N. Slatkin, A carboranyl porphyrin for boron neutron capture therapy of brain tumors (this volume).
13. R. J. North, Radiation-induced, immunologically mediated regression of an established tumor as an example of successful therapeutic immunomanipulation. Preferential elimination of suppressor T-cells allows sustained production of effector T-cells, J. Exp. Med. 164:1652 (1986).

A CARBORANYL PORPHYRIN FOR BORON NEUTRON CAPTURE THERAPY OF BRAIN TUMORS

S.B. Kahl[1], D.D. Joel[2], G.C. Finkel,[2] P.L. Micca[2], M.M. Nawrocky[2], J.A. Coderre[2] and D.N. Slatkin[2]

[1]Department of Pharmaceutical Chemistry, University of California San Francisco, California 94143
[2]Medical Department, Brookhaven National Laboratory Upton, New York 11973

INTRODUCTION

Many porphyrins are known to concentrate in tumor tissue both in vivo and in vitro, but the mechanisms of porphyrin-tumor affinity are unknown. A central theme of boron neutron capture therapy (BNCT) research is the search for boronated substances with high affinity for tumor. There is interest in the synthesis of boron-containing porphyrins and their evaluation for possible efficacy in BNCT. This study presents some modifications of a previously described method[1] for synthesis of a particular nidocarboranyl porphyrin and some preliminary experimental indications of its potential usefulness for BNCT.

METHODS

A transplantable mouse ascites tumor developed in 1952 from a spontaneous mouse embryonal ovarian carcinoma[2,3] has been maintained since 1987 at the Medical Department, Brookhaven National Laboratory (BNL) by serial intraperitoneal (IP) injections of ~10^5 ascites cells into 10-12 week old C3HeB/FeJ mice (Jackson Labs, Bar Harbor, Maine). A progressively expanding, tumor cell-rich ascitic fluid is seen after about one week of occult growth. Tumor cells invade connective tissue and striated muscle beneath the parietal peritoneum, but the visceral peritoneum tends to resist invasion by the tumor. A solitary, non-metastatic, slowly growing tumor nodule appears at the site of subcutaneous injection of ~$2x10^7$ ascites cells.

The $\alpha^3\beta$ atropisomer of meso-tetra (o-aminophenyl) porphyrin (0.157 g; 0.233 mmol), prepared by the general method of Collman,[4] was dissolved under argon in 30 ml of dry, freshly distilled CH_2Cl_2 to give a deep, red-purple solution. To this was added carborane carbonyl chloride (0.053 g; 0.256 mmol) and p-dimethylaminopyridine (0.031 g; 0.256 mmol). The resulting red-purple solution was stirred at ambient temperature, protected from exposure to light with aluminum foil, until thin layer chromatography (Kodak 13181 silica gel) in 1:1 CH_2Cl_2/hexane indicated the absence of porphyrin starting material (~ 2 hours). Thirty ml of distilled water were then added to the reaction mixture and rapid stirring continued for one hour. The mixture was poured into a separatory funnel, the aqueous layer discarded and the organic layer washed again with water. This process was repeated with 5% aqueous $NaHCO_3$ (2X), 0.1N hydrochloric acid, and saturated aqueous NaCl (2X). After drying over Na_2SO_4 and filtration, the solvents were removed by vacuum to yield a lustrous powder. This material was dissolved in a minimal amount of CH_2Cl_2 and passed through a pad of silica gel 60. Removal of the CH_2Cl_2 produced 0.307 g (0.226 mmol; 97.2% yield) of a microcrystalline purple solid. This closocarboranyl porphyrin was shown by HPLC to be 98.7% pure $\alpha^3\beta$ atropisomer of the carboranyl anilide with the remainder being the α^4 atropisomer. It was used without further purification for the cage-opening step.

The closed cage material (0.307 g; 0.226 mmol) was stirred under argon with 27 ml of dry pyridine and 9 ml distilled piperidine for 36 hours at room temperature. Volatile material was then removed by high vacuum. The resultant slightly gummy purple solids were triturated with diethyl ether and filtered. This process was repeated twice. The purple solids were dissolved in minimal acetone (~ 15 ml) and filtered. The filtrate was evaporated, redissolved in acetone, filtered and then evaporated. The solid product was again triturated with ether, filtered , and dried and then placed on a high vacuum line and heated at 100-120° for 8 hours. The iridescent purple piperidinium salt was collected and stored under argon. Ion exchange of a solution of the material in 3:2 acetone/water on a Dowex 50 X 80-200 cation ion exchange column in the K^+ form produced a deep purple solution which was rotary evaporated to remove most of the acetone. The remaining aqueous solution was lyophilized and then pumped at high vacuum with 60-80°C heating for 6 hours. The resultant purple solid weighing 0.305 g (0.208 mmol; 92.0% yield) was stored under argon in the dark at 0°C. (The calculated yield for this material is misleading since it contains significant water of hydration which cannot be removed at reasonable temperatures under vacuum. The material is hygroscopic and must be stored under anhydrous conditions.)

Miniature (~1.3g) osmotic pumps (Alza Corp., Palo Alto, California; Model 2001) were filled with aqueous solutions of the potassium salt of this tetra-anionic porphyrin then implanted beneath the dorsal thoracic skin of female C3HeB/FeJ mice under ether anesthesia. The nominal duration of pump action was 9 days at about 1 µl per hour. However, only ~7.8% (range 6.7-8.5%) of the initial boron content of the pump solution (Exp. C) could be extracted from the pump by prolonged immersion in water after 7 days of subcutaneous infusion in mice. Porphyrin uptake was estimated microscopically by epiillumination of unfixed, air-dried specimens using violet/ultraviolet light from a mercury vapor lamp which was passed through a ~405 nm excitation filter, reflected by a ~455 nm dichroic mirror, with observations of red fluorescence through a ~610 nm barrier filter. Boron uptake was measured in liver and blood by neutron-induced prompt gamma (478 keV) spectroscopy[5] and in tumor by neutron-induced alpha radiography.[6]

A transplantable rat glioma, originally induced by methylnitrosourea,[7] has been maintained in vitro at BNL since 1987 by serial inoculation into Dulbecco's Modified Eagle Medium (DMEM) (Gibco, Cat#320-1965) to which 5% fetal bovine serum, 1% antibiotics (penicillin, 100 IU/ml, amphotericin-B 0.25 μg/ml and streptomycin 100 μg/ml) (Gibco, Cat #600-5240AE) and 1% of L-glutamine (200 mM) were added. Within one month after ~4 mm deep injection of $1x10^4$ cultured glioma cells into the frontal lobe of a Fisher-344 male rat, a 50-200 mg solitary intracranial tumor kills the animal.

EXPERIMENTS

A. The confluent growth of rat glioma cells on 75 cm^2 flat-bottom culture flasks (Corning, Cat #25110) was detached with 2 ml of a 0.5 mg/ml trypsin-0.2 mg/ml EDTA solution (Gibco, Cat #610-5300) and diluted to $1x10^5$ cells/ml with DMEM. One milliliter of the suspension was placed carefully on each of forty horizontal 25 mm-diameter round glass coverslips in 35 mm-diameter polystyrene plastic Petri dishes (Falcon, Cat #3001). The cells were allowed to settle for 15-20 minutes and 1 ml DMEM was added for 24 hours of culture at 37°C under 5% $C0_2$ in air. Thirty-four of the forty coverslip cultures had visibly equivalent cell densities and were selected for a further 24 hours of culture (in the dark) with 2 ml of porphyrin, monomer or dimer in DMEM (30 cultures) or with DMEM alone (4 cultures). DMEM solutions with the highest nominal concentrations of boron (0.22 mg B/ml as porphyrin, 0.24 mg B/ml as monomer and 0.31 mg B/ml as dimer) were filter-sterilized (0.22 μm; Corning Cat#25932) then diluted serially 1:2, 1:4, 1:8 and 1:16 with sterile DMEM in duplicate. After 24 hours, the coverslips were washed twice with 2 ml of Dulbecco's phosphate buffered saline (Gibco, Cat #310-4190). One of each duplicate coverslip cultures was air-dried and mounted on a 1"x3" glass microscope slide with cells upward. The matching coverslip cultures were fixed for 10 minutes in a mixture of PBS and 0.1 ml of methyl alcohol: acetic acid (3:1). This mixture was removed and PBS-free 3:1 fixative added for 10 minutes. The cultures then were stained with 5% Giemsa for 20 minutes and mounted on a microscope slide.

B. About $2x10^5$ ascites cells were injected intraperitoneally (IP) into six four-month old female C3HeB/FeJ mice. Two days later, six osmotic pumps were loaded with concentrated solutions of the K^{4+} porphyrin preparation as follows. Exactly 15.0 mg of porphyrin crystals were dissolved in 1.341 g H_20, then two pumps were filled (Table 1, B1 and B2). The residual solution (0.838g) was diluted with 0.846g H_20 and four more pumps were filled (Table 1, B3-B6). The six pumps were promptly implanted subcutaneously and the mice maintained in a darkened cage with free access to food pellets (Purina Rodent Chow, Purina Mills Inc., St. Louis, MO) and water. Mice B1, B2, B3 and B6 were euthanized with ether at seven days and mice B4 and B5 at eleven days after implantation of pumps.

Table 1. Conditions of in vivo mouse experiments.

Experiment Mouse #	Porphyrin Concentration in pump	Total Porphyrin Loaded in Pump	Total Weight of Mouse (g) Weight on Day After IP Implantation of Pump [day]				Total Porphyrin Delivered to Mouse [day]		Boron Dose Delivered to Mouse
	mg/ml	(mg)	[0]	[4]	[6]	Average	(mg)		(μg/gbw)
B1	11.2	2.38	23.6	30.0	29.8	28.1	2.19	[7]	21.6
B2	11.2	2.57	26.3	30.2	28.1	28.6	2.19	[7]	23.0
B3	5.6	1.25	25.7	31.5	31.2	29.8	1.15	[7]	10.7
B4	5.6	1.24	26.3	30.2	32.0	29.8	1.24	[11]	11.5
B5	5.6	1.23	23.4	31.0	30.8	29.3	1.23	[11]	11.6
B6	5.6	1.24	25.7	29.7	31.5	28.9	1.14	[7]	10.9
			[0]	[4]	[6]	Average			
C1	28.4	6.13	36.2	42.0	44.0	40.2	5.65	[6]	38.9
C2	28.4	6.10	32.1	34.5	32.1	33.3	5.62	[6]	46.7
C3	14.8	3.29	33.0	39.1	44.0	37.6	3.03	[6]	22.3
C4	14.8	3.35	36.0	36.7	37.4	36.6	3.09	[6]	23.4

C. Exactly 31.1 mg of porphyrin crystals were dissolved in 1.065 g of a 0.5% solution of sodium bicarbonate in water. Pumps for mice C1 and C2 were filled (Table 1). The residual solution (0.549g) was then diluted with 0.502g of the same solvent, and pumps for mice C3 and C4 were filled. Ten days before filling and implanting these pumps, recipient mice had been injected IP with 1×10^5 ascites cells. Thirty-nine days before implanting the pump, each of these mice received a single subcutaneous flank injection of $\sim 1.7 \times 10^7$ ascites cells. This produced subcutaneous tumor nodules several millimeters in diameter which were seen when the mice were killed six days after pump implantation.

OBSERVATIONS

Experiment A. (In Vitro)

Rat glioma cells exposed for 24 hours in vitro to initial nominal porphyrin concentrations corresponding to 56, 112 and 224 μgB/ml of culture medium and minimal ambient light showed increasingly severe vacuolization of cytoplasm with progressive attenuation of their tapered cytoplasmic processes. Figure 1 shows a 250x photomicrograph of Giemsa-stained cells exposed to the 56 μg B/ml porphyrin culture medium. Cellular toxicity of the porphyrin is clearly evident at this concentration, which corresponds to approximately 200 mg porphyrin/liter. Toxic effects due solely to inherent porphyrin toxicity would be expected to occur in this general range. We have noted previously that mice can tolerate 80-100 mg/kg doses of this compound, administered as a single-bolus intraperitoneal injection. Neither nuclear nor cytoplasmic abnormalities were evident in the cultures with initial nominal porphyrin concentrations corresponding to 14 or 28 μg B/ml. Although the nuclear membrane appeared normal at each porphyrin concentration used, heterochromatin dispersed or disappeared in porphyrin-exposed cells at 112 and 224 μg B/ml.

Dimer-exposed light-protected cells appeared normal 24 hours after the initial culture medium concentration of 19 μg B/ml, and then the nuclei became increasingly distorted and irregularly lobulated 24 hours after initial concentrations corresponding to 38, 77, 153 and 306 μg B/ml. In Fig. 2, dimer-exposed cells (77 μg B/ml) which were stained with Giemsa are observed at 250x magnification under normal light conditions. At this concentration some nuclei

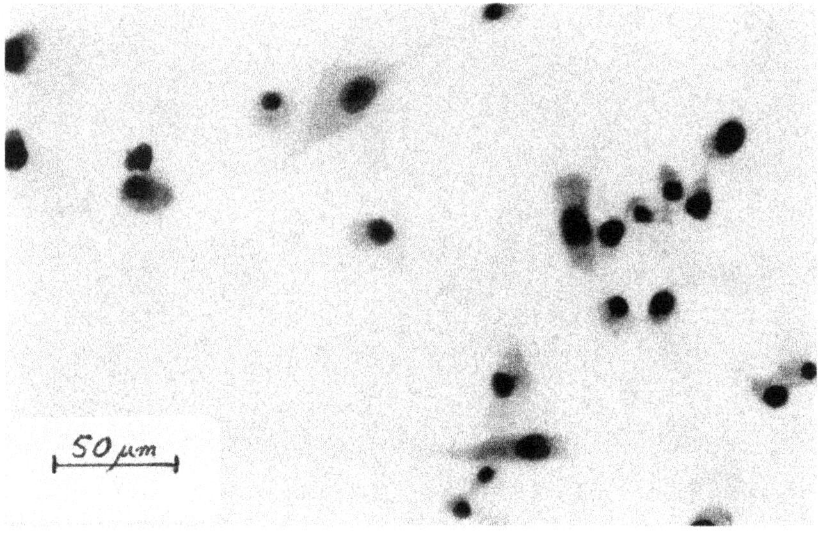

Fig. 1. Giemsa-stained rat glioma cells exposed to 56 μg B/ml porphyrin at 250x magnification.

are noticeably distorted in contrast to the apparently normal nuclei of porphyrin-exposed cells shown in Fig. 1. In contrast to porphyrin-exposed cells, however, cytoplasmic changes were not noted, except at the highest of these dimer concentrations. Unlike porphyrin-and dimer-exposed rat glioma cells, monomer-exposed cells hardly differed from unexposed cells up to the 123 µg B/ml level, as judged by light microscopy, and showed only cytoplasmic vacuolization at 245 µg B/ml.

Microscopic examination of these cultures through a 610 nm barrier filter by violet and ultraviolet-induced fluorescence showed intense cytoplasmic fluorescence in rat glioma cells exposed to the three highest concentrations of porphyrin, and fainter cytoplasmic fluorescence in cells exposed for 24 hours to porphyrin in the 14 and 28 µg B/ml cultures. Figure 3 shows a 100-fold magnification of rat glioma cells exposed to the nido-porphyrin at 56 µg/ml, when illuminated with ~400-450 nm light. Intracellular fluorescence of the cells is evident. At this magnification, fluorescence appears to be more or less evenly distributed throughout the cytoplasm, but does not arise from the nucleus. These results demonstrate that boronated porphyrins, like their non-boronated counterparts, cross the cytoplasmic membrane and remain even after incubation medium has been removed. Nuclear fluorescence from porphyrin-exposed cells was minimal, and no fluorescence whatsoever was seen from any of the in vitro monomer or dimer-exposed cells under the conditions of our fluorescence microscopy system.

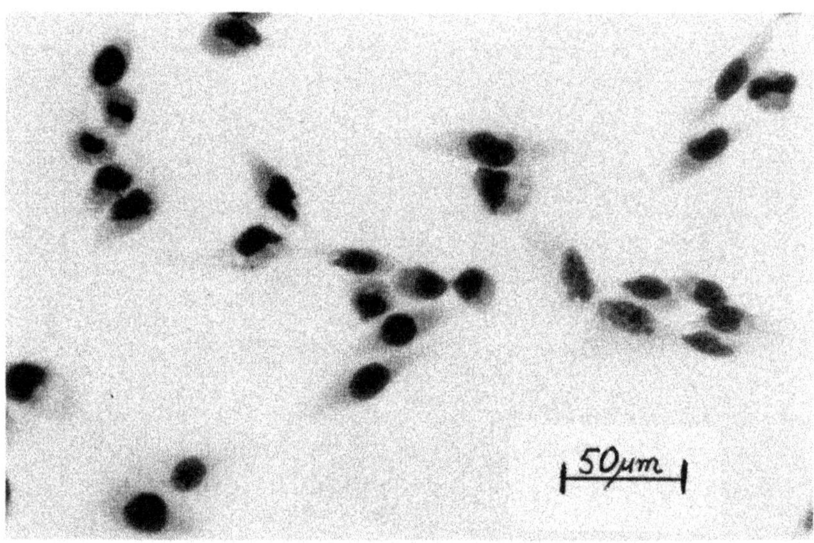

Fig. 2. Giemsa-stained rat glioma cells exposed to 77 µg/ml dimer at 250x magnification.

Experiment B (In Vivo)

This study established the feasibility of performing week-long subcutaneous infusions into mice at total porphyrin doses that yielded up to 23 μg B/gram of body weight (gbw), since the six mice so infused showed no obvious change in behavior, and since their weight gain was as expected during the early stage of ascitic tumor growth. At necropsy, ascitic fluid was sparse but small tumor nodules were seen beneath the parietal peritoneum.

One peritoneal tumor nodule (from mouse B2) was analyzed for boron by alpha radiography. An 8 μm thick cryomicrotome section of the tumor was mounted on a SiO_2 glass microscope slide and air-dried with similarly prepared sections of normal mouse liver and liver containing ~2.5 μg ^{10}B/g and ~5.9 μg ^{10}B/g following 9-day IP infusions of 95 atom % ^{10}B-enriched $Na_2B_{12}H_{11}SH$. The bulk ^{10}B concentrations of the two boronated livers from which reference liver sections were taken were evaluated by the neutron-induced prompt gamma (478 keV) technique. Using a computer program that analyzed a digitized transform of the microscopic images, it was found that the ratio of the average number of tracks over the tumor to that over the 2.5 μg ^{10}B/g reference liver section was 0.7. Analysis of the identical 30 sample areas for each specimen using the same discriminator settings showed that the corresponding ratio of track areas was 0.4. Thus, the nominal average peritoneal tumor nodule boron concentrations calculated by counting of tracks and measurement of track areas were 9 μg B/g and 5 μg B/g, respectively.

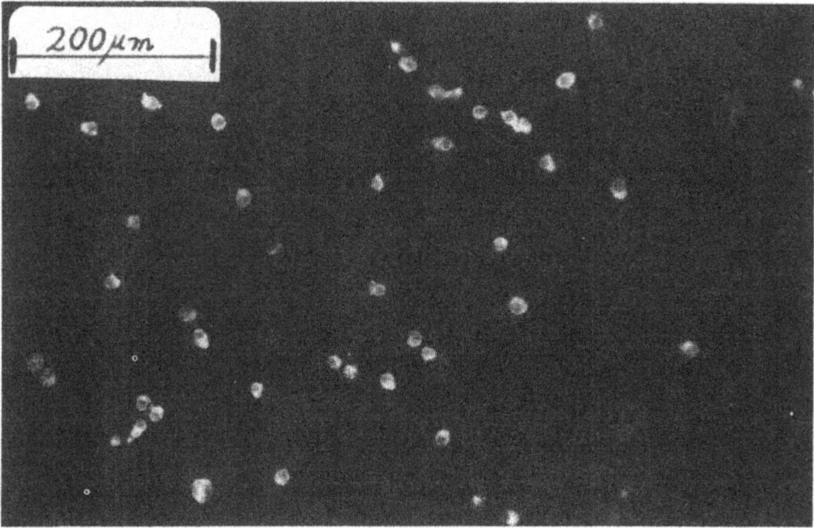

Fig. 3. Rat glioma cells exposed to 56 μg B/ml observed under fluorescence conditions at 100x magnification.

Fig. 4 shows the intense, intracellular fluorescence from air-dried, unfixed ascitic fluid from mouse B6. These cells are probably tumor cells. The pale circumferential zone beneath the plasma membrane and the blebbing of the plasma membrane are probably due to hypoxia in vivo. Similar blebs have been observed in hepatocytes cultured under hypoxic conditions.[7] Experiments are underway to confirm the porphyrin uptake in hypoxic cells. If this is confirmed, boronated porphyrins might be expected to show unusually good potential in treating larger tumors which tend to have hypoxic regions. Figs. 5 and 6 show fluorescence from thin sections of unfixed solid tumor and liver, respectively, from mouse B2 (total dose of boron delivered was 23 μg/gbw) under identical optical conditions. Even at this low total boron dose, the intense fluorescence is easily observed. The fluorescence intensity in hepatocyte cytoplasm is only slightly greater than that of the cytoplasm of tumor cells, suggesting that porphyrin (and boron) concentrations in these cells are similar. The liver boron concentration in mouse B2 was determined by the prompt gamma technique to be approximately 20 μg/g. Since this was approximately the whole body dose "concentration" and since the fluorescence intensity of the tumor was similar to that of liver, we estimate that cytoplasmic tumor boron concentrations approach whole body dose "concentrations" under these conditions of slow subcutaneous infusion.

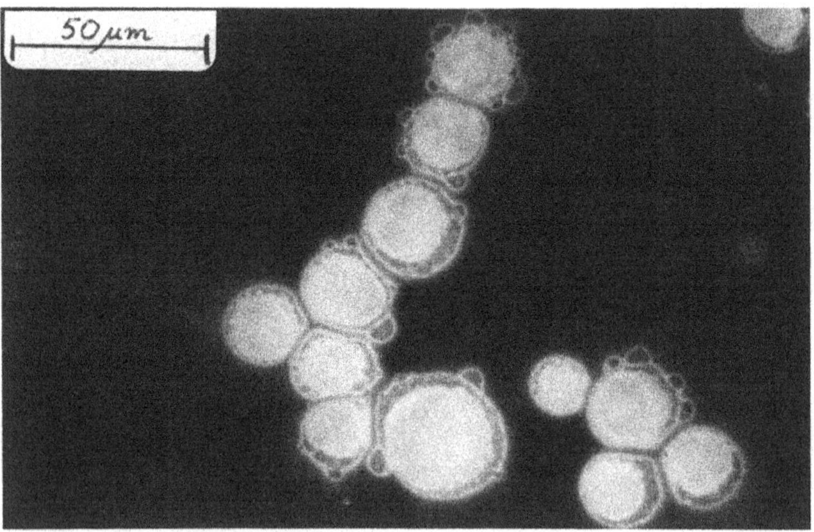

Fig. 4. Ascitic fluid from mouse B6 observed under fluorescence conditions at 400x magnification.

Experiment C (In Vivo)

When the four mice [C1-C4] were killed (6 days after implanting the pump and 16 days after the IP injection of tumor cells), about 3-6 ml of ascitic fluid was obtained and centrifuged promptly at 2000 rpm for 10 minutes at 5°C. Analysis of the packed cell sediment (about 60% by volume) and the protein-rich amber supernate by the prompt gamma technique yielded boron concentrations of ~4 μg/g and ~2μg/g, respectively.

Cryomicrotome sections of the subcutaneous tumor, the liver, the cerebellum and the cerebrum of mouse C2 were mounted on the same SiO_2 glass slide and also observed by fluorescence microscopy. Hepatocyte nuclei showed minimal fluorescence. Little fluorescence was seen outside the hepatocytes except for an extraordinarily intense fluorescence from numerous small (<2μm) perisinusoidal granules. No fluorescence was seen from the cerebellum or from the cerebrum. The intensities of cytoplasmic fluorescence from hepatocytes and tumor cells were comparable. From such qualitative observations of tumor and liver fluorescence, we believe that tumor cytoplasmic boron levels in excess of 40 μg/g are achievable.

Analyses of whole blood and liver specimens removed during necropsy from mice C1-C4 by the prompt gamma technique revealed whole blood boron concentrations of 4, 2, 5 and 4 μg/g, and average liver boron concentrations of 40, 46, 21 and 20 μg/g, respectively.

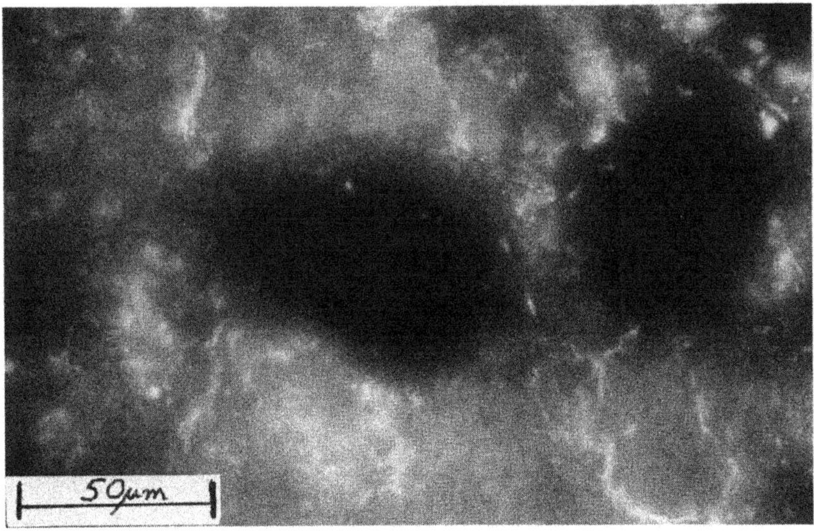

Fig. 5 Tumor thin section from mouse B2 observed under fluorescence conditions at 400x magnification.

CONCLUSIONS

This preliminary study shows that boronated porphyrin can be delivered slowly to mice in a total dose corresponding to as much as 47 µg B/gbw (Table 1, mouse C2) without serious detriment to vital physiologic functions. Moreover, qualitative observations by fluorescence microscopy indicate that concentrations of porphyrin in the cytoplasm of tumor cells and in hepatocytes can approach the whole body dose "concentration," for example in mouse C2, 46 µg B/g in liver after slow delivery of 47 µg B/gbw. Additionally, there is substantial spontaneous clearance of porphyrin from the blood (liver : blood concentration ratio of boron ~8:1).

The in vitro study demonstrates that rat glioma cells have a substantial affinity for the boronated porphyrin, and that the affinity is largely cytoplasmic. The in vitro study also shows that this porphyrin is toxic to rat glioma cells at concentrations that approach those that might be relevant to BNCT. Indeed, it is conceivable that this carboranyl porphyrin might exert some chemotherapeutic inhibitory effect on tumor growth.

Cytotoxic effects of this porphyrin and of the dimer $Na_4B_{24}H_{22}S_2$ apparently occur at comparable concentrations of boron, but are different in kind and in severity. Cytotoxicity from the porphyrin seems to affect the cytoplasm and leads to attenuation of cytoplasm at high concentrations, whereas the dimer seems to affect the nuclear membrane without affecting the cytoplasm.

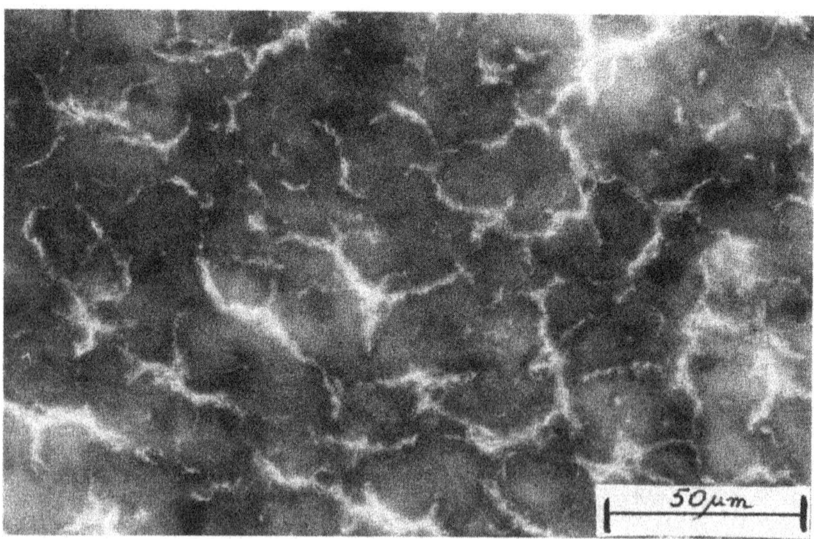

Fig. 6. Liver thin section from mouse B2 observed under fluorescence conditions at 400x magnification.

This carboranyl porphyrin shows considerable promise for use in BNCT of brain tumors since it has substantial affinity for glioma cell cytoplasm, clears spontaneously from the blood, and has no observable affinity for normal cerebellar or cerebral tissue. Whether its undoubted cytotoxicity will prove to be an insurmountable obstacle to its use for clinical BNCT remains to be investigated. The apparent lack of morbidity in mice infused subcutaneously in total doses up to 47 μg boron per gram of total body weight gives us reason to speculate that transient toxicity from therapeutically useful doses of this boronated porphyrin may be tolerated by patients undergoing post-operative BNCT for malignant glioma.

ACKNOWLEDGEMENTS

Work at the University of California, San Francisco, was supported by Grant 37961 from the National Cancer Institute of the National Institutes of Health. Work at Brookhaven National Laboratory was performed in part under contract number DE-AC02-76CH000016 with the U.S. Department of Energy.

REFERENCES

1. S.B. Kahl, Recent advances in the synthesis of boron-containing steroids and porphyrins, in: "Proceedings of the First International Symposium on Neutron Capture Therapy", G.L. Brownell and R.G. Fairchild,eds., Brookhaven National Laboratory, 51730, Upton, NY, 1983.

2. E. Fekete and M.A. Ferringno, Studies on a transplantable teratoma of the mouse, Cancer Res 12:438 (1952).

3. S.E. Order, V. Donahue, and R. Knapp, Immunotherapy of ovarian carcinoma: An experimental model, Cancer Res. 32:573 (1973).

4. J.P. Collman, R.R. Gagne, C.A. Reed, T.R. Halbert, G. Lang, and N.T. Robinson, Picket Fence Porphyrins. Synthetic models for oxygen binding hemoproteins, J. Am. Chem. Soc. 97:1427 (1975).

5. R.G. Fairchild, D. Gabel, B.H. Laster, D. Greenburg, W. Kiszenick, and P.L. Micca, Microanalytical techniques for boron analysis using the ^{10}B $(n,\alpha)^7Li$ reaction, Med. Phys. 13:50 (1986).

6. D. Gabel, I. Hocke, and W. Elsen, Determination of sub-ppm amounts of boron in solutions by means of solid state track detectors, Phys. Med. Biol. 28:1453 (1983).

7. J. Yoshida and H. Cravioto, Nitrosourea-induced brain tumors: An in vivo and in vitro model system, J. Nat. Cancer Inst., 61:365 (1978).

8. B. Herman, A.-L. Nieminen, G.J. Gores, and J.J. LeMasters, Irreversible injury in anoxic hepatocytes precipitated by an abrupt increase in plasma membrane permeability, FASEB Journal, 2:146 (1988).

DISTRIBUTION OF A BORONATED PORPHYRIN IN MURINE TUMORS

S.B. Kahl, B. H. Laster,* M.-S. Koo,
L.S. Warkentien* and R.G. Fairchild*

School of Pharmacy
Department of Pharmaceutical Chemistry
University of California
513 Parnassus
San Francisco, CA 94143-0446

*Medical Department
Brookhaven National Laboratory
Upton, NY 11973

INTRODUCTION

Boron neutron capture therapy (BNCT) as an effective therapeutic technique in the treatment of glioblastoma multiforme, a malignant and lethal brain disease, is largely dependent upon the availability of boronated compounds which demonstrate high tumor-to-normal tissue concentration ratios. The ^{10}boron-thermal neutron reaction [$^{10}B(n,\alpha)^{7}Li$] can successfully induce tumor cell reproductive death provided that the ^{10}B atoms are distributed within or around the cell so that the resultant α-particle will traverse the cell nucleus at least to some extent. It is generally thought that 20-30 μg of ^{10}B/g of tumor could achieve therapeutic results when irradiated with a thermal neutron fluence of $5x10^{12}$ n/cm^{2}.[1,7]

Currently, the boronated compound being most widely considered for the initiation of clinical BNCT trials in the United States is $Na_2B_{12}H_{11}SH$ (BSH), in its monomeric form. This compound is being utilized in human clinical trials in Japan by Dr. Hiroshi Hatanaka with apparent success[2]. While ^{10}B levels in tumors in small animal models approach those required for therapy, it has been difficult to demonstrate

Table 1. Effect of Prolonged Clearance Time on the Tissue Boron Concentration. 26 $\mu g^{N}B$/gbw (total dose) SBK-II Administered i.p. for 2 Days. Boron Distribution in Tissue Determined at 18 and 48 Hours After Final Injection Via Prompt-Gamma Analysis

Tissue	µg B/g tissue	
	18-hour clearance	48-hour clearance
	n = 5	n = 5
Tumor	16.1	19.0
Liver	57.1	42.4
Blood	15.1	11.4
Muscle	8.5	9.4
Brain	<1.0	3.7
Lung	26.5	21.5
Kidney	34.5	28.8
Spleen	32.0	37.5

significant biological efficacy in small animals.[3,8] This same compound in its dimeric form (BSSB) shows even higher ^{10}B levels in tumor and is being evaluated with regard to its possible superiority over the monomer.[4]

Porphyrins such as HPD demonstrate an avidity for tumor, and are being used clinically in photodynamic therapy.[5] Their structure permits a large boron-carrying capacity of up to 4 boron cages per molecule; if tumor uptake is maintained with the boronated analog, boronated porphyrins could become the molecule of choice for BNCT trials.

METHODS

We have recently begun studying the boron distribution provided by a newly synthesized, water-soluble, non-toxic, boronated natural porphyrin (SBK-II). Multiple intraperitoneal injections (6 injections, 0.5 ml each, 3 per day over a 2-day period) with a total boron concentration of 20-50 µgB/gbw were administered to female BALB/cBNL mice bearing a Harding-Passey melanoma subcutaneously in the thigh. Boron distribution was

Table 2. Effect of Prolonged Clearance on Tissue Boron Concentration. Boron Distribution in Tissue of 4 Individual Mice at 9,33 and 43 Days Following I.P. Administration of ≈50 μg ^{N}B/gbw

Tissue	μg B/g Tissue		
	9 days	33 days	43 days
Mouse No.	1	3	4
Tumor	31.7	13.2; 8.5	7.8
Liver	75.0	29.2;39.0	16.0
Muscle	22.5	5.5; 9.8	0
Blood	N.A.	23;4.9	0

determined at various time intervals following the last injection to allow an assessment of tumor uptake and clearance rate for blood and normal tissue. Concentrations of ^{10}boron in tumor and various organs were analyzed by the prompt-γ method.[6] Continuous intravenous infusion techniques were also used to deliver boron to tumor[11], using the KHJJ mammary tumor model in BALB/c mice.

RESULTS

Boron distribution data for 18 and 48 hr post administration are shown in Table 1. There is essentially no decrease in boron levels in tumor between the 18 and 48-hr clearance intervals. These data along with data shown in Table 2, for 9, 33 and 43 days post administration, indicate a long-term retention of boron in tumor. The high levels of boron in liver and blood suggest a possible mechanism, i.e., the redistribution of SBK-II into the circulation enabling the continuous perfusion of tumor.

Boron levels in tissue appear to be proportional to porphyrin dose (Table 3). With the same clearance interval of 18 hours, tissue uptake of the boronated porphyrin is ≈2.5x higher with a doubling of the concentration of the compound, from 25 μg B/g as represented in Column 2, to 50 μg B/g as shown in Column 1.

Continuous intravenous infusions via the tail vein offer great promise as a mode of compound administration. High

Table 3. Porphyrin Dose Vs. Tissue Boron Concentration. Boron Distribution in Tissue Determined 18 Hours After Last I.P. Injection at Two-Different Porphyrin Doses.

Tissue	Dose	
	50 $\mu g^{N}B$/gbw*	25 $\mu g^{N}B$/gbw
	n = 5	n = 5
Tumor	38.6	16.1
Blood	41.4	15.1
Brain	2.1	0

*Boron measurements by prompt γ analysis

levels of boron were found in tissue after a 4-day clearance (Table 4). SBK-II was administered at a boron concentration of ≈7.5 μg/gbw for three (3) days with an external infusion pump delivering ≈85 μl/hr. The compound was synthesized using enriched boron. The analysis of boron concentrations in the tail of the mouse can serve as a checkpoint to evaluate the success of the infusion or its failure due to possible infiltration of the vein. The significance of Table 4 lies in the fact that tumor uptake is close to the equilibrium distribution (administered dose) of 7.5 μg B/gbw. Thus tumor was a greater fraction of the administered dose than that obtained by multiple i.p. administration.

Figure 1 is a neutron capture radiograph (NCR) showing a BALB/c female mouse bearing a KHJJ murine mammary carcinoma on her thigh. Beneath the mouse are a series of whole blood standards with known concentrations of boron. It can be observed that both liver and tumor have boron concentrations somewhere between 30 and 90 μg ^{10}B/g as represented by the last two standards right to left, respectively. The brain, however, remains free of any trace of boron. The apparent heterogeneity of boron within the tumor may be the result of differing ongoing cellular metabolic processes within the tumor. Future studies using tritiated thymidine to define those areas of tumor proliferation as compared with quiescent regions in a double-labeling technique with NCR's should provide additional information on tumor uptake of this compound.[4]

Table 4. Intravenous Infusion Tissue Boron Concentration. 7.5 μg B/gbw* SBK-II Administered to BALB/c Mice Bearing KHJJ Mammary Tumor Over 3 Days. Boron Distribution Determined 4 Days Following Cessation of Infusion Via Prompt-γ Analysis. Data is Average of 3 Mice.

Tissue	μg B/g tissue
Tumor	5.97 ± 1.6
Muscle	4.17 ± 1.97
Liver	13.5 ± 0.54
Blood	1.2 ± 0.54
Kidneys	9.1 ± 2.6
Lungs	4.2 (pooled)
Spleens	10.6 ± 5.4
Brain	< Background (pooled)
Tail	15.3 ± 5

*Enriched boron

Boron distribution data shown above indicate that while the boronated porphyrin SBK-II accumulates in tumor in amounts adequate for BNCT, levels of boron in normal brain are consistently low, regardless of the mode of administration of the compound. The blood-brain barrier, therefore, prevents SBK-II from reaching normal brain cells: This characteristic is highly significant with respect to the possible utilization of boronated porphyrins for the treatment of brain tumors. Further, these data are consistent with those from other experiments showing robust uptake in 7 different tumor models, with little or no porphyrin uptake in normal brain.[9]

The lengthy duration of boron in tumor and liver may imply either an intracellular incorporation, a rebathing of tumor with compound from organ stores or, perhaps, both. Clearly, this phenomenon can prove advantageous for a fractionated regimen of BNCT as the possibility exists that a single administration would be adequate prior to multiple irradiations. Cell culture studies described elsewhere in this symposium give support to an intracellular distribution for boronated porphyrins, thus significantly enhancing the Potential for therapy.[10]

Problems associated with toxicity were not encountered in the studies described above. Nevertheless, toxic levels must be established. In view of the known sensitizing properties of porphyrin to light, animal experiments were carried out in reduced light intensities. Clearly, the sensitizing properties of these boronated porphyrins must be documented. These investigations in conjunction with optimization of dose and delivery systems, and therapy experiments to demonstrate biological effectiveness are under way.

In view of the high and prolonged uptake of boronated porphyrin in tumor, and exclusion from normal brain, as well as

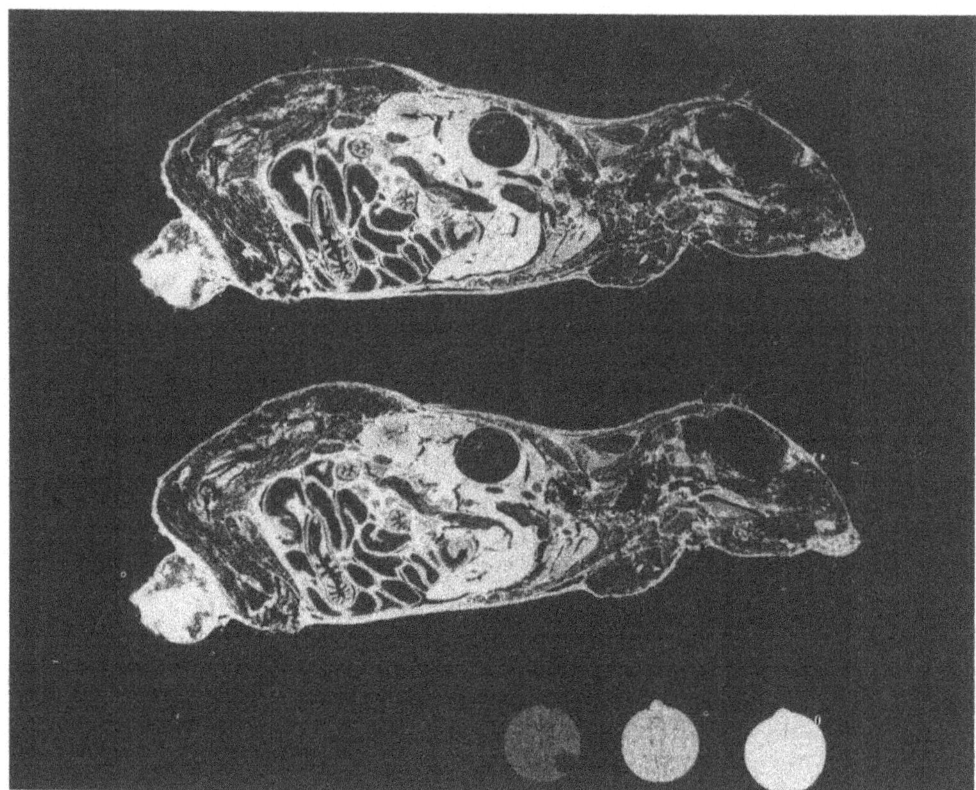

Fig. 1. SBK-II enriched boronated porphyrin administered i.p. to BALB/c female mouse bearing KHJJ mammary carcinoma at boron concentration of 35 μg. ^{10}B/ml (see text).

cell death indicating intracellular location,[10] it is anticipated that this compound will be a strong candidate for clinical application in BNCT of brain tumors.

REFERENCES

1. R. G. Fairchild and V. P. Bond, Current status of ^{10}B-neutron capture therapy: enhancement of tumor dose via beam filtration and dose rate, and the effects of these parameters on minimum boron content: a theoretical evaluation, Int. J. Radiat. Oncol. Biol. 11:831 (1985).
2. "Neutron Capture Therapy", H. Hatanaka, ed., Nishimura Co. Ltd., Japan (1985).
3. D. N. Slatkin, P. Micca, A. Forman, D. Gabel, L. Wielopolski, and R. G. Fairchild, Boron uptake in melanomas, cerebrum and blood from $Na_2B_{12}H_{11}SH$ and $Na_4B_{24}H_{22}S_2$ administered to mice, Biochem.Pharmacol. 35:1771 (1986).
4. D. N. Slatkin, D. D. Joel, R. G. Fairchild, P. L. Micca, M. M. Nawrocky, B. H. Laster, J. A. Coderre, G. C. Finkel, and W. H. Sweet, Distributions of sulfhydryl borane monomer and dimer in rodents and monomer in humans: boron neutron capture therapy of melanoma and glioma in boronated rodents. (This Symposium).
5. T. J. Dougherty, D. H. Boyle, K. R. Weishaupt, B. A. Henderson, W.R. Potter, D. A. Bellmier, and K. E. Wityk, Photoradiation therapy - clinical and drug advances, in: "Porphyrin Photosensitization", D. Kessel and T. J. Doughtery, ed., Plenum Publishing Corp., NY (1983).
6. R. G. Fairchild, D. Gabel, B. H. Laster, D. Greenberg, W. Kiszenick, and P. L. Micca, Microanalytical techniques for boron analysis using the $^{10}B(n,\alpha)^7Li$ reaction, Med. Phys. 13:50 (1986).
7. R. G. Fairchild, J. A. Kalef-Ezra, S. Fiarman, and F. Wheeler, Physics aspects of boron neutron capture therapy: Epithermal neutron beam optimization, Proc. ANS Topical Meeting, Jackson Hole, WY, Sept. 19-21, Vol. II, 423-433 (1988).
8. R. G. Fairchild, et al. Recent developments in neutron capture therapy, Proc. Workshop on Fast Neutron Therapy, Neuherberg and Munich, Oct,. 16-17, 1987 (in press).
9. R. G. Fairchild, D. Gabel, M. Hillman, and K. Watts, The distribution of exogenous porphyrins in vivo, and implications for neutron capture therapy. Proc. 1st Intl. Symp. on Neutron Capture Therapy, Oct. 12-13, 1983. BNL Report No. 51730, pp. 266-275, 1984.

10. B. H. Laster, S. B. Kahl, E. A. Poepnoe, C. Gordon, J. Kalef-Ezra, and R. G. Fairchild, Survival assays with a boronated porphyrin as measured with hamster V-79 cells in culture. (This Symposium).

11. B. H. Laster, E. A. Popenoe, and R. G. Fairchild, Uptake of IdUrd in murine melanoma following multiple-day intravenous infusions, Proc. Workshop on Photon Activation Therapy, BNL Report No. 51997, pp. 17-14, 1985.

SURVIVAL ASSAYS WITH A BORONATED PORPHYRIN AS MEASURED WITH HAMSTER V-79 CELLS IN CULTURE

B. H. Laster, S. B. Kahl* E. A. Popenoe,
C. Gordon, J. Kalef-Ezra, and R. G. Fairchild

Medical Department
Brookhaven National Laboratory
Upton, NY 11973

*School of Pharmacy
Department of Pharmaceutical Chemistry
University of California
513 Parnassus
San Francisco, CA 94143-0446

INTRODUCTION

On the basis of their weight, boron-carrying capacity and propensity for tumor, porphyrins would appear to be the ideal carrier-molecules for use in boron neutron therapy (BNCT). In the past, problems such as toxicity, solubility and/or lability of the boron tag precluded the use of porphyrins for BNCT. However, a newly-synthesized boronated porphyrin appears to have surmounted these problems and, in preliminary *in vitro* studies, SBK-II has demonstrated biological efficacy. Preliminary data will be presented here comparing SBK-II with the monomeric (BSH) and dimeric (BSSB) forms of the sulfhydryl boron hydride currently being considered for use in BNCT clinical trials in the United States.

METHODS

Standard cell culture techniques were used.[1,2] Cells were irradiated in suspension ($\approx 3 \times 10^5$ cells/cc) at the thermal neutron beam of the Brookhaven Medical Research Reactor, and the survival following irradiation was determined by colony assay. The thermal neutron fluence rate density at the center of the 1.5 cm^3 Eppendorf micro-test tube was $2.8x10^{11}$ n_{th} cm^{-2} min^{-1} with associated fast neutron and γ doses of ≈13 and 6.5 rad per minute, respectively. Control cells were irradiated without boron. Cells grown in the presence of the monomer (BSH) or dimer (BSSB) form of $Na_2B_{12}H_{11}SH$, or the boronated porphyrin SBK-II, were exposed to these compounds enriched in ^{10}B for 12 hrs at a concentration of ≈30 μg ^{10}B/g cell medium. Cells were washed (3 times) in PBS, trypsinized, harvested, and then irradiated in boron-free medium ("washed" experiments). In the "ambient" condition, cells were washed in PBS, trypsinized and harvested with all reagents containing 30 μg ^{10}B/g of the appropriate compound, followed by irradiation in the presence of 30 μg ^{10}B/g of the same compound. These steps were followed in order to evaluate the uptake and retention of the compounds in question. Further, it is anticipated that an estimation of the cellular distribution of these compounds can be obtained by comparing survival with that obtained from boric acid (H_3BO_3) where a uniform distribution could be assumed, at least with "ambient" experiments.

RESULTS

The data in Figures 1, 2 and 3 represent the survival (from reproductive death) of V-79 Chinese hamster cells given ≈30 μg ^{10}B/ml of SBK-II, $Na_2B_{12}H_{11}SH$ (BSH) and $Na_4B_{24}H_{22}S_2$ (BSSB), respectively. The top (control) curve in each graph represents the survival of irradiated boron-free cells. The remaining two curves in each graph are indicative of the two different conditions in which the cells were irradiated, ambient and washed.

The establishment of a dose enhancement factor at a particular survival level between boronated cells with compounds having unknown sensitization properties, and unboronated control cells in a mixed irradiation field, would be an inappropriate measurement for comparing biological efficacy. In this situation, the use of D_o (representing the dose required to reduce survival by a factor of 1/e on the linear portion of the curve) would be more suitable as it is less arbitrary and dose-dependent. Since the D_o is proportional to time, we have used T_o (minutes) in this preliminary evaluation of biological efficacy. These results are shown in Table 1, where T_o values were obtained from the slope of each experimental curve.

DISCUSSION

Each curve in Figs. 1-3 has been reproduced, so that the individual slopes represent the results of two or more experiments. A number of results are immediately apparent. For example, washing of the cells appears to remove most of the monomer (BSH) (Figure 2); the dimer (BSSB) (Figure 3) is not washed out of the cells to the same extent. This suggests a longer retention time or stronger binding for the dimer, as is also evident in in vivo studies.[3] However, in the ambient condition, there is little difference between the two forms of the sulfhydryl boron hydride.

The response of the washed boronated porphyrin is ~2-3 times greater than washed dimer and monomer, respectively; the same holds true for the ambient condition as well, to a somewhat greater extent (Table 1).

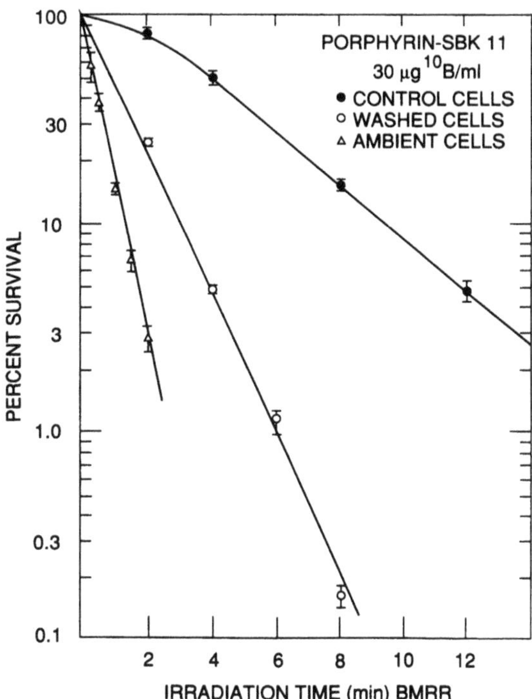

Fig. 1. V-79 Chinese hamster cells given 30 $\mu g^{10}B$ SBK-II for 12 hours prior to neutron irradiation at the BMRR and V-79 controls (·) with no drug exposure.

A direct comparison of T_0's includes the effects of "background" irradiation delivered equally to both boronated and control cells, so that the effect from boron alone is diluted. Measurements are under way with similar concentrations of boron from boric acid, so that by comparing the (inverse of) D_0's, effects of background can be subtracted (assuming no additional sensitization from boric acid).[2] A preliminary evaluation indicates that the distribution of SBK-II is intracellular and that effects are ≈4x greater than that obtained with equal amounts of administered BSH or BSSB.

CONCLUSION

While these results are still preliminary, they clearly suggest an intracellular localization of SBK-II; further, SBK-II demonstrates a significantly greater response than that provided by BSH or BSSB. This could be the result of

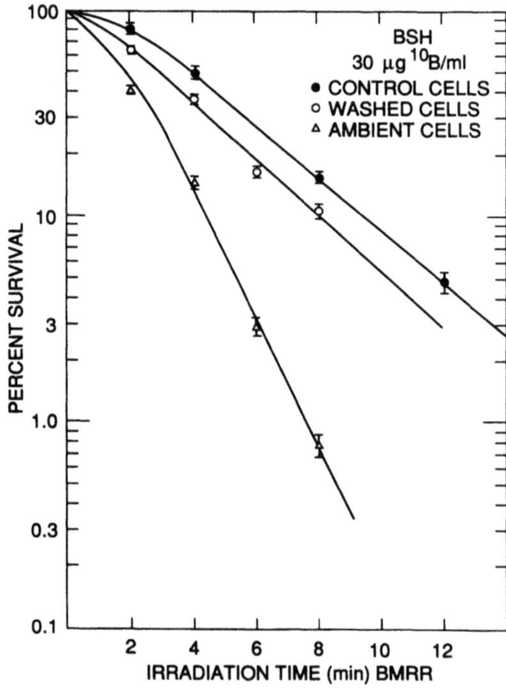

Fig. 2. V-79 Chinese hamster cells given 30 µg ^{10}B/g BSH for 12 hours prior to neutron irradiation at the BMRR, and V-79 controls (·) with no drug exposure.

differences in intracellular site-specificity, or intracellular loading of boron. Data presented elsewhere in these proceedings (Distribution of boronated porphyrin in murine tumors, by Kahl et al.) show uptake of therapeutic levels of boron in tumors of mice. The results of both the in vitro and in vivo studies with the boronated porphyrin SBK-II, strongly suggest that this compound offers promise for clinical trials in BNCT.

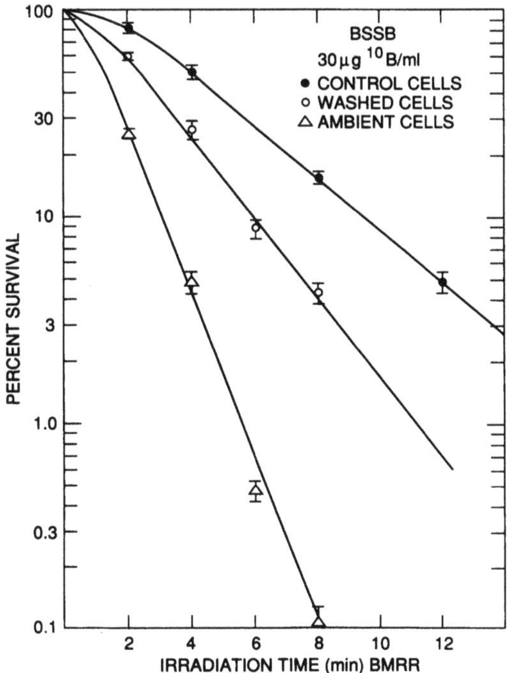

Fig. 3. V-79 Chinese hamster cells given 30 μg $^{10}B/g$ BSSB for 12 hours prior to neutron irradiation at the BMRR, and V-79 controls (·) with no drug exposure.

Table 1. Response of V-79 Cells to Thermal Neutron Irradiation Following Growth for 12 h (1 Cell Cycle Time) in the Presence of 30 μg ^{10}B/g from Various Compounds

	T_o(min)	
Compound	Washed	Ambient
BSH	3.3	1.4
BSSB	2.2	1.2
SBK-II	1.2	0.5

REFERENCES

1. R. G. Fairchild, B. H. Laster, S. L. Commerford, P. S. Furcinitti, B. Sylvester, D. Gabel, E. Popenoe, and S. Foster, Proc. of Workshop on Photon Activation Therapy,Upton, April, 1985, Brookhaven National Lab. Report No. 51997, pp. 1-16 (1986).

2. R. G. Fairchild, H. G. Borner, and B. Larsson, The relative biological effectiveness in V79 Chinese hamster cells of the neutron capture reactions in boron and nitrogen, Radiat. Res. 98:307-316 (1984).

3. D. N. Slatkin, P. Micca, A. Forman, D. Gabel, L. Wielopolski, and R. G. Fairchild, Boron uptake in melanomas, cerebrum, and blood from $Na_2B_{12}H_{11}SH$ and $Na_2B_{24}H_{22}S_2$ administered to mice. Biochem. Pharmacol. 35:1771 (1986).

NEUTRON CAPTURE THERAPY FOR MELANOMA

Jeffrey A. Coderre, John D. Glass, Peggy Micca
and Ralph G. Fairchild

Medical Department
Brookhaven National Laboratory
Upton, N.Y. 11973

INTRODUCTION

The dose-limiting factor in cancer radiation therapy is the tolerance level of normal tissues within the radiation field. In boron neutron capture therapy (BNCT), thermal neutrons interact with boron via the $^{10}B(n,\alpha)^{7}Li$ reaction (Taylor, 1935) to produce short-range (~ 5-9 μm), high-linear energy transfer radiations which have a large relative biological effectiveness (RBE) (Gabel, 1984; Fukuda, 1987). In theory, selective localization of ^{10}B within the tumor should allow most of the dose to be restricted to the tumor (Locher, 1936). The failure of the initial clinical trials of BNCT, carried out between 1953 and 1961 at Brookhaven National Laboratory and the Massachusetts General Hospital (Farr, 1954; Goodwin, 1955; Asbury, 1972) was attributed to two major factors: (i) the use of boron-containing compounds which showed no selective accumulation in tumor and (ii) the rapid attenuation in tissue of the incident thermal neutron beam. The high neutron doses employed resulted in excessive surface tissue exposure; viable tumor was found at depth following the neutron irradiations. The substantial levels of boron in blood during irradiation contributed to the damage to normal brain vasculature (tumor/blood ratio <1).

The development of boron-containing compounds which localize selectively in tumor may require a tumor-by-tumor type of approach that exploits any metabolic pathways unique to the particular type of tumor. Melanin-producing melanomas actively transport and metabolize aromatic amino acids for use as precursors in the synthesis of the pigment melanin. It has been shown that the boron-containing amino acid analog p-borono-phenylalanine (BPA) is selectively accumulated in melanoma tissue, producing boron concentrations in tumor that are within the range estimated to be necessary for successful BNCT (Mishima, 1983; Coderre, 1987). We report here the results of therapy experiments carried out at the Brookhaven Medical Research Reactor (BMRR).

METHODS

Murine Melanoma

Adult female BALB/c mice (~ 15-20 g) in which the Harding-Passey melanoma had been implanted subcutaneously on either the abdomen or the thigh were used. This tumor has been maintained in our laboratory by serial transplantation for over 10 years and is reproducible with respect to melanin content and uptake of melanin affinic agents. Melanin content (0.68% melanin by weight) is analogous to that found in human melanotic melanoma (0.1 to 0.8%; average value, 0.35%) (Watts, 1981). The Harding-Passey melanoma does not metastasize but grows at the original subcutaneous implantation site with a volume doubling time of about 3 days. The subcutaneous location of this heavily pigmented tumor facilitates volume measurements. For therapy experiments, tumors between 30 and 100 mg in size were chosen; this size corresponds to 14-18 days of growth. Tumors which have grown to this size do not undergo spontaneous remission. Mice with untreated tumors or mice with tumors which eventually resumed growth following the irradiation procedures were sacrificed when the tumors became unnecessarily large (approximately 2-3 cm^3). Mice whose tumors did not regrow after therapy were monitored until they became incapacitated by old age near the end of a normal lifespan (~ 18 months).

BMRR Dosimetry

The BMRR is a 5-MW modified, pool-type nuclear reactor designed for biomedical research (Godel, 1960). The BMRR has been the site of numerous BNCT experiments; the irradiations described here were done at the BMRR patient port. Fast neutron and gamma doses were measured directly using standard tissue equivalent and graphite-CO_2 chambers as well as TLD-700 dosimeters (Robertson, 1972; Fairchild, 1966). Contributions from the $^{14}N(n,p)^{14}C$ and $^{10}B(n,\alpha)^7Li$ reactions were calculated from gold foil measurements of thermal neutron flux density and corrected for resonance response by the cadmium difference technique (Beckurts, 1964).

Irradiation Procedures

During irradiations, mice were anesthetized with sodium pentabarbital (65 μg/g body weight via i.p. injection). To evaluate the radiosensitivity of the Harding-Passey melanoma to conventional x rays, mice bearing thigh tumors were irradiated with a Phillips RT-100 superficial x-ray machine using 100 kVp x rays (1.7 mm Al added filtration) at a dose rate of 1000 rad per min. The tumor-bearing region of the thigh was exposed directly, the body and foot were shielded with lead.

For neutron irradiations, the BMRR patient port thermal beam (25 x 25 cm) was restricted to 1.5-cm diameter using an insert of 1:1 ^{6}LiF mixed with epoxy resin molded to collimate the beam at the port center. Additional body shielding was provided by sheets of lithium metal in oil-filled plastic bags. The tumor-bearing leg was extended over the 1.5-cm beam port during irradiation. Neutron exposures ranged from 2.5 to 6.7 x 10^{12} n/cm^2.

Therapeutic Endpoint

The endpoint used to assess the effectiveness of the tumor irradiations was a determination of tumor growth delay or tumor control. Tumor size was measured daily following irradiation. Tumor volumes were estimated by the formula $v = 0.5\ ab^2$, where a and b are the longest and shortest diameters, respectively (Rofstad, 1985). Tumor volumes were normalized to the volume on the day of irradiation, then averaged for each group. Irradiated tumors exhibited a longer volume doubling time and, at higher doses, a lag period of no growth followed by a resumption of growth at a slower rate than unirradiated controls. Tumors showing apparent growth control, following irradiation, were monitored for subsequent regrowth during the residual lifespan of the mouse. Tumor growth control was considered complete only if the mouse lived out its residual lifespan (over 1 year) with no evidence of tumor regrowth.

RESULTS AND DISCUSSION

Distribution Studies

We have recently described the results of our tumor uptake and distribution studies (Coderre, 1987). Using the Harding-Passey melanoma carrying s.c. in BALB/c mice, we have demonstrated that BPA is taken up by melanoma tissue to a much greater extent than by normal tissues. Following a single i.p. injection or a series of injections given over 1 h, the accumulation of boron in melanoma was found to be transient, reaching a maximum approximately 6 h post-injection. The concentrations of boron achieved in tumor ranged from 9-33 μg/g and are within the range estimated to be necessary for successful application of the nuclear reaction $^{10}B(n,\alpha)^{7}Li$ for neutron capture therapy. Boron concentrations in tumor and tissues were determined using either a prompt-gamma spectroscopic technique or by quantitative neutron capture radiography using whole-body sections. Distribution studies with the resolved stereoisomers of BPA indicated that the L isomer is preferentially accumulated in the melanoma compared to the D isomer (see Figure 1). The L isomer of BPA was shown to be targeted to actively dividing tumor cells by simultaneously comparing the boron and [^{3}H]thymidine ([^{3}H]Thd) distribution in tumor (see Figure 2).

Toxicity of BPA

BPA is not toxic. We have been unable to deliver a lethal dose of BPA to mice by normal means. The solubility of BPA at pH values which are tolerated physiologically is about 6 mg/ml. Volume limits the amount that can be administered. At this concentration, i.v. injections are limited to roughly 3 mg (150 mg/kg body weight). Using i.p. injections, we have been able to administer 6 mg (1-ml i.p. injection) or up to 12 mg (four 0.5-ml i.p. injections over the course of 1 h). Even at the highest i.p. dose of 12 mg (600 mg/kg), no toxic effects were observed.

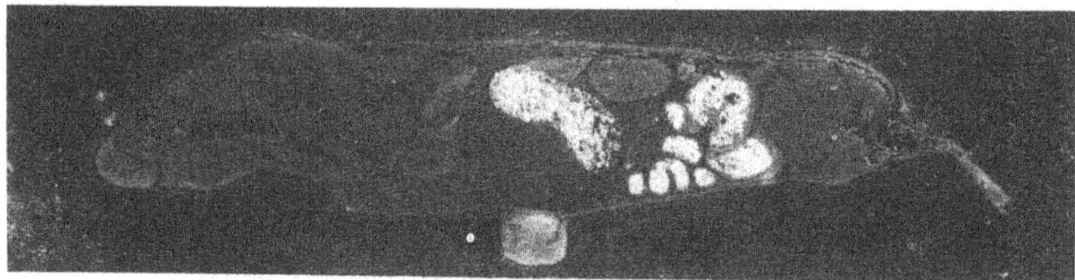

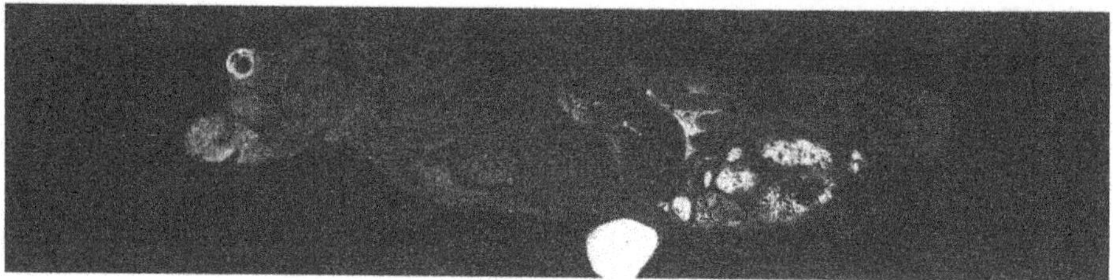

Fig. 1. Distribution of L-BPA vs. D-BPA. Tumor-bearing mice given injections of D-BPA or L-BPA, sacrificed 6 h post-injection; whole-body sections prepared; neutron capture radiograms shown. Top, D-BPA containing natural abundance boron; neutron fluence - 6.0 x 10^{12} n/cm^2. Bottom, ^{10}B-L-BPA; neutron fluence - 1.2 x 10^{12} n/cm^2. Note preferential accumulation of L-BPA in melanoma.

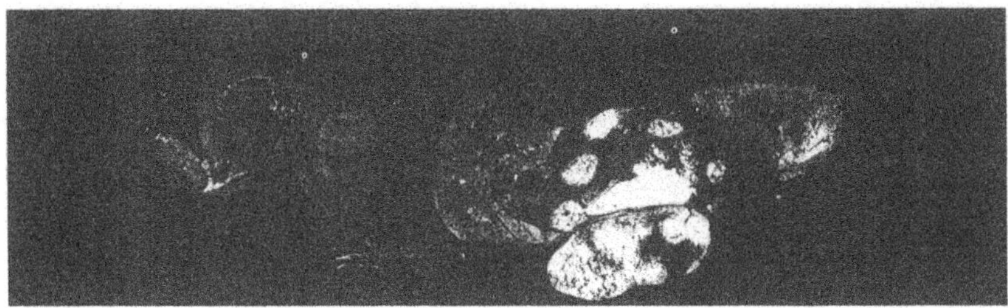

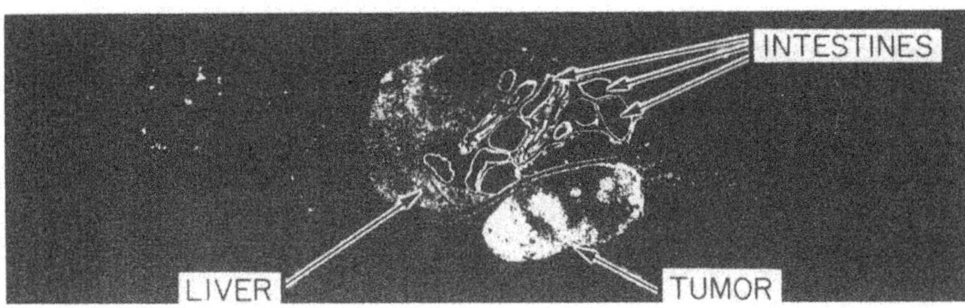

Fig. 2. Double labeling with boron and [^{3}H]Thd. Tumor-bearing mouse given injections of both ^{10}B-L-BPA and [^{3}H]Thd; whole-body sections prepared. Top, neutron capture radiogram prepared from whole-body section. Neutron fluence used to generate this image - 2.4 x 10^{12} n/cm^{2}. Bottom, [^{3}H]Thd autoradiogram prepared from same whole-body section used for neutron capture radiogram. Note highest concentrations of boron in tumor correspond closely with areas of rapid cell division identified by [^{3}H]Thd incorporation.

Oral Dose

Since our distribution data indicated that bolus injections were most effective, we have recently begun using oral administration of BPA as a slurry in water to deliver as much as possible in a single dose. The time course for tumor uptake was similar to i.p. injections; at 6 h post- (oral) injection, the tumor values were maximal. The amount of BPA that can be delivered orally is now increased to a maximum of 40 mg (2000 mg/kg). Even at this high oral dose of 40 mg, BPA was not toxic. This is in contradiction to previously published reports for the LD_{50} of BPA of 1600 mg/kg (Soloway, 1961) and 840 mg/kg (Mishima, 1980) administered i.p. These values were obtained using aqueous solutions of BPA at a pH of 10 and 3, respectively, in order to increase the solubility. The observed toxicities were probably due to the extremes of pH utilized.

Table 1. Boron content of tissues (μg/g) following an oral dose of BPA

No. of Mice	Blood	Tumor	Muscle	T/B	T/M
n = 2	3.1 ± 0.8	23.8 ± 3.2	5.1 ± 0.7	7.7	4.7
n = 5	7.6 ± 2.3	41.1 ± 2.1	8.7 ± 2.1	5.4	4.7

Using a standard dose of 15 mg ^{10}B-L-BPA in 0.5 ml water, sacrifice at 6 h, we have been able to increase the boron concentration in the tumor considerably. Table 1 summarizes these results.

Therapy Experiments

Table 2 summarizes the dosimetry calculations for the mouse leg irradiations at the BMRR. The total dose to the tumor during BNCT depends on the ^{10}B concentrations in the tumor. The contribution to the dose from the $^{10}B(n,\alpha)^{7}Li$ reaction was calculated by assuming 15 μg ^{10}B/g tumor; actual boron concentrations in tumor varied from 15-30 μg/g (Coderre, 1987). Using the dose estimates given in Table 2, exposure times at the BMRR were chosen to give total doses in the therapeutic range. The BMRR operating power was 1 megawatt (MW); exposure times were 3, 6, and 8 minutes (the corresponding fluences were 2.0, 5.0, and 6.7 x 10^{12} n/cm^2, respectively). The doses to normal tissue within the neutron field at these exposure times were 234, 468, and 624 (rad x RBE), respectively. (Absorbed dose in a mixed radiation field is expressed as effective dose (rad x RBE), due to the different relative biological effectiveness (RBE) of the component radiations). The corresponding doses to tumor, assuming a ^{10}B concentration of 15 μg/g, are 1020, 2040, and 2720 (rad x RBE). The whole-body doses were 144, 288 and 384 (rad x RBE).

Preliminary BNCT experiments using BPA and the conditions outlined above indicated that irradiation for 3 MW-minutes produced only transient growth delays, whereas, 6 and 8 MW-minute exposures resulted in significant tumor growth delays (>4 weeks), as compared to irradiated controls, while still holding the whole-body dose within tolerable limits.

Figures 3 and 4 show the results of BNCT experiments carried out at the BMRR with exposure times of 6 and 8 MW-minutes, respec-

Table 2. Dosimetry for mouse irradiations at the BMRR. Irradiations and dosimetry measurements using a ^{6}LiF/epoxy (1:1) collimator with a 1.5-cm cone aperture; reactor power, 1 MW.

Component	Dose Rate (rad/min)	RBE	Effective Dose Rate (radxRBE/min)
Gamma	8	1	8
Fast neutrons	20	2	40
Thermal neutrons	15	2	30
Total	43		78
$^{10}B(n,\alpha)^{7}Li$ (assuming 15 µg ^{10}B/g)	105	2.5	262
Total + ^{10}B	148		340

Flux density, bare port face = 1.93×10^{10} n/cm^2.sec
Flux density, center of aperture = 1.15×10^{10} n/cm^2.sec
Flux density w/mouse leg (i.e., 20% backscatter) = 1.38×10^{10} n/cm^2.sec
Fluence (Φ) (1 minute) = 8.4×10^{11} n/cm^2
$^{14}N(n,p)^{14}C$ dose* (rad) = $(1.84 \times 10^{-11})(\Phi)$ = 15 rad/min
$^{10}B(n,\alpha)^{7}Li$ dose* (assuming 15 µg ^{10}B/g tissue) = $(1.26 \times 10^{-10})(\Phi)$ = 105 rad/min

*Fairchild, 1966

tively. Tumor volumes were normalized to the day of irradiation; each line is the average of 6 mice. Irradiation in the absence of ^{10}B delivers a dose sufficient to delay tumor growth (5 and 6 weeks for 6 and 8 MW-minutes, respectively), but all "neutrons only" controls eventually regrew. In the 6 MW-minute experiment shown in Figure 3, neutron irradiation in the presence of BPA produced growth delays of from 5 to 7 weeks, yet all of these tumors also eventually regrew. At 8 MW-minutes (Figure 4), however, of the 6 BPA-containing tumors, 3 resumed growth after delays of from 7 to 10 weeks, but the remaining 3 showed complete tumor growth control, surviving for over 1 year with no sign of tumor regrowth. Figure 5 shows the individual growth data for the 6 tumors in the "neutrons + BPA" group in Figure 4.

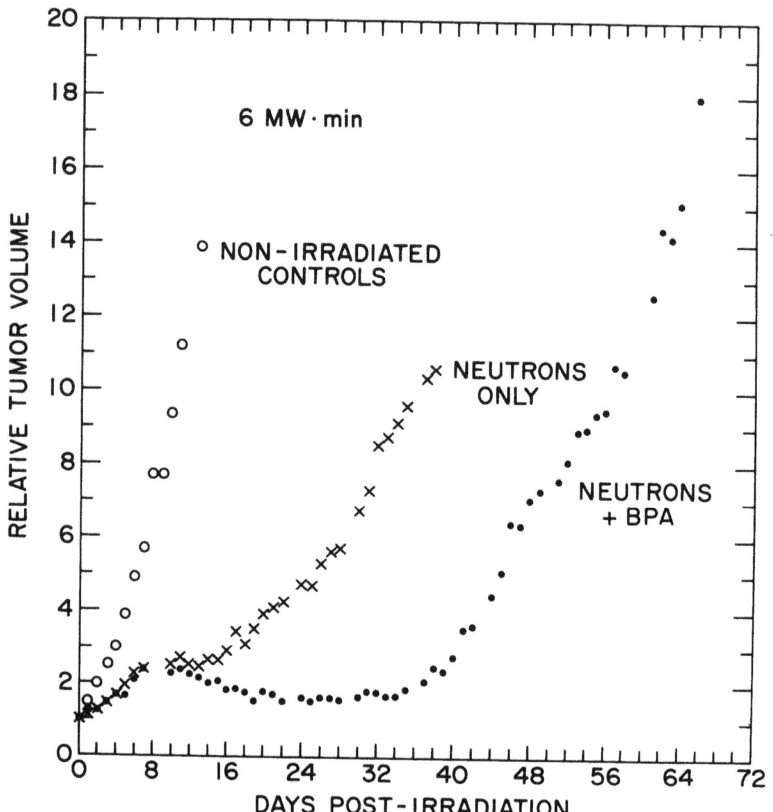

Fig. 3. BNCT at BMRR; neutron fluence - 5.0×10^{12} n/cm^{-2}. BALB/c mice bearing Harding-Passey melanoma subcutaneously on thigh each received 12 mg BPA (four 0.5-ml injections/1 h); irradiated 6 h after final injection. Each line = average 6 mice. Tumor volumes normalized to day of irradiation. Tumor dose, neutrons only = 468 (rad x RBE). Tumor dose, neutrons + BPA = 2040 (rad x RBE). Whole-body dose = 288 (rad x RBE).

The experiments described here show that the response of the Harding-Passey melanoma to BNCT after a fixed course of BPA injections was directly related to the neutron fluence; increasing the exposure time resulted in longer tumor growth delays. At the highest neutron fluence utilized, 6.7×10^{12} n/cm^2 (8 MW-minutes), 3 of 6 treated tumors regressed completely and did not regrow during the remainder of the mouse's lifespan. The calculated absorbed dose for the tumor at this exposure level was 2720 (rad x

Table 3. BNCT using BPA and the Harding-Passey Melanoma in BALB/c Mice

No. of mice	Dose	Neutron Exposure[a]	Positive response[b]
6[c]	12 mg i.p.	6 MW-min	0/6
6[d]	12 mg i.p.	8 MW-min	3/6
8	15 mg oral	8 MW-min	7/8
6	15 mg oral	6 MW-min	5/6

[a]One megawatt minute (MW-min) corresponds to a neutron fluence of 8.4×10^{11} n/cm^2

[b]To be counted as a positive response, the tumors must undergo complete and permanent regression.

[c]Results illustrated in Figure 3.

[d]Results illustrated in Figures 4 and 5.

RBE). This apparently curative dose is in concordance with the observed sensitivity of the Harding-Passey melanoma to 100 kVp x rays. The x-ray dose required to cure 50% of treated tumors was about 3000 rad. The absorbed dose to the tumor in control mice that received no BPA was 624 (rad x RBE). The effect of the BPA treatment was, therefore, to increase the effective radiation dose to the tumor by about 4.4 relative to controls which received no BPA prior to irradiation. The therapeutic gain or ratio of tumor dose to normal tissue dose within the treatment volume was ~ 3.3, assuming a tumor/normal tissue boron distribution of 10 to 1. It should be noted that this radiation enhancement was achieved unevenly over the tumor with the highest effective radiation doses concentrated in the most actively growing areas of the tumor. The growth rates of unirradiated tumors were unaffected by administration of BPA.

Additional Therapy Experiments

Using the oral delivery method for BPA, higher boron concentrations can be achieved in the tumor (25-45 μg $^{10}B/g$). Therapy experiments are summarized in Table 3 which illustrate the greater effectiveness of BNCT following the oral doses of BPA.

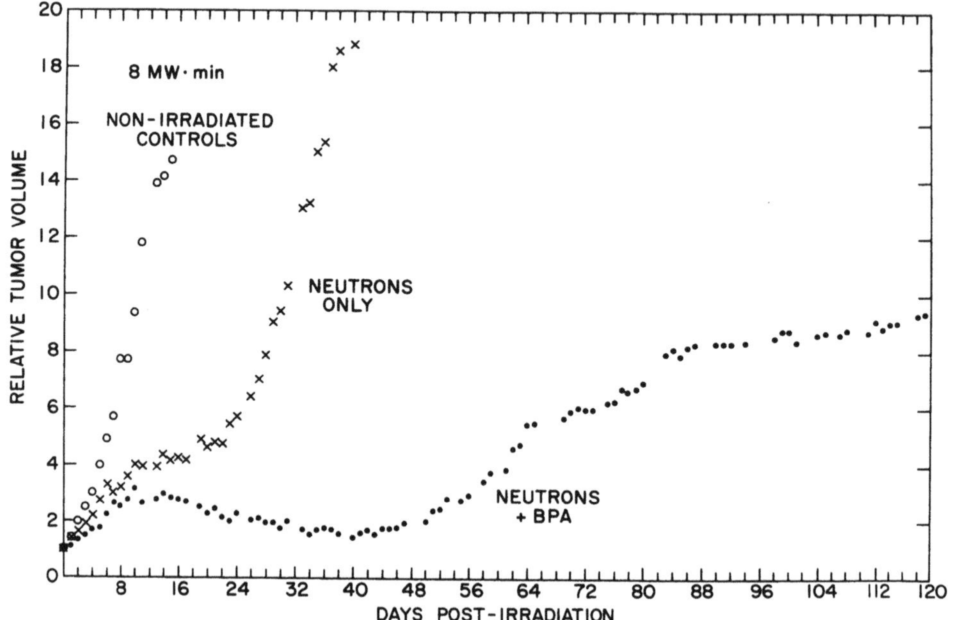

Fig. 4. BNCT at BMRR; neutron fluence - 6.7 x 10^{12} n/cm^{-2}. Experimental details as in Fig. 3, except: tumor dose, neutrons only = 624 (rad x (RBE); tumor dose, neutrons + BPA = 2720 (rad x RBE). Whole-body dose = 384 (rad x RBE).

Dose Fractionation in BNCT

Conventional radiation therapy is given in multiple small doses in order that normal tissues within the treatment volume can repair sublethal damage. This assumes that normal tissues have a greater capacity for repair of such damage than malignant tissues.

Our demonstration of the ability to produce complete and permanent tumor regression of the murine melanoma implanted subcutaneously on the thigh with a single BPA/BNCT treatment enables us to utilize this model for testing the effects of dose fractionation on the effectiveness of BNCT. To date, one experiment has been carried out. All mice received 15 mg of ^{10}B-L-BPA orally 6 h prior to irradiation. Group 1 received BPA followed by 6 MW-min of neutron irradiation. Group 2 received BPA and 3 MW-min, then 2 days later, another full dose of BPA and another 3 MW-min. The results:

Group 1 (6 MW-min)	0/6	complete regression
Group 2 (3 + 3 MW-min)	4/6	complete regression

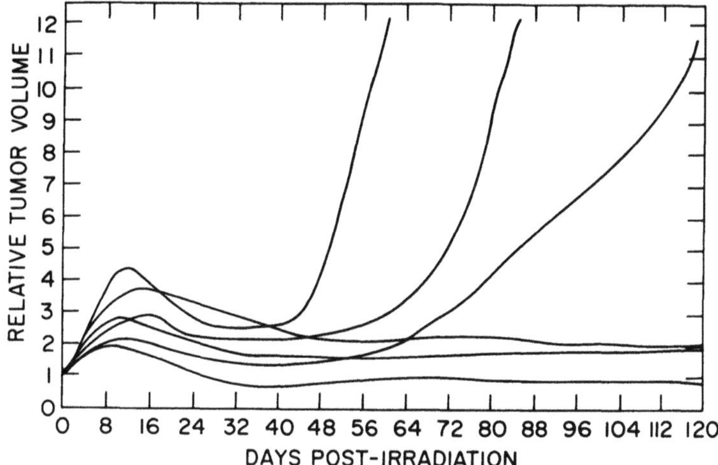

Fig. 5. Individual tumor growth curves from neutrons + BPA group shown in Fig. 4. Of 6 tumors treated, 3 eventually grew, 3 were controlled. Average of 6 lines shown produced neutrons + BPA line in Fig. 4.

These results are preliminary, but the greater effectiveness of the fractionated therapy may be due to the killing of cells in the second irradiation that were somehow missed during the first irradiation. This could be due to a non-uniform boron distribution within the tumor or perhaps to the presence of a latent cell pool.

Boron-containing compounds that show affinity for a wide variety of tumors (such as boronated porphyrins or antibodies) would be ideal for BNCT, but efforts to develop such compounds have not yet been able to demonstrate biological efficacy. It may be that BNCT of a particular type of tumor will require the identification and development of boron-containing compounds with specific affinity for that tumor; such affinity may also provide for favorable distribution within the tumor. BPA is demonstrably the first example of such a compound. As an analog of a melanin precursor, BPA selectively delivers boron to murine melanoma, especially to rapidly growing areas of the tumor, making it possible to obtain ratios of boron in tumor to that in normal tissues in the range of 5 to 15. To our knowledge, such selective accumulation in tumor of a systemically applied boronated compound has not been reported. NCT with the sulfhydryl borane BSH is based primarily on its exclusion from normal brain by the blood-brain barrier, rather than by selective binding. However, high blood boron concentrations from BSH present obvious problems, as it is believed that damage to normal tissue blood vessels is a limiting factor in radiotherapy of brain tumors (Sweet, 1986; Moustafa, 1980).

Investigators in Japan have described the enhanced killing effect of thermal neutrons on melanoma cells *in vitro* that had been preincubated with BPA (Ichihashi, 1982; Itsumi, 1986).

Mishima (1983) has described the use of BPA to effect the apparent cure of a spontaneously occuring melanoma in a Duroc pig and to suppress the growth of the Green melanoma in hamsters, following a single thermal neutron treatment. In the pig experiment, the BPA was administered via two peri-lesional injections at 19 h and 20 min before the irradiation. Mishima has recently carried out the first BNCT treatment of human melanoma using BPA (described at this Workshop), initial results are encouraging.

We have shown that BPA has little or no affinity for either a mammary adenocarcinoma (Coderre, 1987) or the KHJJ murine mammary tumor carried in BALB/c mice (unpublished data). Interestingly, preliminary results indicate that BPA does accumulate significantly in a poorly pigmented B-16 melanoma carried in C57Bl mice (unpublished data). This observation implies that BPA uptake is dependent upon amino acid transport and not upon melanin synthesis. Human melanoma metastases vary significantly in degree of pigmentation (Watts, 1981). If BPA can accumulate in both pigmented and non-pigmented metastatic sites, the chances for successful BNCT will be greatly enhanced.

REFERENCES

Asbury, A. K., Ojemann, R. G., Nielsen, S. L., and Sweet, W. H., 1972, Neuropathologic study of fourteen cases of malignant brain tumor treated by boron-10 slow neutron capture radiation, *J. Neuropathol. Exp. Neurol.*, 31:278.

Beckurts, K. H., and Wirtz, K., 1964, Simultaneous thermal and epithermal foil activation, *in*: "Neutron Physics," Springer-Verlag, New York.

Coderre, J. A., Glass, J. D., Fairchild, R. G., Roy, U., Cohen, S., and Fand, I., 1987, Selective targeting of boronophenylalanine to melanoma for neutron capture therapy, *Cancer Research*, 47:6377.

Fairchild, R. G., and Goodman, L. J., 1966, Development and dosimetry of an "epithermal" neutron beam for possible use in neutron capture therapy. II. Absorbed dose measurements in a phantom man, *Phys. Med. Biol.*, 11:15.

Farr, L. E., Sweet, W. H., Robertson, J. S., Foster, C. G., Locksley, H. B., Sutherland, D. L., Mendelson, M. L., and Stickley, E. E., 1954, Neutron capture therapy with boron in the treatment of glioblastoma multiforme, Am. J. Roentgenol., 71: 279.

Fukuda, H., Kobayashi, T., Matsuzawa, T., Kanda, K., Ichihashi, M., and Mishima, Y., 1987, RBE of a thermal neutron beam and the $^{10}B(n,\alpha)^{7}Li$ reaction on cultured B-16 melanoma cells, Int. J. Radiat. Biol., 51:167.

Gabel, D., Fairchild, R. G., Borner, H. G., and Larsson, B., 1984, The relative biological effectiveness in V79 Chinese hamster cells of the neutron capture reaction in boron and nitrogen, Radiat. Research, 98:307.

Godel, J. B., 1960, Description of facilities and mechanical components, Medical Research Reactor (MRR), Brookhaven National Laboratory Report No. BNL-600, Upton, NY.

Goodwin, J. T., Farr, L. E., Sweet, W. H., and Robertson, J. S., 1955, Pathological study of eight patients with glioblastoma multiforme treated by neutron capture therapy using boron-10, Cancer, 8:601.

Ichihashi, M., Nakanishi, T., and Mishima, Y., 1982, Specific killing effect of $^{10}B_1$-paraboronophenylalanine in thermal neutron capture therapy of malignant melanoma: in vitro radiobiological evaluation, J. Invest. Dermatol., 78:215.

Itsumi, H., Ichihashi, M., Funasaka, Y., Mishima, Y., Ikushima, T., Kobayashi, T., and Kanda, K., 1986, Potentially lethal damage repair of B-16 melanoma cells pretreated with $^{10}B_1$-paraboronophenylalanine after exposure to thermal neutron radiation, in: "Neutron Capture Therapy," H. Hatanaka, ed., Nishimura Co., Ltd., Niigata.

Locher, G. L., 1936, Biological effects of therapeutic possibilities of neutrons, Am. J. Roentg. Radium Ther., 36:1.

Mishima, Y., 1980, Japanese Patent Request, Public Disclosure No. 122720-1980.

Mishima, Y., Ichihashi, M., Nakanishi, T., Tsiyi, M., Ueda, M., Nakagawa, T., and Suzuki, T., 1983, Cure of malignant melanoma by single thermal neutron capture treatment using melanoma-seeking compounds, Proc. 1st Int. Symp. on Neutron Capture Therapy, Brookhaven National Laboratory Report No. 51730.

Moustafa, H. F., and Hopewell, J. W., 1980, Late functional changes in the vasculature of the rat brain after local x-irradiation, Br. J. Radiol., 53:21.

Robertson, J. S., Fairchild, R. G., and Atkins, H. L., 1972, Dosimetry of californium-252, Radiol., 104:393.

Rofstad, E. K., and Brustad, T., 1985, Tumor growth delay following single-dose irradiation of human melanoma xenografts. Correlations with tumor growth parameters, vascular structure, and cellular radiosensitivity, Br. J. Cancer, 51:201.

Soloway, A. H., Wright, R. L., and Messer, J. R., 1961, Evaluation of boron compounds for use in neutron capture therapy of brain tumors. I. Animal investigations, J. Pharmacol. Exp. Ther., 134:117.

Sweet, W. H., 1986, Medical aspects of boron slow neutron capture therapy, Brookhaven National Laboratory, Report No. 51994.

Taylor, H. J., and Goldhaber, M., 1935, Detection of nuclear disintegration in a photographic emulsion, Nature, London, 135:341.

Watts, K. P., Fairchild, R. G., Slatkin, D., Greenberg, D., Packer, S., Atkins, H. L., and Hannon, S. J., 1981, Melanin content of hamster tissues, human tissues and various melanomas, Cancer Research, 41:467.

TUMOR-SEEKING COMPOUNDS FOR BORON NEUTRON CAPTURE THERAPY: SYNTHESIS AND BIODISTRIBUTION

Detlef Gabel

Department of Chemistry
University of Bremen
Bremen, F.R.G.

INTRODUCTION

A successful application of boron neutron capture therapy towards the treatment of human malignancies relies on two prime conditions: the delivery of a sufficient amount of neutrons to the target volume, and the delivery of a sufficient amount of boron to the target cells.

We recently showed that the very short range of the particles generated by the neutron capture reaction in boron renders useless the parameters of dose as they are normally used in radiotherapy (Gabel et al., 1987a). Rather, the energy deposited in a cell nucleus by a given average concentration of boron can vary by a factor of 10 or more, depending on where in relation to the cell nucleus the boron is located. Also, cells not accumulating boron will receive a much smaller dose to the nucleus than will cells that contain boron during the irradiation.

It must therefore be the aim of the chemist to synthesize tumor-localizing compounds that are able to target all tumor cells, and preferentially such compounds that are internalized by the cells. For a realistic chance of a successful therapy, it might be necessary to administer several compounds that accumulate through independent routes, and thus are able to reach all cells of the tumor.

To be able to predict the outcome of a clinical therapy trial with a given boron concentration, it will be necessary to know the location of boron on an intracellular scale. A few methods are described in the literature that would allow such determination, the most notable being that of Kirsch and Brownell (1984).

It is clear, however, that the determination of boron in the tissue by gross analysis, either through prompt-gamma spectroscopy (Fairchild et al., 1984), chemical methods (Kaczmarczyk et al., 1971), or Inductively Coupled Plasma Atomic Absorption Spectroscopy (ICP) (Demers and Allemand, 1981) will give information about boron concentrations that cannot be related to therapeutic success or failure. Especially, these methods require either large samples of a few hundred milligrams to yield reliable data, or, in the case of ICP, whose sensitivity is superior to that of the two other methods, handling the sample is tedious and difficult.

1.IRRADIATE

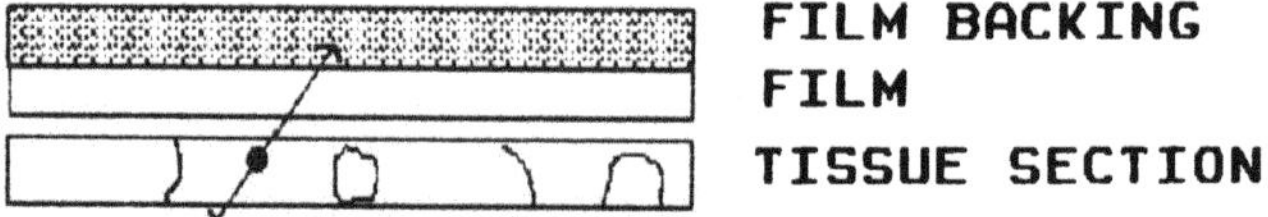

2.ETCH

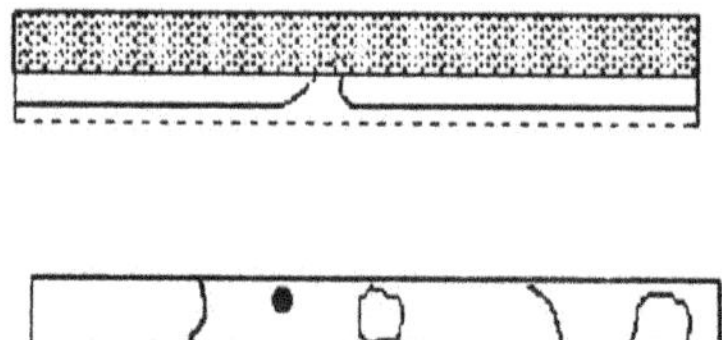

Fig. 1. Principle of QNCR. A cellulose nitrate film (type 115 from Kodak-Pathé) is irradiated in close contact with a section of the material in question. The film is subsequently etched, and the holes are counted opto-electronically.

QUANTITATIVE NEUTRON CAPTURE RADIOGRAPHY

We developed a method that allows for the analysis of boron in tissue sections. This method, Quantitative Neutron Capture Radiography (QNCR), utilizes the selective sensitivity of cellulose nitrate films to the particles generated by the neutron capture reaction in boron (Fig. 1) (Gabel et al, 1987b). The tracks of the particles in the film are made visible by etching, and the area of the tracks then can be evaluated opto-electronically. The area is compared to that of standards that consist of homogenized tissue doped with boric acid at known concentrations.

This method of boron determination is sensitive, simple, and informative. The lower detection limit is limited by the induction of spurious tracks by other particles, especially by fast neutrons. With a pure thermal beam, the sensitivity approaches the natural abundance of boron in tissue (Fig. 2).

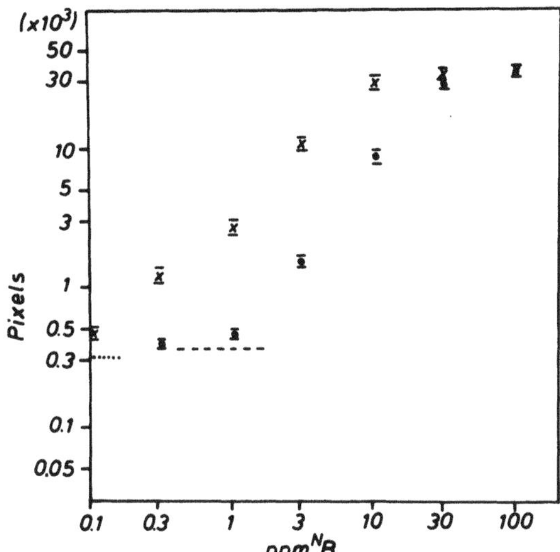

Fig. 2. Area of tracks of boron in liver tissue standards versus boron concentration. The two reactors used were the Medical Research Reactor at Brookhaven National Laboratory, NY, (•) and the Heavy Water Facility at Studsvik, Sweden (x). (Reprinted from Cancer Res. 47:5451, 1987 with permission.)

The spatial resolution of this technique is about 0.1 mm. Although this does still not yet represent the resolution necessary for assessing the success of boron in cell killing, it is far superior to other techniques presently available. Differences in the accumulation of boron within one tissue can readily be visualized and quantified, as illustrated by Fig. 3.

With this technique, we analyzed the distribution of BSH and BSSB, the dimer formed by oxidation, in tumor-bearing mice. Although these compounds show a relative selectivity in the tumor, their accumulation in the tumor is heterogeneous (most being accumulated in the necrotic parts of the tumor). More important, however, is the fact that following an intraperitoneal injection of BSH of 35 mg boron per kg, the boron concentration in the Harding-Passey melanoma transplanted in Balb/c mice is far below the concentrations needed for therapy (Gabel et al., 1987b).

PORPHYRINS

Porphyrins have been implicated frequently as suitable agents for tumor therapy. Their accumulation in a variety of tumors is large and persistent (Fairchild et al., 1984).

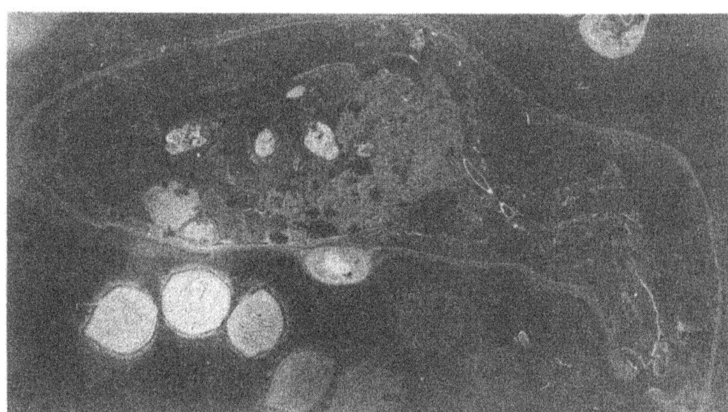

Fig. 3. Neutron capture radiogram of a mouse injected with 35 mg/kg boron-10 in form of $Na_2B_{12}H_{11}SH$ (BSH) 24 hours before death. Brightness represents boron. The high concentration of boron in the central part of the tumor is associated with necrotic tissue. (Reprinted from Cancer Res. 47:5451, 1987 with permission.)

Fig. 4 shows the biodistribution of sulfur-35-labeled tri- and tetrasulfonated meso-tetraphenylporphyrin ($TPPS_3$ and $TPPS_4$), that are among the best tumor-localizing porphyrins (Winkelman, 1962). Uptake in skin and internal organs is high, uptake in brain and muscle is low. Their uptake resembles that of BSH (see Fig. 2).

The high uptake in some of the blood vessels emerging from the heart is of special interest. It has been speculated earlier that the photodynamic tumor killing mediated by porphyrins could be caused by damage to the vascular system (Henderson et al., 1985)

To assess their potential in neutron capture therapy, we synthesized a variety of water-soluble porphyrins with different physico-chemical properties, and analyzed their uptake (Oenbrink et al., 1988).

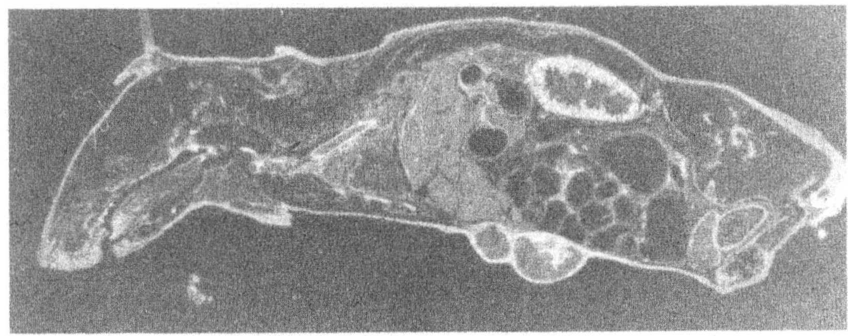

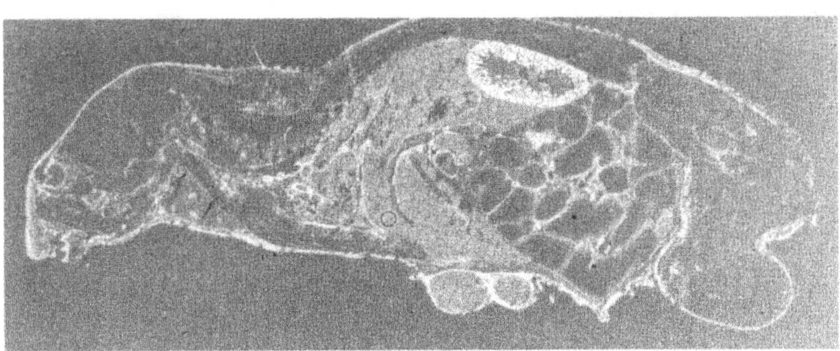

Fig. 4. Autoradiograms of Harding-Passey-tumor bearing Balb/cJ mice injected with $TPPS_3$ (top) or $TPPS_4$ (bottom). The high uptake of $TPPS_3$ in the central part of the tumor occurs in necrotic tissue.

We found a very strong correlation between the hydrophobicity of porphyrins (as measured by their distribution coefficient between octanol and water) and their uptakein cells. The most hydrophobic porphyrin was a boronated porphyrin. Its biodistribution in tumor-bearing animals showed an extremely high uptake in the intestine, liver, and lung, following an intraperitoneal injection. This differential distribution might be caused by uptake in the first cells that are exposed to the porphyrin after injection.

The synthesis of this porphyrin (Oenbrink et al., 1988) is shown in Fig. 5.

BORONOTHIOURACIL

Boronated thiouracil derivatives have been suggested as specific melanoma seekers (Fairchild et al., 1982), and attempts to synthesize such compounds were reported (Allen et al., 1986).

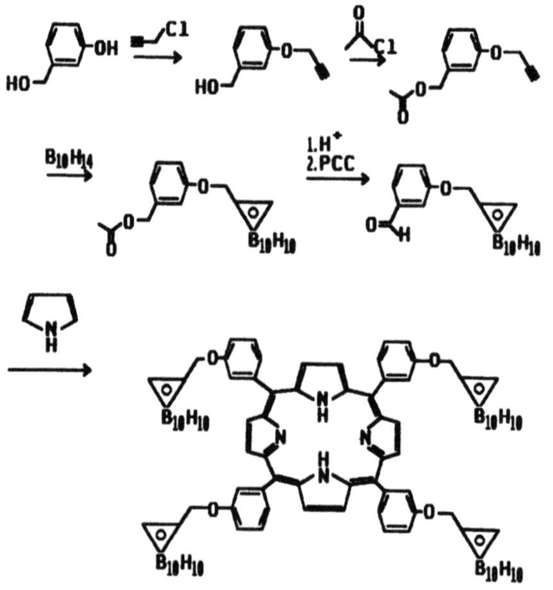

Fig. 5. Synthesis of a boronated porphyrin. After degrading the carborane cage with KOH to the corresponding nido-carborane, the porphyrin is water-soluble in concentrations of more than 20 mg/ml.

Fig. 6. Synthesis of 5-dihydroxyboryl-2-thiouracil.

We recently succeeded in synthesizing of boron-containing thiouracils (Tjarks and Gabel, unpublished). The synthesis of 5-dihydroxyboryl-2-thiouracil (BTU) is described in Fig. 6.

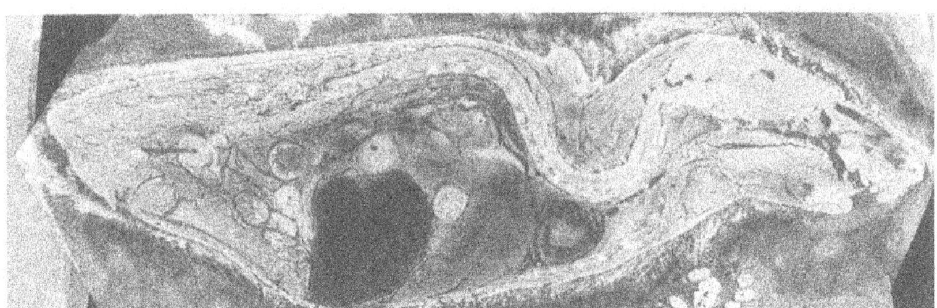

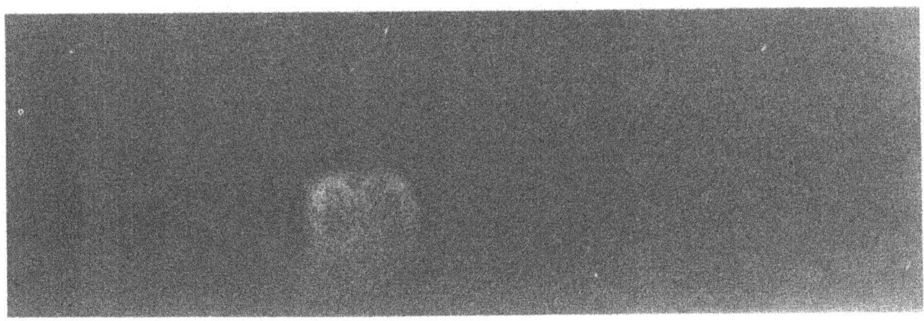

Fig. 7. Whole-body section of a Harding-Passey tumor-bearing mouse and the corresponding neutron capture radiogram. 6 mg of BTU were administered i.p. 24 hours before death.

This compound shows a high degree of accumulation in the Harding-Passey melanoma model in mice as expected. Following a single dose of 300 mg compound (18 mg boron) per kg, tumor accumulations of boron of up to 20 ppm are found after 24 hours. A neutron capture radiogram is shown in Fig. 7. Concentration ratios of 50:1 can be obtained between the tumor and all other organs of the body.

The uptake is persistent in time. After three hours, tumor concentrations of over 100 ppm can be obtained, with a tumor-to-blood ratio of 5:1.

The compound is relatively non-toxic. Single injections of 300 mg/kg are tolerated, as are daily injections of 150 mg/kg over a period of one week. This is in concordance with the relative non-toxicity of other thiouracils used for the treatment of hyperthyroidism.

ACKNOWLEDGEMENTS

I am indepted to my co-workers in Bremen, who had and still have the courage of tackling the difficult task of boron chemistry, and to my friends Börje Larsson and Ralph G. Fairchild, for their continued collaboration. This work was supported by grants from the Deutsche Forschungsgemeinschaft, the Fonds der Chemischen Industrie, the North Atlantic Treaty Organization, the U.S. Department of Energy, the Fulbright Foundation, and the National Institutes of Health.

REFERENCES

Allen, B.J., Brown, J.K., Harrington, B., Izard, B., Linklater, H., Maddalena, D.J., McNeill, J., McGregor, M.J., Mountford, M.H., Snowdon, G.M., Wilson, D.J., Wilson, J.G., Parsons, P., Moore, D., Tamat, S., and Hersey, P., 1986, Neutron capture therapy research for malignant melanoma, in "Neutron Capture Therapy", H. Hatanaka, ed., Nishimura, Niigata.

Demers, D.R., and Allemand, C.D., 1981, Atomic fluorescence spectrometry with an inductively coupled plasma as atomization cell and pulsed hollow cathode lamps for excitation, Anal. Chem. 53:1915.

Fairchild, R.G., Packer, S., Greenberg, D., Som, P., Brill, A.B., Fand, I., and McNally, W.P., 1982, Thiouracil distribution in mice carrying transplantable melanoma, Cancer Res. 42:5126.

Fairchild, R.G., Gabel, D., Hillman, M., and Watts, K., 1984, The distribution of exogenous porphyrins in vivo; implications for neutron capture therapy, in "Proceedings of the First International Symposium on Neutron Capture Therapy", R.G. Fairchild and G.L. Brownell, eds., BNL Report 51730, Upton, N.Y.

Gabel, D., Foster, S., and Fairchild, R.G., 1987a, The Monte Carlo simulation of the biological effect of the 10B(n,a)7Li reaction in cells and tissue and its implication for boron neutron capture therapy, Radiat. Res. 111:14.

Gabel, D., Holstein, H., Larsson, B., Gille, L., Ericson, G., Sacker, D., Som, P., and Fairchild, R.G., 1987b, Quantitative neutron capture radiography for studying the biodistribution of tumor-seeking boron-containing compounds, Cancer Res. 47:5451.

Henderson, B.W., Waldow, S.M., Mang, T.S., Potter, W.R., Malone, P.B., and Dougherty, T.J., 1985, Tumor destruction and kinetics of tumor cell death in two experimental mouse tumors following photodynamic therapy, Cancer Res. 45:572.

Kaczmarczyk, A., Messer, J.R., and Pierce, C.E., 1971, Rapid determination of boron in biological materials, Anal. Chem. 43:271.

Kirsch, J.E., and Brownell, G.L., 1984, Improved methods of neutron-induced track etch autoradiography, in "Proceedings of the First International Symposium on Neutron Capture Therapy", R.G. Fairchild and G.L. Brownell, eds., BNL Report 51730, Upton, N.Y.

Oenbrink, G., Jürgenlimke, P., and Gabel, D., 1988, Accumulation of porphyrins in cells: Influence of hydrophobicity, aggregation and protein binding, Photochem. Photobiol., in the press.

Winkelman, J. 1962, The distribution of tetraphenylporphinsulfonate in the tumor-bearing rat, Cancer Res. 22:589.

BORON-11 MAGNETIC RESONANCE IMAGING AND SPECTROSCOPY; TOOLS FOR INVESTIGATING PHARMACOKINETICS FOR BORON NEUTRON CAPTURE THERAPY

G.W. Kabalka [*,†] P. Bendel [*,Φ], M. Davis[†],
D.N. Slatkin[o], and P.L. Micca[o]

U. Tennessee Institute for Biomedical Imaging,
Departments of Radiology[*] and Chemistry[†],
Knoxville, TN
[Φ]Elscint MRI Division, Herzlia, Israel
[o]Medical Department
Brookhaven National Laboratory, Upton, NY

INTRODUCTION

Boron neutron capture therapy (BNCT) is brachyradiotherapy by heavy charged particles from the $^{10}B(n,\alpha)^{7}Li$ nuclear reaction.[1,2] BNCT depends upon the delivery of boron-10 containing drugs to the targeted lesions; the non-invasive verification and quantification of the boron content is a difficult problem. Clearly, experimental and clinical investigations of BNCT drugs would be greatly improved by the development of a non-invasive method for measuring the boron distribution *in vivo*. For example, such a technique could be used to monitor the course of distribution of a BNCT drug in the liver, kidney, bladder, brain and other organs of a patient scheduled for BNCT of a brain tumor so as to predict the optimum time for neutron irradiation of the brain.[3]

Multinuclear magnetic resonance imaging (MRI) and spectroscopy (MRS) have proven valuable in the localization of tumors, infarcts, and other medically significant conditions.[4,5] MRI and MRS have the capability of providing *in vivo* information concerning the identity, quantity, and environment of drugs and other physiologically important materials. Significantly, the information is provided in three dimensional space which permits precise, non-invasive localization of the agent of interest. Since boron-11 and boron-10 are magnetically active, MRI and MRS are potentially valuable techniques for evaluation of BNCT agents *in vivo*.

We present preliminary MRI and MRS measurements of the sulfhydryl dodecaborane dimer ($B_{24}H_{22}S_2^{-4}$), which include the first boron-11 image of a BNCT agent and the first boron-11 spectrum of a BNCT agent measured in an intact animal.

EXPERIMENTAL

Magnetic Resonance Studies

Imaging and Spectroscopy experiments were conducted using a Gyrex-2T, 90-cm bore, whole-body MR unit operating at 26 MHz for boron-11 and 81 MHz for hydrogen. An octagonal surface coil (12 cm x 12 cm) and a gaussian-shaped excitation pulse of 400 μsec duration was used to create the transverse magnetization. An 82 millisecond acquisition time and a 500 millisecond pulse repetition time were utilized in the boron-11 spectroscopy experiments.

A three-dimensional gradient echo, imaging protocol was employed for the boron-11 imaging studies, with either a TE of 6.4 millisecond or 1.7 millisecond. The image acquisition was two-dimensional since the effective width of the excited section encompassed the entire object and no phase encoding was applied in the slice-select direction. The effective pixel area for the solution phantoms was 3 cm x 3 cm.

Hydrogen MRI measurements were obtained using a 30 cm, Helmholtz saddle coil. The spin echo imaging protocol employed a TR of 2000 milliseconds and the echo times were varied (30, 60, 120, 150 milliseconds).

BNCT Agent

Cesium μ-disulfido-bis(undecahydro-closo-dodecaborate), $Cs_4B_{24}H_{22}S_2$, was the dimeric BNCT agent. It was prepared via oxidation of the monomeric sulfhydryl dodecaborane, $Cs_2B_{12}H_{11}SH$, (Callery Chemical Company, Callery, PA).[6] The sodium salt ($Na_4B_{24}H_{22}S_2$) was obtained by passing the $Cs_4B_{24}H_{22}S_2$ over a Dowex 50xW8 resin.[7] This agent was used to infuse Fisher 344 rats. MR phantoms were prepared using aqueous solutions of the cesium salt containing 0.086 g of boron-11 per milliliter.

Animals

Male, Fisher 344 rats (Taconic Farms, Germantown, NY) weighing ~250 grams received 250 μg of boron per gram of body weight. $Na_4B_{24}H_{22}S_2$ was infused via an intraperitoneally implanted osmotic pump (Alza Corp., Palo Alto, CA) which was rated to deliver 2 mL of solution continuously for 7.3 days. Previous experiments demonstrated that rats infused in this manner attain a boron concentration in the liver approaching 80 μg/gram (8).

Rats with tumors and rats without tumors were used for this study. Tumor-bearing rats bore several subcutaneously implanted gliomas [strain RGC-9].[9,10] The rats were euthanized one week after the pumps were implanted and the carcasses stored at -10°C or lower. The imaging experiments were conducted at ambient temperatures.

RESULTS

The implanted tumor is clearly visible in the hydrogen MRI, Fig. 1.

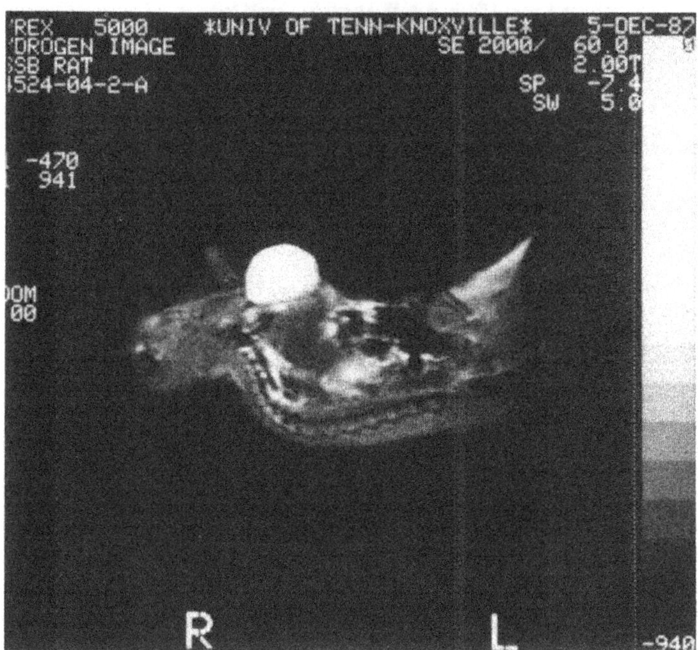

Fig. 1. Saggital MRI of Fisher 344 rat bearing a subcutaneously implanted RGC-9 glioma. The tumor exhibits a long hydrogen T2 relaxation time and appears as bright hemisphere.

The boron-11 spectrum of the dimeric BNCT agent is presented in Fig. 2. This spectrum was obtained using an aqueous solution (phantom) in which the boron-11 concentration approximated a therapeutic dose (86 μg/mL). The total scan time was thirty minutes.

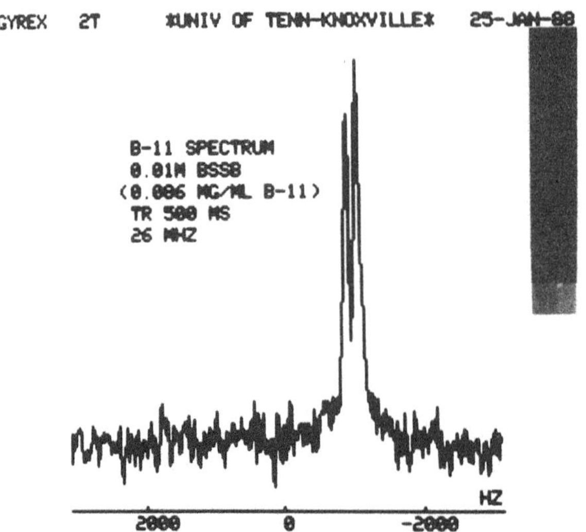

Fig. 2. Boron-11 spectrum of an aqueous 10 mL phantom containing 86 μg/mL of boron-11. A 5 Hz exponential line broadening filter was applied.

Fig. 3 shows the boron-11 spectrum of a BNCT agent in an intact animal.

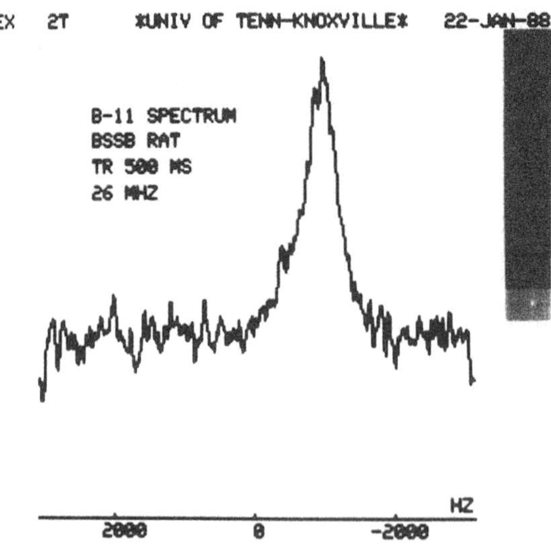

Fig. 3. Boron-11 spectrum of an intact Fisher 344 rat which was treated with the dimer. A 20 Hz exponential line broadening filter was applied.

Fig. 4 is a boron-11 magnetic resonance image of an aqueous phantom containing 86 μg of boron-11 per milliliter of the disulfide BNCT agent. The total imaging time was 10 minutes.

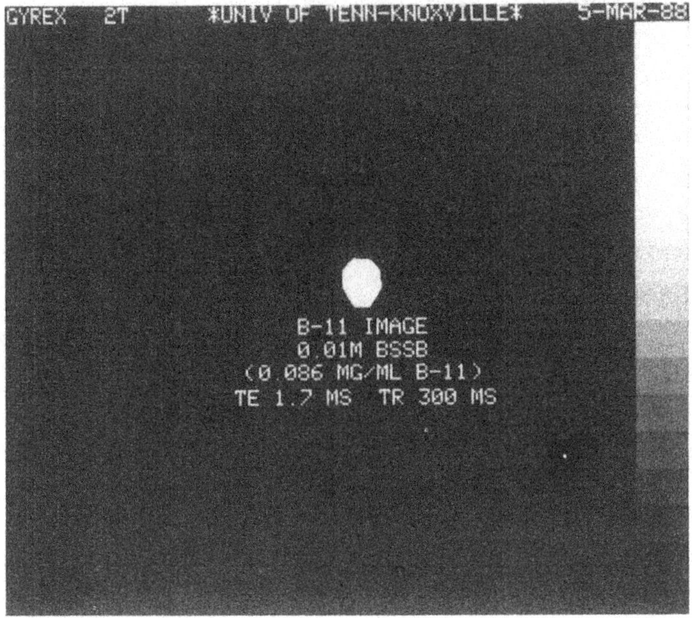

Fig. 4. Boron-11 image of a 10 mL phantom containing an aqueous solution of the dimer with a boron-11 concentration of 86 μg/mL.

DISCUSSION

Magnetic Resonance is a powerful non-invasive technique for the localization and quantification of a number of medically significant structures. The hydrogen MRI, Fig. 1, reveals the implanted tumor in a rat infused with the dimeric BNCT agent. No significant differences in the appearances of tumors in either the control or the treated animals were observed using T1- and T2-weighted protocols. In all cases the tumors exhibited much longer hydrogen T2 relaxation rates than surrounding tissue.

The boron-11 spectrum of the dimer, at somewhat higher than therapeutic levels of boron-11, is presented in Fig. 2. The spectrum is essentially identical to those obtained on analytical instruments. The small peak located 300 Hz downfield of the large doublet, which is due to the boron attached to the sulfur atom, is nearly lost in the baseline of the whole-body MR unit.

The boron-11 spectrum of the BNCT agent in the intact rat, Fig. 3, is less resolved than the corresponding spectrum of the BNCT phantom, Fig. 2. The broadening of the spectrum in the animal is caused by a shortening of the boron-11, T2 relaxation time and not by local inhomogeneity. This was demonstrated by measuring the line width of the hydrogen spectral signal from the rat which turned out to be significantly less than the width of the boron signal. The T2 relaxation time of the boron-11 agent in the intact animal is on the order of one millisecond. The shortened boron-11, T2 relaxation time is presumably due to a decrease in the correlation time caused by attachment of the boron agent to protein. The shorter T2 of the boron-11 is a major obstacle to successful boron imaging.

The first boron-11 MRI is shown in Fig. 4. The image is that of a 10 mL phantom containing the dimer with a concentration of 86 μg/of boron-11 per milliliter. This concentration approximates the therapeutic level found in the livers of rats (8). The image was obtained in the whole-body, 90-cm bore, unit using an octagonal surface coil with a gradient echo protocol.

As noted, the boron-11 T2 relaxation rate of the BNCT agent in the intact animal was on the order of one millisecond, as estimated from the line width and the rate of decay of the signal. Since the shortest echo time that we could achieve using a conventional spin-warp imaging protocol was 1.7 milliseconds, most of the boron signal was lost before acquisition. Moreover, imaging requires much higher sensitivity than spectroscopy because the signal is spread over a larger frequency range. Consequently, we have not been able to achieve a boron-11 image of the BNCT agent in the intact rat.

Boron-11 magnetic resonance holds promise for the quantification of BNCT agents in organs such as the liver and brain by using spectroscopic techniques. Our estimates indicate that, at the level of sensitivity available, we should be able to observe a boron-11 image by using a back-projection protocol that observes the signal immediately after the pulse. Further improvements in sensitivity may be derived from improved coil design and polarization transfer, using the boron hydrogen coupling.

ACKNOWLEDGEMENTS

We wish to thank the Department of Energy [DE-FG05-86ER60434] for supporting this research. We also wish to thank J. DeVinney, D. D. Joel, and M. M. Nawrocky for technical assistance.

REFERENCES

1. H. J. Taylor and M. Goldhaber, Detection of nuclear disintegration in a photographic emulsion. Nature 135:341 (1935).
2. G. L. Locher, Biological and therapeutic possibilities of neutrons, Am. J. Roentgenol. 36:1 (1936).
3. W. H. Sweet, The uses of nuclear disintegration in the diagnosis and treatment of brain tumor, N. Engl. J. Med. 245:875 (1951).
4. C. L. Partain, A. E. James, F. D. Rollo, and R. R. Price, "Nuclear Magnetic Resonance Imaging," W. B. Saunders, New York (1983).
5. P. D. Esser and R. E. Johnston, "Technology of nuclear magnetic resonance," The Society of Nuclear Medicine, New York (1984).
6. G. R. Wellum, E. I. Tolpin, A. H. Soloway, and A. Kadzmarczyk, Synthesis of μ-disulfido-bisfundecahydro-closo-dodecaborate and of a derived free radical, Inorg. Chem. 16:2120 (1977).
7. D. Slatkin, P. Micca, A. Forman, D. Gabel, L. Wielopolski, and R. Fairchild, Boron uptake in melanoma, cerebrum and blood from $Na_2B_{12}H_{11}SH$ and $Na_2B_{24}H_{22}S_2$ administered to mice, Biochem. Pharmacol. 35:1771 (1986).
8. D. N. Slatkin, D. D. Joel, R. G. Fairchild, P. L. Micca, M. M. Nawrocky, B. H. Laster, J. A. Coderre, G. C. Finkel, C. E. Poletti, and W. H. Sweet, Distribution of sulfhydryl borane monomer and dimer in rodents and of monomer in humans: nuclear reactor irradiations of melanoma and glioma in boronated rodents, in "Neutron Capture Therapy," R. G. Fairchild, A. D. Woodhead, and V. P. Bond, eds., Plenum Press, New York (in press).
9. H. H. Schmidek, S. L. Nields, A. L. Schiller, and J. Messer, Morphological studies of rat brain tumors induced by N-nitrosomethylurea, J. Neurosurg. 34:335 (1971).
10. P. Benda, K. Someda, J. R. Messer, W. H. Sweet, Morphological and immunochemical studies of rat glial tumors and clonal strains propagated in culture. J. Neurosurg. 34:310 (1971).

SELECTIVE THERMAL NEUTRON CAPTURE THERAPY AND DIAGNOSIS OF MALIGNANT MELANOMA: FROM BASIC STUDIES TO FIRST CLINICAL TREATMENT

Yutaka Mishima, Masamitsu Ichihashi,
Susumu Hatta, Chihiro Honda, and Akihiro Sasase
and Keizo Yamamura

Department of Dermatology
Special Institute of Cancer Neutron Capture Therapy
Kobe University School of Medicine
Kobe, 650 Japan

Keiji Kanda and Tooru Kobayashi

Research Reactor Institute, Kyoto University
Osaka, 590-04 Japan

Hiroshi Fukuda

National Institute of Radiological Sciences
Chiba, 260 Japan

BASIC AND PRECLINICAL STUDIES

As melanoma genesis occurs in pigment cells, accentuated melanogenesis concurrently occurs in principle[1]. Thus, harnessing this accentuation of melanogenesis, we developed a new mutually-dependent two-step therapy, in which melanogenesis-seeking compounds first specifically target melanoma cells, enabling the powerful second step to selectively destroy the targeted cells. Our new thermal neutron capture therapy[2,3,4,5] (NCT) uses a ^{10}B-dopa (melanin substrate) analogue, $^{10}B_1$-p-boronophenylalanine ($^{10}B_1$-BPA) which accumulates preferentially in melanoma cells[6,7]. The cells then are irradiated with thermal neutrons to induce the $^{10}B(n, \alpha)^7Li$ reaction which releases energy of 2.33MeV to a distance of 10~14μ, the diameter of melanoma cells. Extensive in vitro and in vivo radiobiological analysis[8] confirmed the highly enhanced killing effect of $^{10}B_1$-BPA. Measurements of the accumulating capacity of $^{10}B_1$-BPA into melanoma cells in vitro and in vivo using both chemical and prompt gamma ray spectrometry[7] assay showed its high affinity for these cells[9].

We first successfully eradicated Greene's melanoma transplanted into Syrian golden hamsters[5]. These results led us to conduct pre-clinical studies[6] using spontaneously occurring melanoma in Duroc pig skin. Three cases of melanoma, from 4.6 to 12cm in diameter were cured by perilesional injection of $^{10}B_1$-BPA, followed by a single irradiation of $1.3\text{-}2.6 \times 10^{13} n/cm^2$. The treated melanomas ulcerated and then consistently regressed, finally disappearing between 65 and 115 days after irradiation[10]. No substantial side effects were observed. In a control study, we cured one half of a melanoma lesion when irradiation was limited to one side only.

The acute and sub-acute toxicity[11] as well as pharmaco-dynamics of $^{10}B_1$-BPA have been studied in relation to its therapeutic dosage requirements. The LD50 for female mice was found to be 710mg/kg, several times the projected dosage for treatment of human melanoma.

We also studied clinical dosimetry of the absorbed radiation energy using a human phantom[12] with skeletal bone and melanoma to evaluate the precise dosage and distribution of total absorption of thermal neutrons and gamma ray in melanoma and various important areas, such as genitals and eyes, the entire human body for safe sapplication of this therapy. Protection of non-melanoma areas of the body was found to be easily achieved[12].

Further pre-clinical studies using human melanoma transplanted into nude mouse[13] were found to be a useful model for analyzing the differential effects of, and obtaining an optimal result for, each type of melanoma.

FIRST HUMAN MELANOMA TREATMENT BY OUR SELECTIVE THERMAL NEUTRON CAPTURE THERAPY

After clarifying the necessary findings in preparation for the first clinical trial, we applied our new therapy for the first human case.

Human Melanoma Treated

In 1984, the patient had subungal melanoma of the acral lentiginous type on the medial portion of his right toe. The lesion was amputated, along with the first metacarpal bone and the second proximal phalanx. This primary lesion demonstrated Clark invasion level[14] 5 and Bagley high-risk categorisation.

The post-operative course was uneventful, until in February, 1987 a subcutaneous tumor was noticed on the patient's left occipital region. The tumor was very firm and not movable, showing rather marked vertical growth. Xerography of the lesion was taken on June 26, and CT of the lesion showed possible invasion of the cranial bone. After careful examination of the lesion with a neurosurgeon, it was concluded that if the tumor was melanoma, it was inoperable since melanoma should be removed en bloc with a wide margin of normal surrounding tissue, and this tumor was positioned immediately above the junction of the transverse, sagittal and occipital sinus.

So far no additional metastases had been detected by ^{67}Ga scintigram, CT and other diagnostic techniques, although the possibility of their presence could not be ruled out. After obtaining approval from KUR and Kyoto University Medical Ethics Committees, we then carried out a confirmatory diagnosis and an estimation of $^{10}B_1$-BPA accumulating capacity, using neutron activation analysis.

Prompt Gamma Assay

The principles of this in situ diagnostic method, developed in cooperation with our physicists Drs. Kobayashi and Kanda[15], are based on the fact that each $^{10}B(n, \alpha)^7Li$ reaction releases a 478 KeV gamma ray. Thus, if we measure this prompt gamma emission in relation to the constantly present hydrogen atoms, we can assay ^{10}B concentration in the target tissues. We administered 100mg ^{10}B-BPA·HCl per kg of body weight by perilesional injection 17 and 4 hours before beginning the assay irradiation, as we planned to administer in the actual treatment of the melanoma lesion. Therefore we injected 640mg of $^{10}B_1$-BPA both times into each of ten perilesional points 4cm distant from the tumor's margin. The time course of ^{10}B administration and its concentration value in blood also were obtained. The values were confirmed by performing a parallel chemical assay which gave close correspondence. The estimated values of the ^{10}B assay of the melanoma lesion, the covering skin and the blood showed the concentration of ^{10}B in melanoma to be sufficiently high for successful neutron capture therapy. ^{10}B concentration in melanoma was found to be in the range of 24µg/ml while those of blood and skin were 1 and 3µg/ml respectively. The results are summarized in Fig. 1.

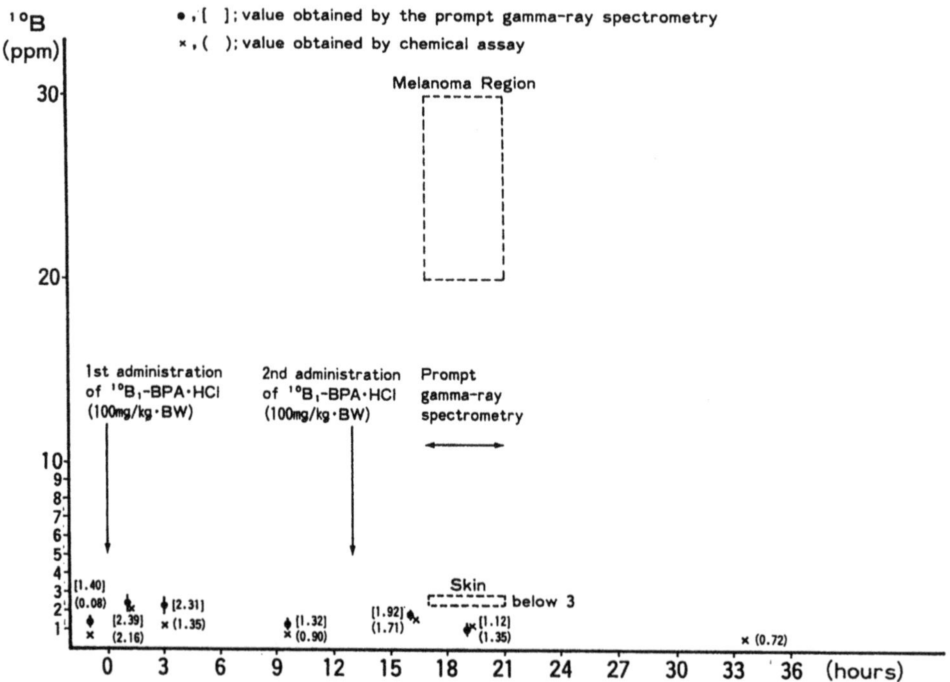

Fig. 1. Pre-treatment prompt γ assay of ^{10}B concentration in melanoma, blood and skin of the first human melanoma patient treated by our selective neutron capture therapy (NCT).

Radiation Dosimetry with Phantom

We worked out the precise, optimum setting of our patient's melanoma in front of the neutron guide tube by first using a human skull with a melanoma model. To determine optimal irradiation doses of thermal neutrons for the cure of melanoma without serious damage to the covering skin, the absorbed energy of the $^{10}B(n, \alpha)^7Li$

reaction, $^{14}N(n, p)^{14}C$ reaction and gamma ray has to be estimated. The absorbed energy from $^{10}B(n, \alpha)^{7}Li$, which is the main cause of tumor killing in this therapy, is determined both by ^{10}B accumulation and thermal neutron distribution in melanoma. However, the surface dose can only be predetermined by short irradiation (as for radiation dosimetry). In addition, thermal neutron distribution in the tumor varies according to the size and shape of the tumor and surrounding tissue. To measure the thermal neutron fluence in the tumor, gold wire was inserted horizontally as well as vertically every 1cm in depth into the life-size phantom of this patient's melanoma on the scalp. Core and secondary gamma rays were measured by TLD placed on the surface of the tumor. The actual isodose curves of thermal neutron and γ-ray obtained are shown in Fig. 2. Based on a Relative Biological Effectiveness(RBE) of 2.5 for the $^{10}B(n, \alpha)^{7}Li$ and $^{14}N(n, p)^{14}C$ reactions, total rem values at the points A, B_1, B_2, B_3, B_4 are 1665, 4815, 3295, 1050 and 630 rem respectively.

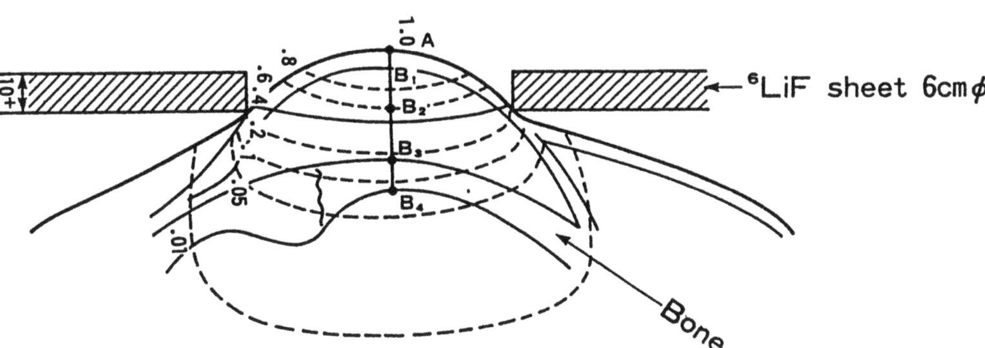

Fig. 2. Clinical dosimetry of first human melanoma lesion which was subsequently treated by our NCT method.

Absorbed Dose Estimation

The Total absorbed doses of $^{10}B(n, \alpha)^{7}Li$ and $^{14}N(n, p)^{14}C$ reactions as well as core and secondary γ-rays were estimated by using an RBE of 2.5 for the first two reactions. The total absorbed dose obtained in skin and at various depths in the melanoma, together with our earlier findings on ^{10}B concentrations with prompt γ assay and from radiation dosimetry with a phantom model of the melanoma lesion and total body human phantom were used to determine the optimal and most effective radiation dose which could be given without sacrificing safety.

Therapy Procedure

To determine the final duration of irradiation we first irradiated for 30 minutes to obtain the actual neutron fluence. This was found to be $1 \times 10^9 n/cm^2 \cdot sec$ at 100kW. Two major factors then had to be considered. The first was the skin and vessel tolerance dose of 1800rem. The second was the dose to cure the melanoma, about 4000rem. Since this was the first treatment of human melanoma by NCT and because of the position of the proliferating melanoma just above the large sinus, patient safety was considered to be our first priority, although we also wanted to have good suppression of melanoma growth. If the melanoma had not been completely cured by a single treatment, a second treatment would have been given.

Thus we took the schedule of irradiating with 1×10^{13} neutrons/cm^2 at the melanoma surface and we irradiated for 2 hrs 19 mins in the same position. The collimation in place around the lesion left an irradiation area of 6.5 x 6.7 cm corresponding exactly to the melanoma margins.

Result

The clinical appearance of the melanoma on Sept. 16 approximately 2 months after treatment compared with just before treatment of July 10(Fig. 3) showed marked regression of melanoma(Fig. 4), an elevation of 7.5mm compared to 21mm on July 10 being measured by caliper. Regression continued unabated, resulting in the disappearance of the patient's symptoms of double vision, nausea and headaches.

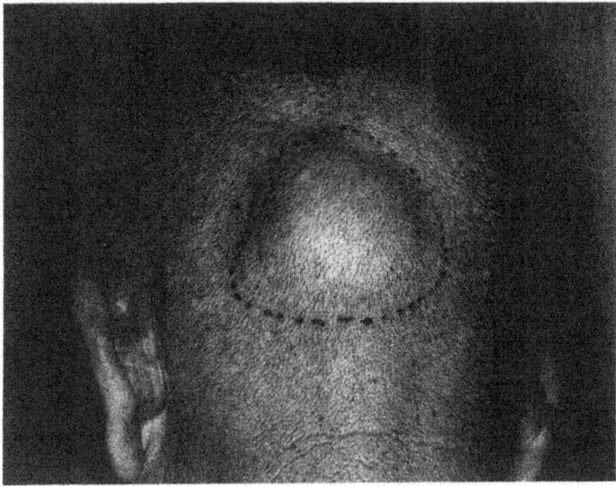

Fig. 3. Clinical appearance of the melanoma lesion before NCT.

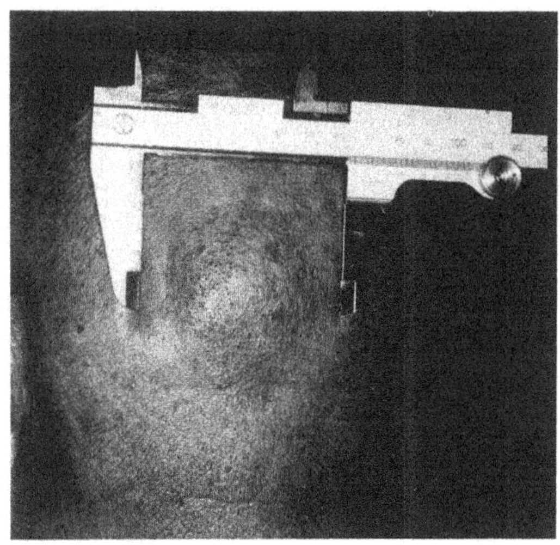

Fig. 4. Marked regression of the NCT-treated melanoma lesion which was clinically observable.

Fig. 5 shows the growth and regression curve of the treated melanoma, which displayed a time-course of regression almost identical to that of our successfully treated 12cm-diameter Duroc pig melanoma[6]. In both cases, the melanoma volume regressed very rapidly to approximately 1/10 of its original value over the two months following irradiation and has further regressed, though at a somewhat reduced rate, up to the present.

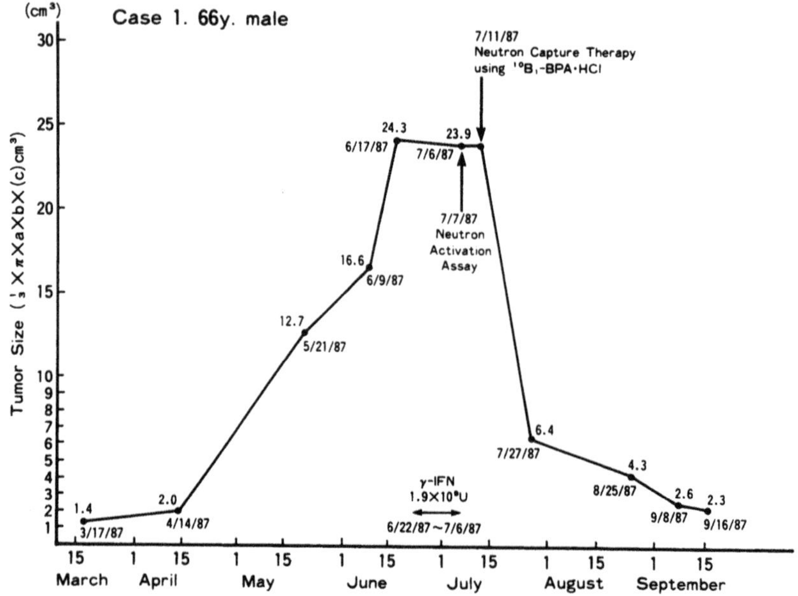

Fig. 5. Rapid proliferation and abrupt regression of malignant melanoma before and after NCT.

REFERENCES

1. Y. Mishima, M. Ichihashi, K. Hayashibe, M. Ueda, S, Hatta, Y. Funasaka and G. Imokawa, Control of melanogenesis and melanoma oncogenesis, in: "Advances in Pigment Cell Research", Proc. of 13th Int. Pig. Cell Conf., Tucson, Arizona, Oct. 5-9, 1986. Alan R. Liss, New York (1988).
2. Y. Mishima and T. Shimakage, Thermal neutron capture treatment of malignant melanoma using ^{10}B-dopa and ^{10}B12-chlorpromazine compound, in:"Pigment Cell", Vol.2:394, V. Riley, ed., S. Karger, Basel (1976).

3. T. Nakanishi, M. Ichihashi, Y. Mishima, T. Matsuzawa and H. Fukuda, Thermal neutron capture therapy of malignant melanoma:in vitro radiobiological analysis, Int. J. Radiat. Biol. 37:573 (1980).
4. Y. Mishima, M. Ichihashi, T. Nakanishi and T. Nakagawa, Selective thermal neutron capture therapy of cancer cells using their specific functional differentiation, Kyoto University Research Reactor Institute(KURRI)-Technical Report 195:3 (1980).
5. Y. Mishima, "Selective Thermal Neutron Capture Treatment of Malignant Melanoma Using Its Specific Metabolic Ability", KURRI-Technical Report 260 Y. Mishima, ed.(1985).
6. Y. Mishima, M. Ichihashi, T. Nakanishi, M. Tsuji, M. Ueda, T. Nakagawa and T. Suzuki, Cure of malignant melanoma by single thermal neutron capture treatment using melanoma seeking compounds:^{10}B/melanogenesis interaction to in vitro /in vivo radiobiological analysis to preclinical studies, in:"Proc. 1st Int. Symp. Neutron Capture Therapy", BNL51730:355, R. G. Fairchild, G. L. Brownell, eds., U.S.Government Printing Office (1984).
7. K. Yoshino, M. Okamoto, H. Kakihana, T. Nakanishi, M. Ichihashi and Y. Mishima, Spectrophotometric determination of trace boron in biological materials after alkali fusion decomposition, Anal. Chem. 56:839 (1984).
8. M. Ichihashi, Y. Mishima, M. Ueda, K. Hayashibe, S. Hatta, Y. Funasaka, H. Fujiwara and K. Yoshino, Selective lethal effects of $^{10}B_1$-paraboronophenylalanine on mouse and human melanoma cells in thermal neutron capture therapy enhanced by tyrosine and phenylalanine deficiency, in:"Neutron Capture Therapy", Proc. 2nd Int. Symp. Neutron Capture Therapy, H. Hatanaka, ed., Nishimura Co., Ltd., Niigata, Japan (1986).
9. K. Yoshino, M. Okamoto, H. Kakihana, Y. Mori, Y. Mishima, M. Ichihashi, M. Tsuji and T. Nakanishi, Studies on melanoma-seeking agent, ^{10}B-p-boronophenylalanine·HCl, KURRI-Technical Report 260:233 (1985).
10. Y. Mishima, M. Ichihashi and S. Hatta, Malignant melanoma cure by selective thermal neutron capture therapy, American Nuclear Society Transactions 53: 33 (1986).
11. K. Taniyama, H. Fujiwara, T. Kuno, N. Saito, H. Shuntoh, M. Sakaue and C. Tanaka, Acute and subacute toxicity of ^{10}B-paraboronophenylalanine,

Proc. 2nd Japan-Australia Workshop on Neutron Capture Therapy for Malignant Melanoma, Pig. Cell. Res.(1988), in press.
12. H. Karashima, J. Hiratsuka and Y. Mishima, Clinical dosimetry using human phantom with skeleton bone for thermal neutron capture therapy, in:"Neutron Capture Therapy", H. Hatanaka, ed., Nishimura, Niigata, Japan (1986).
13. H. Tamauchi, K. Tamaoki, M. Ueda and Y, Mishima, Therapeutic effect of thermal neutron capture therapy on human melanoma growing in nude mouse, KURRI-Technical Report 260:91 (1985).
14. W. H. Clark, Jr., L. From, E. H. Bernardino and M. C. Mihm, The histogenesis and biologic behavior of primary human malignant melanomas of the skin. Cancer Res. 29:705 (1969).
15. T. Kobayashi and K. Kanda, Microanalysis system of ppm-order ^{10}B concentrations in tissue for neutron capture therapy by prompt gamma-ray spectrometry, Nuclear Instruments and Methods 204:525 (1983).

WORKSHOP SUMMARY OF MODERATORS' REPORTS

WORKING GROUP ON TUMOR COMPOUND AND COMPOUND DELIVERY SYSTEMS

a. It is considered desirable to demonstrate biological efficacy in animal tumor models for $Na_2B_{12}H_{11}SH$ (BSH) and other prospective compounds before the clinical trials.

b. No effort should be spared to analyze the physiological effects and tumor-targeting behavior (pharmacokinetics) of BSH, its dimer, and possible new compounds, first in animal systems and then in initial clinical trials.

c. NCT following Hatanaka's procedures is to be regarded as a "benchmark" representing an acceptable state-of-the art at present. However, we should take the opportunity to improve knowledge and techniques and to employ these improvements in the initial clinical trials.

d. P-boronophenylalanine had biological efficacy in melanoma test systems and may have therapeutic value; it may be a candidate for clinical trials.

WORKING GROUP ON OPTIMIZATION OF RADIATION DOSE DELIVERY

Thermal and Epithermal Beams

a. Epithermal neutrons are superior to thermal neutrons in providing better penetration, possible skin sparing and obviating any need for surgery to correct for poor thermal neutron penetration.

b. Parallel opposed beams, or any other beam combination, would be desirable to improve the homogeneity of the dose.

c. To reproduce the data reported from Japan, the parameters should be optimized for human irradiations (i.e., beam energy, number and orientation and dose and compound delivery).

Fractionation

a. Historically, fractionation has been shown to be advantageous in radiation therapy.

b. The large and unavoidable low-LET component to normal tissues from irradiation with epithermal beams strongly suggests that fractionation would increase the tolerance of normal tissue.

c. Experimental and clinical data show that the blood-brain barrier is highly radio-resistant and that doses as high as 20 Gy (acute irradiation) are necessary to significantly alter its permeability. This is true also for doses of high-LET radiation that would be equally effective. Therefore, concern about alteration of the blood-brain barrier is probably unjustified for the fractionation schemes considered.

d. Four to six fractions are recommended as a reasonable compromise.

e. If a single protracted (low-dose rate) irradiation would be applied, extending the duration of the exposure to achieve full repair of sublethal damage would raise practical difficulties, so that fractionation is preferred.

f. If four to six fractions were used, the duration of the fractions (i.e. 1 min, 10 min, 60 min) would not significantly influence the brain's tolerance: short sessions are preferable for the comfort of the patients.

g. In view of the inexperience with epithermal beams in humans, a protocol of dose escalation should be followed.

Uniform Boron Incorporation

a. The basic requirement for successful NCT is a uniform incorporation of boron compound in tumor cells.

b. It is expected that new boron compounds with appropriate diffusion ranges, combined with repeated administration associated with fractionated irradiation, will improve homogeneity of boron distribution.

General

Before starting clinical trials in the United States, it is advisable that such trials be reviewed and coordinated with other neutron capture therapy projects by a small international group of individuals such as those brought together in the current workshop.

MODERATORS' REPORT AND DISCUSSIONS

WORKING GROUP ON TUMOR COMPOUND AND COMPOUND DELIVERY SYSTEM

Moderators: Sara Rockwell
Department of Therapeutic Radiology
Yale School of Medicine
333 Cedar Street
New Haven, Connecticut

Borje Larsson
Department of Radiation Science
Uppsala University
Box 531 - S-75121
Uppsala, Sweden

The purpose of this section is to present an account of the discussions of the two working groups. First is a report by the moderators of the tumor compound group followed by a general discussion. Second is a report by moderators of the dose rate group followed by a discussion.

We are thankful to the Department of Energy, who gave us the funds to hold this workshop. Our gratitude also goes to the moderators for donating their time.

GLIOBLASTOMA

The working group began its deliberations with a general discussion of glioblastoma, which is being intensively considered as an appropriate disease for the resumption of clinical trials of neutron capture therapy (NCT). A major reason for considering the initial resumption of NCT with glioblastoma is the global experience that established therapeutic regimens have little to offer patients with grade IV glioblastomas. Because of this, it is impossible to neglect the intriguing and encouraging reports from H. Hatanaka in Tokyo of an increased survival and improved quality of life for some glioma patients treated by NCT. The working group also noted that the principle of NCT holds promise as a technique which may have great utility in other areas of radiation oncology and neurosurgery; this area was reserved for later deliberation, which is reviewed below.

There are several factors which raise problems in the design and implementation of clinical trials assessing the efficacy of NCT in glioma. First is the problem of interpreting Hatanaka's reports of his experience with NCT. These reports do not lend themselves readily to evaluation in terms of clinical trials. This is partly due to the fact that the result of treatment of grade III-IV glioblastomas are difficult to evaluate even in carefully designed clinical trials. Data from a non-randomized series of patients, with all of the patient selection problems inherent in such a situation, are extremely difficult to evaluate. Comparisons between Hatanaka's patients and American glioma patients are more difficult because data on some factors used to stage American patients (e.g., Karnofsky status) are not available for all of Hatanaka's patients and because there are epidemiological factors (e.g., age-specific incidence rates) which suggest differences in the biology of the disease in the Japanese and European/American populations. Another difficulty is that the pathologic staging of brain tumors (notably, the differentiation between stages III and IV) is difficult and subjective; staging is of extreme importance because of the great variation in prognosis with stage. The working group discussed the importance of evaluating critically the individual grading of Hatanaka's NCT patients, a discussion which implies no criticism of the records from Tokyo, but rather a recognition of the difficulty and importance of the task. The working group also discussed the difficulties inherent in assessing whether the favorable results found in Hatanaka's experience reflect the NCT *per se* or whether other factors (e.g., the parameters of the neutron radiotherapy; good surgical technique) played a role in producing the observed long-term responses.

A second problem is that the negative experiences from the NCT trials during the 1950's and 1960's in the United States have resulted in an exceptional scrutiny of plans for new approaches towards clinical trials of NCT. For psychological and political reasons, preclinical evaluations of the safety and potential efficacy of NCT will need to be of a much higher quality than is generally required for Phase I-II studies of new regimens for treating glioblastomas. Some workshop participants expressed the concern that a premature or poorly conceived clinical trial of the efficacy of NCT, which resulted in a negative result or in excessive patient toxicity, could cause a potentially valuable therapeutic modality to be abandoned for years or decades.

A third problem in implementing trials of NCT is that of knowing which factors are critical in effecting the successful application NCT. Hatanaka's treatment regimen involves surgical excision of operable tumor, followed by the infusion of $Na_2B_{12}H_{11}SH$ (BSH), 30-80 mg ^{10}B/kg into the carotid or vertebral artery over 1-2 hours, 16 hours prior to irradiation of the exposed tumor bed in the anesthetized patient with thermal neutrons at a dose rate requiring an irradiation time of several hours. The workshop participants discussed the desirability of changing many of these parameters. However, it is not known which factor or factors in Hatanaka's treatment regimen are responsible for the reported efficacy of this treatment (the thermal neutron irradiations _per se_, the low dose rate, the nonhomogeneous dose distributions, the pharmacological action of BSH, or, as the working hypothesis of this conference presumes, the ^4He, ^7Li and gamma radiations resulting from neutron capture in ^{10}B). As stated succinctly by W.H. Sweet, "We understand so little of what the crucial factors are in the results of Hatanaka."

Moreover, there is no adequate animal model for glioblastoma that would permit a complete evaluation and refinement of all of the many parameters which might influence treatment efficacy in this complex situation. The available transplanted rodent brain tumors have significant limitations as models for human glioblastoma multiforme. The known biological differences between human gliomas and the transplanted rodent tumor lines and the artificial tumor/host relationship resulting from injection of tumor cells into the rodent brain both limit the utility of the available rodent models. The physiological differences between rodents and people raise problems similar to those encountered in other pharmacology studies. The small size of the rodents and the shape of the rodent head create unique problems during neutron irradiations, as they lead to excessive whole-body radiation doses and to high radiation doses to normal tissues which would be outside the radiation field in human patients. The discussants, therefore, felt that animal studies would be of limited value in improving Hatanaka's NCT protocols. This is not to say that _in vitro_ studies and experiments with tumors and normal tissues in rodents are of little importance in the further development of new agents, principles, and regimens of NCT. Such studies will be absolutely essential for the initial evaluation of the biological, radiobiological, and cytotoxic effects of new boronated compounds; for toxicological, pharmacological, and biodistribution studies of new compounds, and for studies demonstrating the efficacy of such compounds as agents for NCT. Animal studies would also be extremely useful in basic research projects examining such subjects as the mechanism of NCT damage to normal tissues and glioma, and the variation in the efficacy of NCT with the ^{10}B dose, the duration of irradiation, and the radiation fractionation pattern. The use of dogs with spontaneous gliomas may also be of value in some preclincial studies. It was pointed out during the discussion that dogs with such brain tumors are more common than was appreciated.

The question was raised whether metastatic melanoma in the brain should be treated and used as a clinical model for primary brain tumors. Some discussants felt that this might be a valuable approach to initiating NCT of intracranial tumors, because of the fact that several seemingly efficient melanoma-seeking compounds have been invented. (This issue was discussed later in the workshop; the discussion is summarized in Section 4 below).

The general discussion was concluded with a consensus that it seems inevitable that clinical trials will soon be initiated at one or more sites in the United States or Europe to evaluate the possible merits of NCT for advanced glioblastoma. The working group expressed the feeling that this endeavor should be based on the support from the international community of scientists, oncologists, and neurosurgeons now engaged in NCT research and development. Adequate statistical analyses and clinical surveys should be an integral part of this program. As far as the pharmacokinetics of the boron compounds are concerned, no effort should be spared to analyze the physiological and tumor-targeting behavior of BSH, its dimer, and possible new compounds, both in animal systems and in initial clinical trials. These studies would include examinations of the microscopic distribution of boron within the tumors and the normal tissues which will be irradiated. The heterogeneity of the ^{10}B distribution in the tumor will ultimately limit the efficacy of NCT in killing the tumor cells and will therefore limit the ability of this approach to cure the cancer. The microscopic distribution within normal tissues will be critical in determining the nature and severity of the toxicities resulting from the NCT. Mention was made of the potentials of positron emission tomography and track-etch autoradiographic techniques for studying drug distributions on macroscopic and microscopic levels, respectively.

The factors raised in the discussion summarized above formed the framework used to answer questions formulated by the organizers of the workshop.

Should Dr. Hatanaka's NCT regimen be replicated exactly in trials to be initiated in the near future?

The working group felt that Hatanaka's experience with NCT for glioblastoma could be accepted as a benchmark, at the time of the workshop, representing the present state of the clinical art. However, the consensus of the group was that new clinical trials with this modality should not attempt to repeat Hatanaka's protocols exactly but rather should use all of the data which is becoming available to improve the NCT regimens and to optimize the treatment of patients in the trials. It would seem reasonable to believe that considerable improvements in NCT regimens should be attainable within the near future. Among the points mentioned as worthy of consideration were optimization of the neutron energy, dose distribution, total dose, and fractionation patterns to be used; obtaining an understanding of the role of endothelial cell lesions in normal tissue damage; and detailed considerations of the boronated compounds to be used (including detailed studies of the macroscopic and microscopic distribution of ^{10}B in tumors and normal tissues).

As some members of the working group involved in the radiologic aspects of NCT wondered how the neurosurgical community would view these procedures, the neurosurgeons in the working group were asked whether they would be willing to accept NCT _ad modem_ Hatanaka in its present form and recommend it to their own patients. These five individuals formulated a consensus statement which stated that: "Boron neutron capture therapy is considered to be a potentially effective method of treating primary CNS malignant tumors. At our present level of understanding, clinical trials should be entered into with caution. Improved understanding of pharmacokinetics, compound distribution, and beam delivery will be necessary prior to recommendations being made that clinical therapeutic trials should be initiated." This statement also reflects the opinions of many of the participants in the working group.

Should the pharmacokinetics of BSH be investigated as a function of the mode of administration, length of administration, time between end of administration and irradiation, and amount of boron administered?

Yes. Such investigations are already in progress at various centers in experimental animals and in patients and should certainly be continued. Boron distributions should be studied both macroscopically (using PET, SPECT and possibly NMR, if the NMR techniques can be developed adequately) and microscopically (using high-resolution autoradiographic techniques to assess distribution in biopsy samples). It is also desirable to know more about the various factors that influence tumor uptake, blood clearance, and intracellular localization of the boronated compounds.

Of what quality should the pharmacokinetic data of an optimized administration be before clinical trials are feasible?

The working group felt that good human pharmacokinetic data were essential to the success of the clinical trials. The homogeneity of ^{10}B distribution within the tumor cells will determine the efficacy of NCT, as only a small number of resistant cells would be sufficient to prevent eradication of the tumor. Conversely, the distribution of ^{10}B in normal tissues (particularly the peritumor vasculature) will determine the nature and amount of normal tissue damage resulting from the treatment. Both factors must be assessed before the safety and efficacy of the treatment can be predicted with adequate certainty.

Would the dimer ($Na_4B_{24}H_{22}S_2$) be more advantageous than the monomer ($Na_2B_{12}H_{11}SH$)?

Possibly. Toxicity tests and pharmacokinetic studies must be performed before this question can be answered.

Is the dimer toxicity prohibitive relative to that of the monomer?

The working group lacked sufficient data to answer this question. Data on animals suggest a greater toxicity for the dimer, but the working group was not aware of detailed comparisons of the distributions, toxicities, and therapeutic efficacies of the two compounds which would allow this question to be answered rigorously.[1] Even if the dimer were more toxic than the monomer, as appears likely, it could theoretically prove superior for NCT if it also produced higher and/or more uniform ^{10}B tumor levels in tumors and therefore resulted in greater antineoplastic efficacy. Boron "cocktails" also could be considered to reduce the toxicity for a given amount of boron.

What significance, if any, with respect to clinical trials should be attached to the failure to date to demonstrate biological efficacy in animals of either monomer or dimer?

---

[1]An invited paper on the toxicity of monomer vs dimer in mice is included in this volume.

The working group was uncertain that the statement implicit in the question is true. Studies with intracerebral glioma transplants in rats reported at the meeting by R.F. Barth reported an increased duration of survival after treatment with the monomer plus neutron irradiation relative to that obtained with radiation alone. These studies suggest that the monomer increases the anti-neoplastic effects of neutron irradiation in this animal model system. It is certainly correct, however, that the efficacy of NCT has been difficult to demonstrate in animal models. The reasons for this and the implications of this fact should be considered carefully.

On the other hand, there are many studies which show uptake of high amounts of boron, more or less preferentially, in transplanted tumor models. Extrapolation from experiments examining the effects of the ^{10}B concentration on the response of cells irradiated *in vitro* suggests that the ^{10}B concentrations found in these model tumors should be sufficient to enhance the efficacy of radiotherapy with slow neutrons. These studies therefore provide indirect evidence that a significant neutron capture dose could be delivered to these tumors. It was also noted in the discussion that rodent studies of NCT efficacy have often been limited by radiation reactions in normal tissues which receive intensive irradiation in the rodents, but which are outside the irradiated field in patients.

OTHER COMPOUNDS AND TUMORS

This phase of the workshop started with a general discussion of the preclinical model studies known to the working group and of the first clinical experiences with NCT in melanoma reported by Dr. Mishima at the workshop.

The group discussed the merits of melanoma as a candidate for the next clinical trials with NCT. The importance of studying more than one kind of tumor, more than one anatomical site, and more than one boron-containing compound in NCT trials were emphasized as critical factors in choosing to study a second malignancy. The fact that there is at least one compound available (p-boronophenylalanine) which has been shown to localize in tumors and to produce therapeutic efficacy in transplanted mouse and hamster tumor systems and spontaneous swine tumors provides a strong basis for predicting that therapeutic gain might be obtained clinically with this approach.

The aims of the initial clinical studies in Japan are to study the distribution of p-boronophenylalanine and to examine the efficacy of NCT using this compound in producing local regression and palliation of cutaneous melanomas in selected patients with advanced recurrent or metastatic disease. An encouraging response was noted in the first patient. Treatment of other Japanese and Australian patients in Japan is planned by Mishima who emphasized his philosophy that these initial clinical studies must be focused and must be limited to situations in which there is no other effective therapy, the safety of the NCT regimen is assured, and the benefits of effective therapy are significant and obvious.

The working group considered the extension of NCT to melanoma to represent a first step in the application of this modality to use in the treatment of other neoplastic and non-neoplastic diseases. Eventual applications to such conditions as leukemia (in the purging of marrow for transplant), arteriovenus malformation of the brain, and possibly arthritis and other autoimmune diseases were discussed. The possible use of NCT as an adjunct to fast neutron radiotherapy also was mentioned. The working group also discussed the concept that NCT should not be envisioned as a single agent but rather as one of several modalities which might be applied in concert to obtain optimal treatment of an individual patient. Mention was made of the fact that some boronated compounds have other therapeutic effects which might be used along with NCT (e.g., the photosensitizing effects of boronated porphyrins in phototherapy; the cytotoxic effects of boronated antibodies or boronated anticancer drugs). The potential use of targeted boronated compounds in diagnostic imaging was discussed.

The importance of detailed pharmacokinetic data, on both a macroscopic and a microscopic level, was emphasized for all possible applications of NCT. The use of the noninvasive, quantitive imaging techniques, which are now being developed to permit dynamic studies of the distribution of boronated compounds in individual patients, might prove exceedingly valuable in tailoring the therapy of individual patients. The combination of these biodistribution data with the detailed analyses of microscopic distribution, available through studies of biopsy material with high-resolution autoradiographic techniques and other microanalytical techniques, should provide pharmacologic data which will greatly enhance the evaluation of new boronated compounds and the design and implementation of NCT regimens in the clinic. These techniques might also be used to evaluate combinations of compounds, to ascertain whether some combinations could be used to minimize heterogeneity in the distribution of ^{10}B within tumors and to evaluate the effects of physiological modifications on the biodistribution of the boronated compounds.

Should p-boronophenylalanine be used in the initial clinical trials with malignant melanoma?

The working group considered this to be a moot point, as clinical trials with this compound in this disease have recently started and were reported at the meeting by Mishima. The fact that p-boronophenylalanine was shown to accumulate with some selectivity in animal melanomas and the fact that this compound was efficacious in increasing the effects of neutron radiotherapy in a mouse model system were mentioned as factors suggesting that this approach might be especially promising.

Would melanoma metastatic to the brain be a viable system in which to initially evaluate NCT in humans?

The working group generally agreed that cutaneous melanoma represented a better system for initial clinical trials with melanoma than did brain metastases. There are several reasons for this conclusion. First, the prognosis for melanoma patients with multiple brain metastates is very poor; even if disease in the brain could be controlled, such patients would succumb to metastases in other vital organs. Because of this, some members of the group felt that these patients might make poor candidates for such a clinical trial. Second, some members of the working group expressed concern about the potential risks for such patients, because the chemical relationship between the melanoma-seeking compounds and neurotransmitters could theoretically lead to an accumulation of the melanoma-seeking compounds in nervous structures and therefore lead to brain damage after NCT. Several participants also expressed the opinion that there was merit in studying NCT in a clinical situtation in which the response of the tumor and the damage to normal tissues could be observed continuously and closely. The study of both the tumors and the dose-limiting normal tissues is difficult with intracranial tumors but straightforward with cutaneous melanomas. Therefore, it was felt that studies of cutaneous melanomas had several clinical and scientific advantages as the first step in the application of NCT to this disease.

The committee based its discussions of melanoma primarily on a consideration of this disease *per se* and discussed the best approach towards applying NCT to melanoma. In this respect, the discussions of this working group differed significantly from those of working group I, which considered the combination of a melanin-seeking compound and intracranial melanoma as a model for NCT treatment of glioma and noted the potential advantages of metastatic melanoma for initial studies of intracranial malignancy.

Should biological efficacy be demonstrated in animals for any compound considered for clinical use?

Yes, in principle and also because this would probably be required by the regulatory agencies. Efficacy in animals has already been reported both for the $Na_2B_{12}H_{11}SH$ monomer in transplanted gliomas and for p-boronophenylalanine in transplanted melanomas. In essence, this provides a benchmark to which other compounds must be compared. Before efficacy studies could be begun in patients, clinical studies demonstrating adequate boron levels and microscopic distributions in the tumors and acceptably low boron concentrations in normal tissues within the irradiated field would also be necessary.

Are there better compounds on the horizon?

Data on several exciting classes of compounds were presented at the conference. The working group felt that several of these approaches offered exciting possibilities for future applications in NCT, including boronated porphyrins, boronated monoclonal antibodies, boronothiouracil, boronated phenothiazines, and other classes. The working group discussed the need for additional studies of the biodistributions, toxicities, and efficacies of these compounds in animal systems.

DISCUSSION

Ryabukhin: When techniques were mentioned for determining boron *in vivo*, it was said that positron emission could be used. I think it should not be positron emission techniques but rather single-photon tomography (SPECT), because there are no positrons in neutron capture by boron. Did I understand it correctly, or perhaps you meant something else.

Larsson: We meant something else: Labeling of the boron compounds with positron emitters, without changing the structure of the boron compound.

Ryabukhin: I thought that you were talking about the determination of boron by prompt gamma. In this case, in principle, you can try to use SPECT.

Larsson: Maybe we can include neutron activation, but what we said about positron emission tomography is still true.

Madoc-Jones: I am surprised about your feelings regarding metastatic melanoma in brain, because I think that if you consider cutaneous metastatic melanoma on the trunk or in the extremities, there may be well-established, very good conventional surgery or local radiation that may be very effective. You will have to compete against those methods to be sure that ethically you can go with the new modality. In certain circumstances, there may be a problem there. I understand that it is easier to follow in terms of an endpoint, but that could pose a problem. When I think of brain metastasis and melanoma, one could almost turn the argument the other way around and say that in the case of metastatic melanoma in the brain, there really is no good conventional therapy, so you do not have that problem. I would have thought, therefore, that it would be reasonable to go with the new modality, even if there is some extra risk involved.

Rockwell: Could Dr. Allen respond to that? He was making the strongest case for the approach of extremity melanoma.

Allen: The class of patients at the Sydney Melanoma Clinic we are considering for this trial are a group for which conventional therapies were unsuitable. It is a very small class that underwent trials such as chemotherapy, immunotherapy and localized heating of the limbs. These patients had very intensive but unsuccessful treatment, and neutron capture therapy could easily provide a superior modality for them.

A second point is that only a thermal neutron beam is required for treating the superficial melanoma. I think that this is a major factor in supporting clinical trials with superficial melanomas, because I think we all agree ideally that until we have a keV or an epithermal neutron beam, one would not have the optimum neutron delivery system for deep-seated tumors of any sort.

Madoc-Jones: I have no disagreement with any of that. I am thinking in terms of an epithermal beam. May I make one other point? In our group, we also discussed the question of treating arterial-venous (A-V) malformations, for which there is already very excellent conventional treatment, not only with the protons, for example, at the Harvard Cyclotron, but also using a gamma pencil, which is said to be very effective. It does not make a lot of sense to me to be going ahead with this very complex way of treating a benign disorder that is already very effectively treated.

Larsson: The very reason for this project (and it actually is a project now) is that with the gamma unit, we have not been able to treat the larger heavy malformations. When heavy malformations are above 2 1/2 to 3 cm in size, they are extremely difficult to treat, either with protons or photons. The idea is to add a little of the dose to the pathological vessels to prepare the ground for the localized irradiation with protons or photons, making use of the sigmoid response function. I would consider that a typical case of adjuvant therapy, which is simply motivated by the fact that we have had very poor results in that area. Boron therapy is not for the small malformations which can be effectively treated now.

Sweet: I must join Madoc-Jones in challenging the concept that the proton beam would be unsuitable for large A-V malformations. The larger they are, the more massive the pools of blood and the more difficult they are to manage by any form of radiation; but that is the fundamental advantage of the proton beam over the focused photons using the Leksell apparatus. Two and one-half centimeters is not the upper limit of effective treatment by protons at the Harvard Cyclotron. As I commented to our group, Kjellberg recently treated his 1,000th case, a good many of whom had lesions that were larger than the 2-1/2 to 3-cm maximum for the gamma unit.

Larsson: We are aware of these accomplishments at Harvard and have worked with the proton beam ourselves. But the clinicians at Stockholm and Uppsala do not share this point of view.

Riaboukhine: I would like to continue this discussion on superficial melanoma or metastasis of melanoma to the brain. First, I think that we could add to the statement about superficial melanoma; mainly, that neutron capture therapy might be a method of choice in the case of tumors with signs of localized dissemination. Sometimes there are small, black dots, which are very difficult to deal with, either surgically or with conventional radiation therapy. A second point is that I do not see any contradiction between application of neutron capture therapy for both superficial melanoma and its metastasis, not only to the brain but to other tissues as well. I think that in our tests, we would take the following approach: If a patient were treated by neutron capture therapy for melanoma in an extremity and the outcome was good, then this patient would be a candidate for future treatment of distant melanoma metastasis with the same technique. I think it is much easier to defend that approach before any ethical committee rather than taking a patient whose prime tumor was treated by something else and treating his or her metastasis by neutron capture.

Mishima: First of all, "superficial melanoma" should not be confused with the medical term "superficially spreading melanoma" (SSM). The four major types of melanoma can be classified as superficially spreading melanoma and lentigo-malignant melanoma which spreads horizontally, while nodular melanoma and acral lentiginous melanoma proliferate predominantly in a vertical direction. These four types of melanoma exhibit distinctly different characteristics and have different prognoses.

Therefore, in general, when we discuss melanomas in the skin, we should call them cutaneous melanomas rather than superficial melanomas, which is easy to confuse with SSM. This is a small but important point. To establish NCT not only in prolonging the life of patients in an advanced stage of melanoma for whom no other effective therapy exists, but also subsequent to the success of the initial clinical trials, we must compare therapeutic data with conventional therapy, including multidiscipline surgery with immuno-chemotherapy. After demonstrating the superiority of NCT, then we can treat the primary melanoma on the face or extremities for example, without disfigurement.

Today melanoma specialists have a practical concept, that is, tumor thickness, for evaluating the chances of survival of a patient. If a patient has a melanoma 3-mm thick, then the probability of 5-year survival is less than 50%. Of 1,000 people treated for melanoma, 500 will die. For research purposes, we are dealing with the remaining 500 people, and we should consider boron neutron capture therapy. We should approach 99.9% survival of the patients using NCT. Why do 500 people die from a 3 mm tumor? They die because of subclinical satellite metastases, which already exist around the primary lesion, which surgeons cannot recognize and for which chemotherapy and immunotherapy are insufficient. However, our NCT can irradiate a much larger area, and melanoma-seeking ^{10}B compounds can eradicate metastases at the cellular level.

Bond: How well do your data indicate that it is the satellite cells that are responsible for the metastases?

Mishima: We have shown at the cellular level in the radiobiological studies, as well as with a small animal study, and a preclinical study and human study, and in prompt gamma and chemical assays, that the highly metastatic melanoma cells usually have the accentuated property of synthesizing melanin polymers within the premelansome by the action of oxidated enzyme tyrosinase, which attracts DOPA. In 10% or some small proportion of the cases, there is amelanotic melanoma in few of the metastatic lesions. But even these amelanotic lesions attract about 50% paraboronophenylalanine compared to melanotic melanoma. A second point is to educate the public to accept NCT as a "new" modality. It is very important to demonstrate this new modality with the best case. We discussed this approach with the Australian group led by Allen. Let us say that we have operated on the primary lesion. Around the scar, there is a great deal of superficial metastasis, but still not beyond stage II (metastasis is limited up to regional lymph nodes and no further), but let us say that there are 100 cutaneous metastases. You operate again when the disease recurs. We can see such a patient quite often, as melanoma specialists. These patients and their families endure a great deal of pain. These cases are also good target melanoma lesions for NCT.

WORKING GROUP ON OPTIMIZATION OF RADIATION DOSE DELIVERY

Moderators: Andre Wambersie

Catholic University of Louvain
Medical Faculty
Avenue Hippocrate 54, B-1200
Brussels, Belgium

Ludwig E. Feinendegen

Institut fur Medizin
Der Kerforschungsanlage Julich GmbH
Postfach 1913, D-5170 Julich I
West Germany

INTRODUCTION

For a long time, it has been the dreams of radiotherapists and oncologists to have molecules or drugs which could seek and specifically reach and destroy cancer cells. These molecules or drugs could be toxic in several ways:

- chemically
- because they are labelled with an appropriate radionuclide
- because they can be made toxic in the cancer cell

Boron compounds can become toxic through thermal neutron irradiation, causing the $^{10}B(n,\alpha)^{7}Li$ reaction.

The latter is the rationale of boron neutron capture therapy (NCT). There are at least three clinical situations where selective toxicity at the cellular level may be attainable:

1. For brain tumors which destroy the blood-brain barrier (BBB), normal cells of the central nervous system (CNS) are protected by the BBB from toxic compounds present in the blood.
2. Some tumors with a specific metabolism through which a toxic component can be selectively incorporated (for example, synthesis of melanin in melanomas).
3. Tumors against which monoclonal antibodies or polyclonal antibodies can be prepared, for instance, some bronchogenic carcinomas, prostatic adenocarcinomas, and breast tumors.

The particular problem of brain tumors has been well known for many years. Already in the 1950's and 1960's, two NCT programs were started in the United States. Later, the technique was extended in Japan.

In recent years, significant progress has been made in the two other clinical situations, utilizing specific tumor metabolism and antibodies. Mishima presented his data on the treatment of melanoma in animals and in humans. He uses p-boronophenylalanine, which is incorporated into melanin pigment and, thus, concentrates in tumor cells. It is encouraging to see that research in this direction has reached the stage of clinical application. The progress in the field of monoclonal and polyclonal antibodies is also very fast: there is no need to emphasize the huge amounts of effort and money invested in that direction. Monoclonal and polyclonal antibodies are used today for diagnosis and tumor localization.

Neutron capture therapy will always have specific advantages over treatments which simply consist of injecting chemically toxic compounds or drugs labelled with a radionuclide. NCT encompasses two steps: injection of the boronated compound, and neutron irradiation. They are independent, can be applied separately and combined in different ways. Regarding the first step, the uptake of an appropriate boron compound in organs or tissues that will not be exposed to the neutron beam (for example, bone marrow, intestine, liver and kidney) is unimportant. The boronated compounds, in general,can be non-toxic by themselves. With respect to the second step, an optimal time between injection and irradiation can be selected. We know that the boron concentration varies with time in a different way in tumors, blood or normal tissues.

We shall concentrate on the treatment of brain tumors. However, some aspects of the discussion also could relate to the other applications of NCT. In the treatment of brain tumors, we shall consider successively the main problems which were discussed in our working group:

1. Neutron energy

2. Fractionation

3. Uniform incorporation of the boron compounds

NEUTRON ENERGY: THERMAL OR EPITHERMAL NEUTRON BEAMS

Ideally speaking, the neutron flux should be as homogeneous as possible over the volume of tissue to be treated. In this respect, some of the approaches currently used in external photon therapy can be applied to NCT:

1. For an optimal beam penetration and possibly some skin sparing, epithermal neutrons (or 2 keV neutrons) are superior to thermal neutrons; they provide a maximum thermal flux density between 1 and 4 cm in depth.

2. In many cases, a combination of several radiation beam directions could improve the neutron fluence distribution (for example, parallel opposed beams for centrally located tumors, parallel opposed beams with different weighting factors for laterally located tumors, and three-beam combinations).

To improve the homogeneity of the dose, the methods used in external beam therapy with photons could be applied. With photons a dose homogeneity of $\pm$10% is currently recommended over the target volume; some researchers aim at $\pm$5%.

It is recognized that positioning of the patient with reactor beams could raise specific problems. For certain beam orientations, the difficulties are much greater than with modern linear accelerators with isocentric mounting.

For superficial tumors, the poor penetration of thermal neutron beams is less of a handicap. However, it implies a surgical intervention with skull reflexion and an irradiation under general anesthesia. Here, fractionation is hardly possible and the only method for reducing damage to normal tissue is the protraction of the irradiation over several hours (low dose-rate irradiation). The Japanese experience showed that a protracted treatment in a single session of 4-8 hours can be tolerated. This could be explained by the fact that, due to the poor penetration of the thermal neutron beam, only a superficial part of the brain is heavily irradiated. In conventional photon therapy, for example, for skin tumors limited in size, a small number of large fractions is sometimes applied for practical reasons, although it is recognized to be less than ideal from a radiobiological point of view.

With respect to the clinical experience from Japan, a desirable demand for reproducing the data must be weighed against the need to employ, for human use, the most recent available facilities, modalities and basic research data.

FRACTIONATED VERSUS SINGLE PROTRACTED IRRADIATION

Historically, the benefit of fractionation in radiotherapy has been evident for many decades, and most of the attempts made to reduce the fraction number were disastrous. This fact should be kept in mind when developing the NCT fractionation scheme, although it is recognized that the situations are not identical.

The following discussion applies only to using epithermal and not to thermal neutron beams for the reasons discussed above (need for surgical intervention with skull reflexion, general anesthesia).

Acute Tolerance of the Brain

Fractionation improves acute tolerance. Acute reactions could be dangerous and should be feared mainly when large volumes and deep-seated volumes have to be treated. However, as discussed before, a greater tolerance is observed for irradiation of brain tumors laterally located and tumors of small size.

Improvement of the Late Tolerance to the Gamma Irradiation

Besides the alpha irradiation originating from the boron compound, the epithermal neutron beam produces an unavoidable irradiation of the brain consisting of a low-LET and a high-LET component. In actual situations, the neutron flux to be used depends on the boron concentration. Typically a thermal neutron fluence of 3×10^{12} n/cm (produced by an epithermal neutron fluence of 1×10^{12} n/cm^2) delivers to the brain about 0.6 Gy high-LET and about 6 Gy low-LET radiation. For gamma rays, it is well known that the tolerance dose is increased when the dose per fraction is reduced and that some benefit is still observed, especially for late effects, for fractional doses smaller than 2 Gy. From that point of view, fractionation contributes to protecting the normal brain, but the benefit of this factor depends on the total gamma dose. Fractionation also improves the tolerance against the high-LET component, but to a much lesser extent.

Modification of the Blood-Brain Barrier

One concern when using fractionated irradiation is that the first fraction would modify the permeability of the BBB so that boron compounds could then be incorporated into normal brain tissue. A survey of the experimental and clinical data indicates that the BBB is highly radio-resistant and that doses at least as high as 20 Gy (acute irradiation) are necessary to significantly alter BBB permeability. This finding seems to be true also for high-LET radiations. Therefore, concern about alteration of the BBB is probably unjustified for the fractionation schemes which will be discussed below. Nevertheless, the available modern equipment, such as NMR and PET, should be used to substantiate the existing experimental data on the alteration of BBB in patients for various molecules and compounds, and for various fractionation schemes.

Fractionation and Boron Compound Distribution

Since each fraction presently demands the administration of the boron compound, it can reasonably be assumed that the homogeneity of the distribution of the boron compound will be improved after repeated administration, and that boron will reach all parts of the tumor as a result of redistribution in the cell compartments, changes in tumor structure and local perfusion, as discussed below.

Practical Aspects of Fractionation

Fractionation versus continuous low dose-rate irradiation. For the low-LET component of the radiation, fractionation and protracted (low dose-rate) irradiation both allow for repair of sublethal damage and would improve the tolerance of normal tissue in a similar way. However, to achieve full repair of sublethal damage with a single protracted irradiation, the duration of the exposure would be excessive and would raise practical difficulties.

Fraction number. To increase the tolerance of normal tissue to the gamma component of the irradiations, a fraction number between 4 and 6 can be considered acceptable. For the current NCT schemes, this would imply a gamma dose per fraction not greater than about 2 Gy, and there is no substantial benefit in further reducing the dose per fraction. For NCT facilities having a larger gamma component from external sources, the fraction number could be increased accordingly, to avoid doses per fraction much greater than 2 Gy.

In view of the novelty of using epithermal neutrons in humans, a dose escalation protocol should be followed.

Overall time. For repair of sublethal lesions in slowly proliferating tissues, between 8 to 12 hours is needed. Therefore, the interval between fractions could be 1 to 2 days: this is a compromise between a reduction of the overall time to avoid tumor cell proliferation and a longer interval to allow for greater changes in tumor structure and local tumor perfusion.

Duration of sessions. From a radiobiological point of view, in relation to the gamma component, little sparing of normal tissue from intracellular repair is to be expected as long as the individual fractions are about 2 Gy or less. Thus, there is little reason to choose exposure durations of an hour or more versus a few minutes, other than to increase the patient's comfort with shorter sessions.

As far as the characteristics of the reactors are concerned, and assuming typically 6 fractions of 2 Gy:

- a duration of exposure for 1-2 minutes would require 10^{10} $n.cm^{-2}.s^{-1}$, and only one reactor in the United States could answer the demand;

- a duration of exposure of about 10 minutes would require 10^9 $n.cm^{-2}.s^{-1}$, and about six reactors in the United States could be made to deliver this;

- a duration of exposure of about 1 hour would require 10^8 $n.cm^{-2}.s^{-1}$, and about 20 reactors in the United States could be available for this.

UNIFORM INCORPORATION OF THE BORON COMPOUND

A uniform incorporation of the boron compound into or near all cancer cells is the basic requirement to fully cure a tumor by NCT. Three different types of clinical situations are schematically identified in Figure 1: [a] No previous surgery - In the "tumor volume," the viable cancer cells are mixed with non-viable cancer cells, necrotic areas, blood vessels and eventually some normal tissue. Some viable cancer cells also exist in the safety margin surrounding the tumor volume. [b] After "incomplete" surgical reaction, some gross tumor tissue is left [as in situation A]. Subclinical involvement by isolated cancer cells or microscopic clusters of cancer cells is also present. In addition, vascularization has been altered by previous surgery. [c] After "radical" surgery, in principle, there is only subclinical involvement but the local vascularization has been altered by previous surgery. There are many obstacles preventing uniform incorporation, such as tumor structure and local tumor perfusion (Fig. 1); they have some similarity to those factors involved when using hypoxic cell sensitizers in photon therapy. It is difficult to prove that boron compounds reach all cancer cells, and, in that respect, autoradiographic studies have well known weaknesses:

- They analyze only a sample of the tissue, as do all histological methods.

- Even in a given section, a small fraction of the cells could escape analysis. However, high resolution autoradiography may improve the situation.

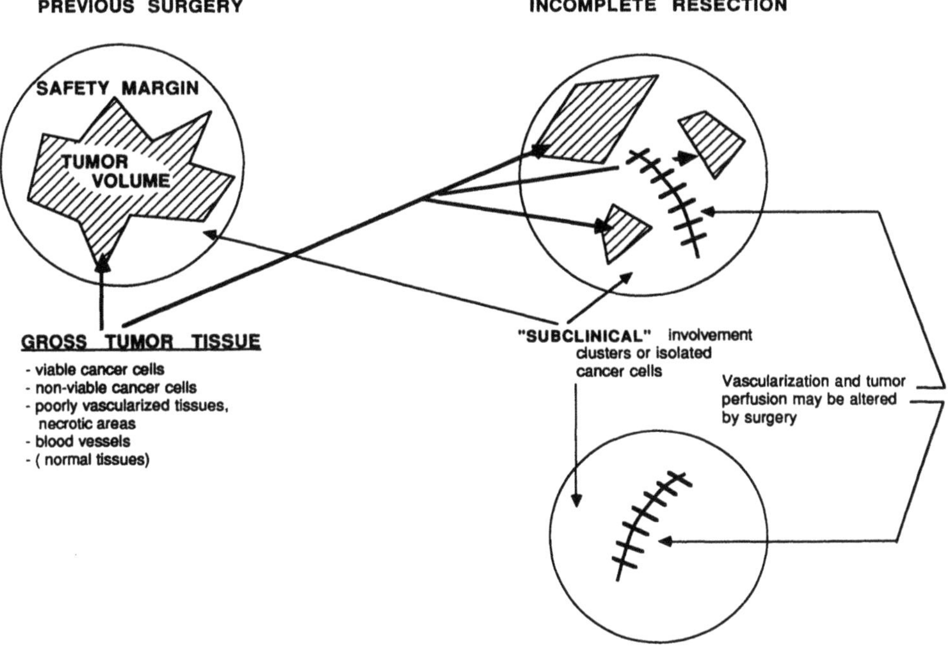

Fig. 1. The challenge of NCT in treatment of glioblastoma in brain is to incorporate boron compounds in all viable cancer cells.

Another experimental approach which was proposed at the previous BNL Workshop on NCT treats different types of animal tumors with NCT and compares the observed rate of tumor control with that expected, assuming a uniform boron distribution. One perplexing problem is the difficulty evidently encountered in proving biological efficacy with the monomer and dimer forms of the sulfhydryl boron hydride in small animal tumor models. Similar troubles have not been encountered with p-boronophenylalanine; for melanomas in BALB mice, the tumor control rate after NCT indeed was comparable to that expected, assuming a uniform boron distribution.

New boron compounds, with appropriate diffusion ranges, are expected to improve the present situation and repeated administrations of the compound associated with fractionation therapy may finally result in all tumor cells being exposed to alpha particles.

In conclusion, when evaluating the effects of high-LET particles originating from the boron neutron capture, the classic concepts of target volume, treatment volume and irradiation volume developed for external beam therapy can no longer be applied. Even the concept of absorbed dose, which involves integration over a macroscopic volume of a large number of elementary events has to be adapted for BNCT.

It is recommended that the effects of the different NCT modalities, which were discussed above, be monitored by *in vivo* observation methods such as radionuclide uptake, PET, MRI, so that eventually the optimal treatment can be tailored to the individual tumor. In NCT, as always in radiation therapy, the therapeutic results must be judged in the light of possible host-tumor effects.

Finally, it is considered advisable that, before starting clinical trials in the United States, such trials be reviewed and coordinated with other NCT projects by a small international group composed of individuals such as those brought together in the current workshop.

DISCUSSION

Zamenhof: At the beginning of your presentation, you mentioned that typical numbers for an epithermal beam for a generated thermal neutron fluence of ~3 x 10^{12} n/cm^2 were ~3,000 (rad x RBE) for a tumor loaded with boron, and I think you said that was ~4 times the normal tissue dose; presumably that value was calculated with a certain boron concentration in mind. Since today we are talking about the BSH compound when we make these estimates, those approximate concentrations are intuitively recognized as being 40-60 μg/g. Two years from now when many other compounds will be available which may have very different accumulation levels, it may not be obvious to the reader where that number came from unless you put into parentheses what boron concentration that dose assumed.

Wambersie: I agree with your comment, of course, and I think I said that this dose depends on the boron concentration. With a ^{10}B concentration of 35 μg $^{10}B/g$ and an RBE of 3.3 the dose from ^{10}B would be 3000 (rad x RBE) with a thermal neutron fluence of 3×10^{12} n/cm^2.

Ryabukhin: I would like to add that this depends not only on the boron concentration but on the diameter of the beam. For different beams, the difference is very substantial.

Zamenhof: Yes, I agree with Dr. Riaboukhine, but I think we are talking about different order effects. You are probably talking about effects of a factor of 2 either way, whereas with an unknown boron concentration, you could be talking about two orders of magnitude.

Soloway: The question of the breakdown of the blood-brain barrier potential with fractionated doses might have a clear benefit because there might be some tumor cells in normal tissue that would escape the boron compound reaching those cells. Having some breakdown of the barrier might permit the compounds to achieve higher concentrations there, become incorporated and then, over a period of time, leach out of the normal brain. Thus, even if there is some breakdown in the blood-brain barrier, it may not be altogether undesirable for localization.

Hopewell: We discussed this problem of the breakdown of the blood-brain barrier quite extensively, and we should make the point that with the doses of fraction we are talking about, or the equivalent single doses in terms of photons, there really is no evidence of any acute breakdown of the blood-brain barrier. I can see the advantage, but I do not think it will happen.

Allen: With relation to the hypoxic cell effect for highly fractionated radiotherapy, the effect seems to disappear. We seem to be talking about quite small fractions in neutron capture therapy. Is there any expectation that there still might not be a significant hypoxic cell effect, and therefore perhaps a significant variation in the uptake of boron compounds into the tumor cells?

Larsson: We discussed this aspect very carefully. I believe we have to take into account the passive diffusion range of the compound, as well as the active uptake of the compound into the cell. The diffusion range is important and varies considerably from drug to drug. With the advent of newer compounds.

Rockwell: Perhaps I could comment on the hypoxic cell sensitizer trials and the experimental work. The cell culture studies on which the sensitizer trials were based used very high concentrations of hypoxic cell sensitizers and showed very spectacular enhancement ratios. In the initial animal trials with single doses, it was possible to get millimolar concentrations of sensitizer into the animal tumors and good sensitization was obtained. As we move toward fractionated studies in the animals, it became clear that there was a maximal total dose of sensitizer that the animals could tolerate, and that it was not possible to use these high doses repeatedly in the animals. In fact, when tumor control studies were done in the animals with fractionation regimens at a maximally tolerated dose of sensitizers, the sensitizer enhancement ratios fell to about 1.1 to 1.3 (depending on who did the trials). This work was done with large radiation doses per fraction. Extrapolating from these studies to predict what one might expect to do in the clinical situation, many of us in the radiobiology community questioned whether a significant enhancement of radiation response could be expected in the proposed clinical trials with hypoxic cell sensitizers and questioned whether some of the trials should have been done with the existing agents using the regimens that were proposed. I think, in retrospect, we were correct in raising these questions. I do not think that that same limitation would necessarily apply to the boron neutron capture therapy trials.

Mishima: I enjoyed Wambersie's beautiful summary and discussion of the fractionation, but I would like to point out that fractionation in NCT and current radiotherapy is different. I think the administration of ^{10}B compounds in fractions is very important. I discussed with Coderre his findings and our experiments with animals and humans and the compounds used. If we can achieve a uniform distribution of ^{10}B compounds, then hypoxic cells and cell cycles are less important because we are using high-LET particles and great amounts of energy at the cellular level, resulting in no cellular repair.

The ^{10}B atoms in melanoma cells are located in the innumerable melanosomes that occur in each cell. Each melanosome is about 0.6 μm in diameter and contains countless ^{10}B atoms in the melanin polymers. When irradiated, lithium atoms and gamma rays randomly hit their own and neighboring nuclei within a distance of 9 microns. The ^{10}B atoms can exist at the center of the cell, next to the nucleus, and also at the periphery. Melanosomes are synthesized in the golgi complex near the nucleus, but as they mature from steps 1 through 4, the melanosomes move to the periphery of the cell. Therefore, you can have a small amount of heterogeneity in the distribution of ^{10}B compound. Thus, lack of homogeneity is not as critical as may be thought.

Feinendegen: We discussed that problem, too, and I think that all that you said is right, but, in the group's opinion, there were three reasons for applying the fractionated scheme of radiation for brain tumors. One is the sparing of normal tissue. Second, as you pointed out, is the chance of repeat administration of the compound to assure an optimal distribution of the compound eventually to all tumor cells to be reached by an alpha particle. Third, it also was thought that one could increase the tolerance level of the blood-brain barrier. I think that if you take these reasons together, then the fractionation scheme is very well justified despite the fact that, for your case, indeed, a single exposure with the compound homogeneously distributed in the tumor leading to cure is the right thing to do.

Bond: Dr. Mishima, what is your ratio of melanaffinic compound in the tumor to that in the adjacent normal tissue?

Mishima: I forgot to emphasize last night that during the preclinical study with my patients, I used one administration of ^{10}B compound one day before, and a second administration in the morning 6 hours before irradiation. Then we irradiated in the afternoon. I showed that the tumor-to-blood ratio is, under optimal conditions, about 15 times higher.

Dorn: At the risk of sounding like a voice crying out from the Idaho wilderness, a couple of comments on fractionation and the blood-brain barrier. First, I am in complete agreement that the data and, certainly, our instincts would suggest that fractionation is probably the best way to go. I think we would certainly hope so, because it will allow several additional reactors to be used and more treatments to be undertaken. However, I do not think that the conclusion that the blood-brain barrier is an unjustified concern is really appropriate. In fact, there are data in the literature showing that doses under 2000 Gy in a single exposure causes a breakdown in the blood-brain barrier. Further, the breakdown increases as the number of fractions increases. Experiments in this direction might turn out to be very useful. I would lean a little more heavily toward doing some preclinical animal studies to try to get a better perspective on this, specifically with respect to the boron compound. Second, with regard to incorporation of the boron compound, the statement was made that with fractionation and repeated injections, we could expect a better uptake of the boron compound. I have two brief comments. One, I think that we have to be careful, since steroids are used liberally in the treatment of brain tumors, and we do not know whether their use improves or worsens the uptake of the boron compound. Two, there is at least one paper in the recent literature suggesting that an ionizing radiation component may decrease the tumor uptake of substances; in other words, the passing of substances from the blood through what would be termed the blood-tumor barrier. I think that this might need to be further characterized. In fact, fractionation and its impact on the uptake of boron in the tumor may play a role.

Barth: I understood that Dr. Mishima said his compound was injected around the tumor (peritumorally) and not given systemically. If you think that this compound does preferentially localize in the tumor, why did you inject it peritumorally rather than systemically?

Mishima: I was waiting for such questions. I did an experiment some years ago injecting the compound at different distances from the melanoma--1, 2, 3, 5, 6 and 7 cm. At present, we have avoided i.v. injections in humans because the ^{10}B-BPA solution must be very highly acidic for complete solubility, we did the experiment on pigs. For humans, we injected into areas 4 cm away from the tumor's margin. The compound goes in by two ways: by perfusion and by circulation in the blood. In our first melanoma patient, when the blood concentration of ^{10}B was about 1 to 2 ppm, the concentration in the tumor was around 25 ppm (10-30). If the distance of the perilesional injection to the margin of the tumor is greater, the ^{10}B concentration in the melanoma would be a little lower. To synthesize a compound in the laboratory is very expensive. Therefore the compound is given as perilesional injections 4 cm away from the tumor, since amounts are insufficient to give systemically for a 70 kg patient, even though our compound preferentially localizes in the melanoma.

Without hydrochloric acid, it is very difficult to dissolve our present compound, but we found that since the stomach is at pH 1.5, there is good solubility. We gave the compound to hamsters by stomach tube, and there was good accumulation in the melanoma. We did the same with the pig, and also had good accumulation. Although we need a large amount of the compound, since we are getting more funds, next time we are planning to administer the compound by mouth.

Barth: Did you ever try to give the disodium $B_{12}H_{11}SH$, the sulfhydryl compound, peritumorally? Did you ever try to give ^{10}B-enriched boric acid peritumorally? What kinds of differences did you see?

Mishima: A tremendous difference. We found that non-specific ^{10}B boric acid gave only the same level in the blood as in the tumor in our experimental systems.

Barth: Was there a difference with the sulfhydryl compound?

Mishima: I have not tried that compound.

Gabel: I would like to raise one point concerning the homogeneous distribution of boron compounds in tumors. I think it is very clear from our work and from the work from Idaho that if there is one cell in a tumor that does not pick up boron, this cell will receive only about a 50% dose compared with the other tumor cells; this is a tremendous reduction in dose. I think that a multiple exposure of the tumor cells to the drugs and subsequently to the neutron beam, might kill more cells. A second point is that I am not quite sure for what we are aiming. What was done clinically in Japan was to get the boron to the tumor cells; this killed the tumor, because there was quite a lot of boron in the blood. Perhaps what actually happened was that the blood vessels in the tumor were damaged to such a degree that the tumor died because of insufficient blood supply. I think this possibility might be kept in mind, at least for basic studies. Perhaps a low boron level in the blood, at least for the BSH compound, may not necessarily be a benefit but might be a disadvantage.

Sweet: What is the evidence for your statement that multiple administrations of the boron compound are likely to lead to a more homogeneous distribution, with a greater number of the tumor cells having taken up the compound on day 3, or a different group of tumor cells on day 3 than day 1. I know of only one study we ourselves made that has a bearing on that question. We gave a substantial dose of boron to one patient and then, during his operation, obtained about 12 to 15 different tumor samples. There was a tremendous variation in the boron concentration from one sample to another. When this patient died 10 or 12 days later, we sampled again at post-mortem; if anything, there was an even larger variation from sample to sample in the boron content. This is a tremendous problem and I am not aware of any evidence that giving the boron on different days is going to help significantly to solve it.

Feinendegen: May I answer that directly? It might be a misunderstanding to use the term homogeneous. What is to be understood is that through successive applications, a successive heterogenous distribution will, due to the changes in the heterogeneity, eventually reach all tumor cells. The changes in heterogeneity are being brought about by the alteration of tumor structure and local perfusion.

Sweet: Have you evidence to that effect?

Feinendegen: There is some evidence that, following radiotherapy, the structure and the perfusion in the tumor changes, and it is hoped that through these structural and local perfusion changes and repeated heterogeneity in distribution, eventually all tumor cells will be reached.

Sweet: If I could make a further comment, what the neurosurgeon does the first time around--which has been referred to in an unattractive way as debulking--is to do his or her best to remove all grossly apparent tumor tissue so that what is left is not likely to be subject to so much variation in concentration as the main tumor mass. Again, we have absolutely no evidence whatsoever to substantiate that hope.

Wambersie: I would like to answer on two points. First, I want to mention that hypoxic cells are another example illustrating the difficulty of incorporating a drug into all the cancer cells. It is true, however, that the situation is not identical in NCT. Second, regarding the comment of Mishima on the choice between one fraction and several fractions, I agree that one fraction would be ideal. Also, in conventional photon therapy, it would be much easier to treat a patient in one session of 10 minutes. Unfortunately, the whole clinical experience from over several decades indicates that it does not work.

Parts of the tumor cell population are resistant at each fraction. This could be due to the fact that some cells are in a resistant phase of the mitotic cycle, or because there is a lack of blood supply in some parts of the tumor and some proportions of the cells become hypoxic or do not incorporate a sensitizer (in the case of BNCT, would not incorporate the boron compound). During the course of a fractionated irradiation, these factors are altered: cells progress in the mitotic cycle, tumor structure and local perfusion are modified, reoxygenation takes place. These changes reduce the risk of missing some resistant parts of the tumor cell population.

Wielopolski: I have two comments with regard to Sweet's comment. Because of the more stochastic nature of the boron uptake by multiple infusions, there is a better probability of better coverage, not in cell uniformity but just in coverage in a larger number of cells. Also, regarding the modification or modulation of the possible boron uptake and the sensitivity of the absorbed dose due to boron, it was mentioned but not emphasized that *in vivo* monitoring before the treatment or during the treatment should be done either by MRI or prompt gamma.

Zamenhof: First, in response to a comment made by Wielopolski, I do not know of any evidence that the boron uptake by tumor cells is governed by stochastic rules. We agree that the activation of boron by neutrons is stochastic, but the uptake is probably not. Gabel commented that a possible explanation of some of Hatanaka's successes was that the boron in the blood was destroying the tumor vasculature and thereby starving the tumor. If that is the case, and assuming the uniform distribution of boron through all blood compartments, why would one not have observed a vasculature effect on normal tissue? Two further comments: one is, that in terms of giving direction and encouragement to people working on developing better compounds either for brain tumors or for melanoma, I think it might be worthwhile to officially recognize a paper by Gabel and Fairchild et al., that showed quite conclusively--albeit on a theoretical basis--that if one compares the boron around a cell against that within a cell against that within the nucleus, one gradually and substantially increases the bioeffectiveness of the boron reaction. I think that by putting this into our recommendations, we would recognize the fact that ideally we should be seeking compounds that are not only tumor affinic but ones which are affinic for the nucleus of the tumor cell and maybe even for DNA.

My last comment is that we here appear to have a very effective consensus regarding the direction for neutron capture therapy. Sometime in the future, someone will be ready to consider treating the first patient in the United States by neutron capture therapy. I think we are all working toward that same end, and we should all be working together. I suggest that whoever is in this position should present his or her proposal to a group such as ours to provide an extended amount of time for discussion so that we may reach a congressional-type consensus regarding the suitability of carrying forward with the treatment. If something should go wrong, this would then prevent people from turning around and saying, "Well, we do not think you should have treated the patient in the first place."

Bond: In regard to your comments on dosimetry, that point was recognized in Wambersie's summary and indirectly in his comments with respect to the unsuitability of absorbed dose.

Larsson: The importance of a homogeneous boron uptake is obvious. As an illustration of this general problem in NCT, I choose an autoradiograph of radioactive antibodies as they are targeting on tumor-associated antigens in a cell spheroid derived from a human colorectal carcinoma cell line (Fig. 1). Such a tumor cell spheroid simulates quite well a volume of intercapillary tumor tissue. We know, by parallel experiments, that the antibodies, at the time of freeze-fixation, have had time to penetrate the spheroid and so the severe inhomogeneity in uptake is mainly a result of variations in the cellular antigen expression, or in the efficacy of internalization of the antibody complex formed. It seems quite likely that the different metabolic activity and cell proliferation activity at various depths in the spheroid could lead to a nonuniform uptake, but on top of that there is also an obvious and strong variation between cells at the same radius. The latter phenomenon may be dependent on the nonuniform genetic constitution of cells in the colony or on variations as a function of the position of the cells in the cell cycle. It should be noted that the cells, in the spheroid here chosen as an example, are known to express the antigens in an extremely heterogeneous way.

Soloway: One of the reasons for multiple injection is that we really do not know, certainly in the case of the sulfhydryl compound, why it localizes. We know that once in the tumor cell, the compound does not equilibrate as readily with the blood. So multiple injections might result in higher incorporations of the compound. With respect to some of the amino acids, it would seem to me that in a rapidly proliferating tissue, there will be incorporation which will depend on the cell cycle. If the problem of adminstering the compound that Mishima spoke about was due to the problems of formulation, such as the acidity of the material, there are ways of dealing with that. For example, we dissolved compounds in albumin and simply adjusted the pH down to normal without getting any precipitation. There are techniques one can use if there is a question of solubility of the material without causing any trauma to the vasculature.

Wielopolski: I would like to answer Soloway's comment. The phenomenum of uptake is controlled by the local dynamics or physiology. If we could count the cells with boron uptake, we would end up with some sort of distribution; if one could

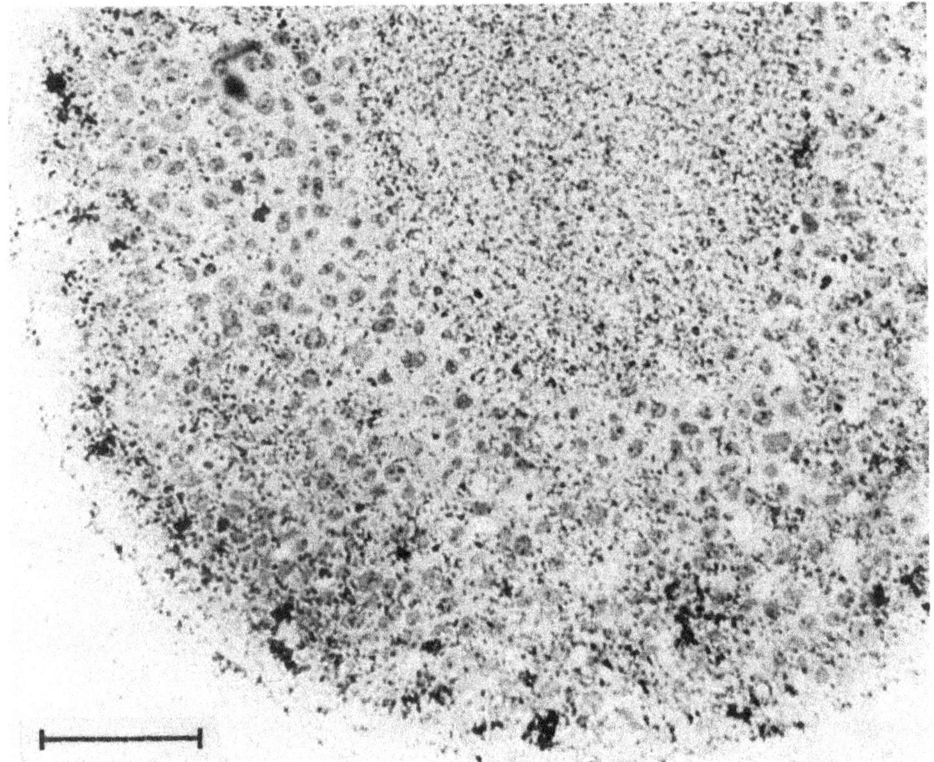

Fig. 1. Example of an autoradiogram of a HT29 spheroid incubated for 8 hours with 125-I-38S1 anti-CEA antibodies. After incubation the spheroid was fixed in formalin, embedded and sectioned in methacrylate and finally processed for autoradiography. The photographed section was stained with haemotoxylin. The labelled cells were arranged in clusters preferentially in the peripheral regions of the spheroid. Nearly no positive cells were seen close to the necrotic areas.
The bar indicates 100 μm.
(Personal communication: Jorgen Carlsson, Inst. Radiation Sciences, Uppsala University, Sweden)

repeat the experiment it would be modified by neutron radiation ionization and other phenomena resulting in another distribution. In this sense and not in a classical sense, it will be stochastic all the way but will result in some variable distribution.

Rockwell: This is not a question so much as a comment on this general subject of blood flow and its variability within tumors. There has been a great deal of renewed interest in this area in animal tumors because of the problem of oxygen distribution, and there is now an accumulating body of data on transplanted tumors in animals, on human tumors xenografted into nude mice, and on spontaneous tumors in animals that proves that there is variability in blood flow through individual tumor blood vessels. These studies were made with time-lapse cinematography on individual blood vessels. Studies also were done where two dyes were injected into an animal at different times. In addition to areas where both dyes were present the tumors also contained areas reached by only one or the other of the two dyes. There also were studies done with NAD/NADPH fluorescence in these tumors, which point to the same conclusion that within tumors and, indeed, even within microscopic tumors and residual disease, there is variation in blood flow through individual blood vessels that may affect the distribution of dyes and, by the same token, other compounds as well.

Gabel: I would like to make one suggestion that falls into the vein of what Zamenhof said. I think there was a general consensus that a study of the pharmacokinetics of BSH should be carried out. I would like to urge this panel, as it represents the majority of all people who are interested in trying to coordinate these studies, to ensure that these studies are not needlessly repeated. Unsuccessful studies may be carried out in different places and successful studies often are not known until a subsequent workshop takes place. Indeed, there should be a working group to coordinate these studies, to serve as a central mailbox and perhaps also give some input. I suggest that this could be done at Brookhaven in the United States, for instance, and at Bremen in Europe. Such a coordination is necessary and desirable, and should be taken up in the final recommendations.

Ryabukhin: I completely agree with what Zamenhof and Gabel have just said. I would like to see a group such as that in the Soviet Union, before the first Soviet patient is treated with neutron capture therapy, which could discuss preclinical preparations to such treatment. It is not only the problem in the United States or Western Europe, but it is a problem for any group preparing for the clinical applications of neutron capture therapy.

My second point is that we should regard the heterogeneity of incorporation just as a rule. Homogeneity would be the exception, but in general, we have to live with heterogeneity. There are many arguments for that, like those which Dr.

Rockwell just gave. Let us take, for instance, a well-known phenomenon such as the incorporation of tracer iodine into thyroid follicles; iodine is incorporated very heterogeneously.

Mishima: In regard to international cooperation, we have been doing government-to-government work with an Australian research group and the Japanese group. Of course, I am waiting to cooperate in whatever way is necessary for the benefit of humankind. One short comment about Professor Larsson's comment. There is a necrotic area and ^{10}B-paraboronophenylalanine requires metabolic activity. However, the $^{10}B_{12}$ chloropromazine does not require metabolic activity. In the test tube, isolated melanin granules and chloropromazine will bind by π electron interaction within the nucleus or melanin. For a necrotic area, we can accumulate ^{10}B chloropromazine.

Durrant: I wish to support the idea set forth by Zamenhof and Gabel that there should be a cooperative group. There is a precedent to follow: in 1985, a consensus group was held on the treatment of breast cancer. One of the objectives of that group was to provide guidance as to what should be standard treatment. The most valuable result was the consensus on development of clinical trials from that time onward. I can see a group such as playing a similar role in guidance in the future.

Madoc-Jones: I would like to have some clarification on the question of fractionation and the number 4 to 6 fractions. It was my understanding, while listening at the workshop, that the number 4 to 6 came out of a discussion by Hopewell, and it would be justified on the basis of the small benefit in protecting normal tissue from the effect of the high-LET radiation. If there were a substantial gamma component, this might justify further fractionation from 6 to maybe 10 or more. That was not the conclusion I heard in the report, and therefore, I would like to clarify that.

Wambersie: I said, in the report, that a fraction number of four to six can be considered as acceptable to increase the normal brain tolerance for the gamma component. Assuming a typical BNCT scheme delivering a total dose of about 6 Gy gamma irradiation, four to six fractions would correspond to a gamma dose per fraction smaller than 1.5 Gy. Of course, if the total gamma dose would be much larger than 6 Gy, higher fraction numbers should be considered.

The tolerance dose for normal tissues increases when increasing the fraction number (i.e. reducing the dose per fraction). However, for brain late tolerance, when the dose per fraction becomes smaller than about 1.5 Gy, there is no further increase in tolerance when further reducing the dose per fraction. For neutrons, the effect of fraction size is less important.

Mishima: Many people have asked me about administration of ^{10}B-paraboronophenylalanine. We have already started to give this compound by mouth and a single oral administration of ^{10}B, although it is a hydrochloric acid compound, to Greene's melanoma-bearing hamster, gives selective uptake that results in the accumulation of 20-25 ppm of ^{10}B in the melanoma.

Larsson: I would like to mention the coupling between systemic treatment with radioactive cell seekers and boron neutron capture therapy. One very important issue is the demonstration by scanning techniques of the microscopic behavior of compounds. We are particularly interested in growth factors and antibodies. We found that there is a potential in the use of boron as a tracer for basic medical studies in human beings because then one has a stable tracer, the boron-10; in addition, one can radiolabel the same boronated molecules with positron emitters which can then be used as radiopharmaceuticals. We find selenium-73 valuable, for example, and the combination of selenium-73 and boron makes a very nice entity, in principle, because it makes it possible to outline the behavior of the molecules, both in terms of macroscopic behavior in the body and microscopic behavior. It is important to have a label on the same molecule, because otherwise one will always debate whether the two populations of molecules will behave differently. This is one very important way to make tracer studies at tracer diagnostic levels by double-label compounds. I would be very interested in getting in touch with persons having the same kind of philosophy, particularly when it comes to growth factors and antibodies.

Zamenhof: I would like to suggest to Larsson that maybe he should inform the public about the status of the International Society for Neutron Capture Therapy and the proposed newsletter. I think we should all become members if we are not already, and the newsletter may be a very good vehicle for exchanging information rapidly.

Gabel: I did not want to make this a "commercial" but perhaps I should. There is an International Society for Neutron Capture Therapy, and the membership in this Society is a one-time lifetime fee of 20 international response coupons, which I think everyone could nearly pay out of his or her own pockets (a rather small cost). This Society tries to keep its members up to date with current points and publishes a newsletter twice a year which lists new publications in the field, draws attention to meetings such as this one, and conveys notices on what has come out of these meetings, addresses of contact, etc. It is also trying to publish an index of all known papers on neutron capture therapy back to 1940 or 1936 when this was originated. By doing so, we can definitely promote and cross-fertilize our efforts. Those who wish to become members should send 20 international response coupons plus a very short c.v. to Hatanaka in Tokyo, who is the secretary of the Society, and then notify the president of your membership in order to receive the regular mailings.

BLOOD-BRAIN-BARRIER IMPAIRMENT AFTER IRRADIATION: IMPLICATION IN BORON NEUTRON CAPTURE THERAPY

V. Grégoire, André Keyeux and André Wambersie

Université Catholique de Louvain
Unité de Radiobiologie et de Radioprotection
1200 Brussels, Belgium

INTRODUCTION

The rationale of boron neutron capture therapy (BNCT) in brain tumors rests on the assumption that the boronated compounds will not be incorporated in the normal CNS protected by the tight blood-brain barrier (BBB) but will enter the tumor at the level at which the BBB is impaired.[1]

If fractionation is to be used in BNCT, or if BNCT would follow external radiotherapy, the question is: To what extent could the fractions (or the previous treatment) alter the BBB? To answer this question, it is necessary to assess the integrity of the BBB after different levels of absorbed dose and different time intervals.

A brief summary of the structure and physiology of the BBB in the normal brain and tumor will be presented first, followed by a review of the published data concerning alteration of the BBB after cerebral irradiation.

STRUCTURE AND PHYSIOLOGY OF THE BLOOD-BRAIN-BARRIER

The BBB separates the brain and cerebrospinal fluid from the blood flow and plays a major role in the homeostasis of the central nervous system.[2]

Already in 1909, Goldman showed that Trypan Blue was excluded from the rabbit brain when injected intravenously but not when given intracerebrally.[3] This observation supported the concept that the BBB was an exclusionary interface separating brain from blood. This concept was progressively abandoned, and it is now well established that the BBB acts as a regulatory interface; it governs the composition of the microenvironment of the neurons in controlling the exchange of ions, metabolites and metabolic products between blood and brain.[2]

The BBB is composed of thin capillaries surrounded by a continuous basement membrane which is, in turn, surrounded by glial cells covering approximately 85% of the capillary surface (Fig. 1).[2] Electron microscopic study shows that endothelial cells are connected to each other by tight junctions which form a continuous layer without fenestration.[4] The junctions restrain intercellular diffusion; transport from blood to neural cells must then traverse the endothelium. It was suggested by many authors that the BBB is not so much a physical as a chemical barrier involving the endothelia of the brain capillaries.[2,5] Different mechanisms such as simple diffusion, active transport with specific enzymes or receptors, facilitated diffusion or ionic channel, account for transport of ionic and non-ionic substances from blood to neurons.[2] However, the rate and pathway of entry depend on the molecular weight and electric charge of the substance, their lipidic solubility, the polarity

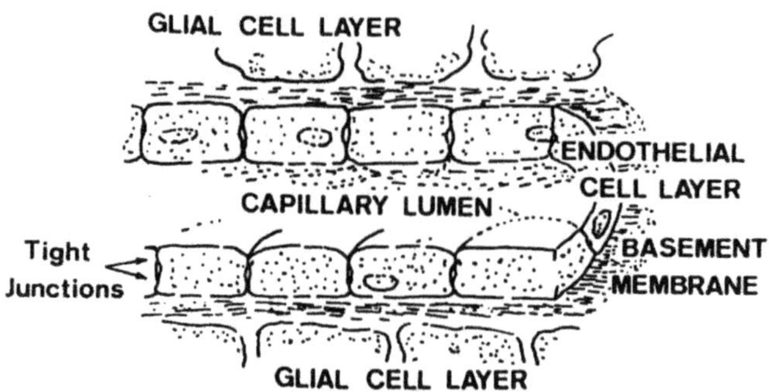

Fig. 1. Schematic view of the blood-brain-barrier. Thin capillaries are surrounded by a continuous basement membrane and glial cells. The endothelial cells are connected to each other by tight junctions which restrain intercellular diffusion. (Redrawn from Rapoport[2]).

of the endothelium and the hemodynamic conditions of the subject.

Breakdown or lack of the BBB facing brain tumors was suggested by many authors. In glioblastoma, Long demonstrated the absence of the BBB by the use of fluorescein protein tracers; these tracers could enter the brain through open endothelium junctions and fenestrated capillaries as observed with electron microscope.[6] Ushio found a greater uptake for tritiated methotrexate (MTX) in glioma and other brain tumors as compared with normal cerebral tissue.[7] More recently, Bar-Sella et al. correlated an increase in ^{99m}Tc pertechnetate uptake in various brain tumors, with the absence of tight junctions rather than fenestration in capillary endothelium.[8] Hypoxic or anoxic conditions due to capillary compression by the tumor mass could explain the impairment of the BBB. Furthermore, specific angiogenic factors released by the tumor could stimulate the anarchic proliferation of the capillaries.[2]

BLOOD-BRAIN-BARRIER IMPAIRMENT AFTER CEREBRAL IRRADIATION

Late brain damage after cerebral irradiation at high doses is well documented. This effect is characterized by BBB breakdown, edema and necrosis; it is generally irreversible and dose-related.

On the other hand, there are little data suggesting early brain damage and BBB impairment after cerebral irradiation at doses relevant in therapy.

We will consider successively early (Table 1) and late (Table 2) brain damage for different dose levels after single or fractionated irradiations. Early damage is that occurring in the days or weeks after irradiation, while late damage appears after several months or years. For the present discussion, single doses higher than 20 Gy are considered as "high doses." "Moderate doses" which are more relevant in radiotherapy, correspond to doses of 20 Gy or less in a single dose or fractionated doses in daily fractions of 2-3 Gy.

Early Effects

After doses higher than 20 Gy, an early alteration in the BBB permeability is generally observed (Table 1). After whole brain irradiation at a single dose of 15000 R, which causes the death of the rats, Pitcock demonstrated, using electron microscopy, membrane alteration such as swelling of the glial cells associated with edema as soon as five minutes after irradiation;

occasionally, there was swelling of the endothelium cells after 18 and 21 hours.[9]

Lundqvist et al. irradiated rat brain on a small field (5-7 mm in diameter) with 200 MeV protons at dose level of 50, 70, 100 and 150 Gy. By measuring the distribution of ^{99m}Tc pertechnetate, they showed an increased uptake in the irradiated area from the second day after irradiation with a maximum after 20-30 days, and then a decrease in the uptake which reached its normal level after 50-60 days.[10]

Remler and Marcussen studied the BBB breakdown using EEG recordings after injection of penicillin (a convulsant drug), which normally does not pass the BBB. Cats were irradiated on a small square field (5 mm) with alpha particles produced at the Lawrence Berkeley 184-inch cyclotron, at a single dose of 60 Gy; BBB impairment was observed as early as one day after irradiation, but the barrier was restored within about 60 days.[11]

After irradiation of one hemisphere in cats at a dose of 20 to 30 Gy, Schettler and Shealy, using isotopic methods (^{203}Hg neohydrin), did not show any alteration in the BBB permeability, at least up to 46 hours.[12] Using the same method, Blomstrand et al., confirmed that after 3000 R the BBB permeability is not altered from 1 hour to 4 months after irradiation, but the irradiation may increase the vulnerability to acute blood pressure as soon as 1-2 hours after irradiation.

Several studies investigated the BBB permeability after smaller dose of radiation.

Griffin et al. showed an increase uptake of MTX up to 6 days after whole brain irradiation at 20 Gy in mice; this effect could not be detected after 5, 10 and 15 Gy.[14]

Storm et al. demonstrated an increase MTX concentration in the brain of the rat exposed to 20 Gy whole brain irradiation; this change in BBB permeability lasted for 9 days post-irradiation.[15]

Levin et al. studied the early variation of the BBB permeability coefficient of ^{14}C-urea, ^{3}H-galacticol (a small hydrophylic compound isomere of manitol) and of two chemotherapeutic agents (bleomycine and ^{3}H-VM26) after a single or a daily fractionated irradiation of the whole rat brain with 230 keV x-rays at dose levels ranging from 2 to 30 Gy. An increased permeability coefficient was observed for galacticol from 3 to 24 hours post-irradiation, whatever the dose level; for urea, a slight increase of transcapillary transport was observed after

Table 1. Early Blood-Brain-Barrier Alteration after "High" and "Moderate" Doses.

AUTHORS	IRRADIATION MODALITIES	DOSES AND FRACTIONATION	METHODS OF INVESTIGATION	BBB ALTERATION
Pitcock	x rays whole brain	15000 "R" 1 fraction	electron microscopy	altered histology
Lundqvist et al.	200 MeV protons, small field	50-150 Gy 1 fraction	isotopic: ^{99m}Tc per-technate	yes
Remler and Marcussen	α particles small field	60 Gy 1 fraction	EEG after penicillin injection	yes
Schettler and Shealy	x rays half brain	20-30 Gy 1 fraction	isotopic: ^{203}Hg neohydrin	no
Blomstrand et al.	x rays half brain	30 Gy 1 fraction	isotopic: ^{203}Hg neohydrin	no
Griffin et al.	x rays whole brain	20 Gy 5-15 Gy 1 fraction	MTX uptake	yes no
Storm et al.	x rays whole brain	20 Gy 1 fraction	MTX uptake	yes
Levin et al.	x rays whole brain	2-30 Gy 1 fraction or daily frac-tion of 2 Gy	isotopic: ^{14}C-urea ^{3}H-galac-ticol ^{3}H-VM26 bleomycine	yes (4 Gy & 5 x 2 Gy) yes no no
Jarden et al.	x rays whole brain	2-6 Gy 1 fraction	PET $^{82}RbCl$	no

Table 2. Late Blood-Brain-Barrier Alteration after "High" and "Moderate" Doses.

AUTHORS	IRRADIATION MODALITIES	DOSES AND FRACTIONATION	METHODS OF INVESTIGATION	BBB ALTERATION
Remler et al.	α particles small field	20-60 Gy 1 fraction	EEG after bicuculline injection	yes
			Blue Evans staining	yes
Caveness	x rays whole brain	15-20 Gy 1 fraction	histology autoradiography	yes
	x rays small field	35 Gy 1 fraction	isotopic: ^{24}Na ^{57}Co DTPA ^{111}In transferrine	yes yes yes
Keyeux et al.	x rays whole brain	20 Gy 1 fraction	isotopic: $Na^{99m}TcO4$	no
Edwards et al.	x rays whole brain	36 Gy 2 Gy daily	isotopic: ^{14}C-urea ^{3}H-galacticol ^{24}Na	 no no no
Nakasaki et al.	x rays whole brain	40, 60 and 80 Gy; 2 Gy daily	histological examination	altered histology

4 Gy and 5 x 2 Gy. In no case was the BBB permeability for bleomycine and VM26 altered by irradiation.[16]

In six patients with metastatic brain tumors, Jarden et al. found no increase in permeability for rubidium chloride (^{82}Rb) using Positron Emission Tomography (PET) at 60 and 90 minutes following whole brain irradiation at 2 to 6 Gy.[17]

Late Effects

In another study, Remler et al. evaluated BBB breakdown in rats by the presence of epileptic spikes following injection of bicuculline methiodide (a convulsant drug), which does not penetrate the healthy BBB; the animals were irradiated with alpha particles, using the technique previously described at different single doses ranging from 20 to 60 Gy. BBB alteration was observed in all of the animals. The frequency and the latency period from irradiation to the time of onset of BBB breakdown was correlated with dose. After 60 Gy, 83% of the animals presented BBB breakdown with a peak incidence of 98 days post-irradiation; after 30 Gy, BBB alteration only appeared in 45% of the animals at 178 days. These results were consistent with those obtained in similar conditions, by the same authors, with Blue Evans dye staining.[18,19]

After whole brain irradiation of monkeys with a single dose of 20 MV x rays, Caveness observed edema, necrosis and vascular alteration (endothelial hyperplasia and telangiectasia) after 15 and 20 Gy using histological and autoradiographic criteria. There was a correlation between the dose and the degree of brain damage, and also between the dose and latency period. Twenty-four weeks after single brain irradiation at 35 Gy on the right occipital lobe of the monkey, he demonstrated increased blood-to-brain transfer constants for [^{24}Na]tracer sodium, [^{57}Co]diethylaminetriaminepenta-acetic acid (DPTA) and [^{111}In]transferrine. He suggested that the BBB breakdown was related to the size of the molecule administered.[20]

On the other hand, using isotopic counting, Keyeux et al. did not observe any BBB breakdown up to 18 months after whole brain irradiation of rats with 250 kV x rays at a dose of 20 Gy, even for small solutes such as sodium pertechnetate ($Na^{99m}TcO4$).[21]

After fractionated irradiation, Edwards et al. did not find any significant difference in the permeability of the BBB in rats for ^{3}H-galacticol, ^{14}C-urea and ^{24}sodium at 6, 10 and 12 weeks post-irradiation (defined as "early-delayed" effect); the rats were irradiated on the whole brain with 230 kV x rays to a total dose of 36 Gy delivered in 18 daily fractions of 2 Gy four times a week.[22]

Nakagaki et al. performed a histological study in monkeys at 6 and 12 months after fractionated irradiation of the whole brain (2 Gy a day, 5 times a week) to a total dose of 40, 60 and 80 Gy. After 40 Gy, only a discrete effect could be detected, while at 60 and 80 Gy marked vascular lesions could be seen, that were directly related to dose level.[23]

DISCUSSION

Many data have accumulated about BBB damage after irradiation but the studies differ according to dose level, irradiation modalities, biological systems and criteria, or latency period of observation. However, some conclusions can be drawn.

For doses smaller than 20 Gy given as a single dose or in fractionated doses in a daily fraction of 2-3 Gy, which are relevant in therapy, there is little evidence suggesting early impairment of the BBB.[14,15,16,17]

However, some data of Levin et al. suggest that there is a breakdown in BBB but only for small substances such as galacticol or urea (molecular weight of 182 and 60, respectively).[16,24] By contrast, in no case increased uptake of large chemotherapeutic drugs such as bleomycine (molecular weight = 1,100) VM26 (molecular weight = 820) or MTX (molecular weight = 455) was observed.[14,15,16]

An early cerebral edema appearing a few hours after the first fraction of radiotherapy for brain tumor, which healed after manitol perfusion, was reported by some authors.[25] This edema could be explained by an increase in the permeability for sodium ions (molecular weight = 58, similar to urea), which normally pass the BBB mainly through a specific channel.[2]

Nevertheless, the fact that the permeability for relatively small solutes such as ^{203}Hg (molecular weight = 200) or ^{82}RbCl (molecular weight = 120) is not increased suggests that irradiation may produce complex membrane effects; it may not open the tight junctions between the endothelium cells through which the large molecules could pass but may affect in different ways the specific transport mechanisms of ionic and non-ionic solutes.[2,16] Alterations in BBB permeability do not seem directly related to the lipophilicity of the solutes; urea and galacticol are hydrophylic metabolites with a log P (octanol/water partition coefficient) of -2.8 and -3.1, respectively, while VM26 is much more lipophylic with a log P of +2.8.[24]

CONCLUSION

In conclusion, there is no evidence indicating that irradiation at dose levels relevant in conventional radiotherapy or in BNCT will affect the BBB permeability for the boronated compounds. This conclusion is especially true since the second and third generation of boronated compounds are large complex macromolecules with high molecular weight.[26,27]

Nevertheless, since in BNCT, normal brain is irradiated not only with gamma rays but also with thermal or epithermal neutrons as well as with alpha particles, one cannot exclude different radiobiological effects on the BBB.

As far as late radiation damages in normal tissue are concerned, it has been suggested that vascular lesions play a major role in their development.[28,29,30] In brain, structural and functional alterations of the BBB could act as the primary event leading to edema and necrosis of cerebral tissue.[31] These effects are irreversible and are not related to the degree of early radiation damages which are transitory and which heal after a few days or weeks.

Most of the experimental data demonstrate that brain damage occurs at doses greater than 20 Gy in single dose or 60 Gy in conventional fractionated scheme. The comparison of the data obtained after single and fractionated doses are consistent with an α/β value of 5, without taking into account cell proliferation.[32]

There is evidence that the level of the late biological damage is dose-related for single as well as for fractionated irradiations.[19,20] Finally, the delay period for late damage seems to be inversely related to the dose level.[19,20]

REFERENCES

1. W. H. Sweet, Medical aspects of boron-slow neutron capture therapy, in "Workshop on Neutron Capture Therapy," R.G. Fairchild and V. P. Bond, eds., Brookhaven National Laboratory, Upton, New York (1976).
2. S. I. Rapoport, "Blood-Brain Barrier in Physiology and Medicine," Raven Press, New York (1986).
3. E. E. Goldman, Die aussere und innere Sekretion des gesunden und kranken Organismus im Lichte der "vitalen Farbung," Beitr Z Klin Chir. 64:192 (1913).
4. M. W. Brightman, Morphology of blood-brain interfaces, Exp. Eye Res. (Suppl. 1) (1977).
5. M. W. Brightman and T. S. Reese, Junctions between intimately opposed cell membranes in the vertebrate brain. J. Cell Biol. 10:648 (1969).
6. D. M. Long, Capillary ultrastructure and the blood-brain-barrier in human malignant brain tumors, J. Neurosurgery. 32:127 (1970).
7. Y. Ushio, T. Hayakawa, and H. Mogami, Uptake of tritiated methotrexate by mouse brain tumors after intravenous or intrathechal administration, J. Neurosurgery. 40:706 (1974).

8. B. Bar-Sella, D. Front, R. Hardoff, E. Peyser, B. Borovich, and I. Nir, Ultrastructural basis for different pertechnetate uptake patterns by various human brain tumors, J. Neurol. Neurosurg. Psychiatry. 42:924 (1979).
9. J. A. Pitcock, An electron microscopic study of acute radiation injury of the rat brain, Lab. Invest. 11:1 (1962).
10. H. Lundqvist, K. Rosander, M. Lomanov, V. Lukjashin, G. Shimchuk, V. Zolotov, and E. Minakova, Permeability of the blood-brain barrier in the rat after local proton irradiation, Acta Radiol. Oncol. 21:4 (1982).
11. M. P. Remler and W. H. Marcussen, Time course of early delayed blood-brain barrier changes in individual cats after ionizing radiation, Exp. Neurol. 73:310 (1981).
12. T. Schettler and C. N. Shealy, Experimental selective alteration of blood-brain barrier by x-irradiation, J. Neurosurg. 32:89 (1970).
13. C. H. Blomstrand, B. Johansson, and B. Rosengren, Blood-brain barrier lesions in acute hypertension in rabbits after unilateral x-ray exposure of brain, Acta Neuropath. Berl. 31:97 (1975).
14. T. W. Griffin, J. S. Rasey, and W. A. Bleyer, The effect of photon irradiation on blood-brain barrier permeability to methotrexate in mice, Cancer. 40:1109 (1977).
15. A. J. Storm, A. J. Van der Kogel, and K. Nooter, Effect of x-irradiation on the pharmacokinetics of metrotrexate in rats: alteration of the blood-brain barrier, Eur. J. Cancer Clin. Oncol. 21:759 (1985).
16. V. A. Levin, M. S. Edwards, and A. Byrd, Quantitative observations of the acute effects of x-irradiation on brain capillary permeability: Part I, Int. J. Radiation Oncology Biol. Phys. 5:1627 (1979).
17. J. O. Jarden, V. Dhawan, A. Poltorak, J. B. Posner, and D. A. Rottenberg, PET measurement of blood-to-brain and blood-to-tumor transport of 82-Rb: effect of whole-brain radiation therapy and dexamethasone treatment, Acta Radiol. Scand. 72:125 (1986).
18. M. P. Remler and W. Marcussen, Late effects of alpha radiation to the CNS on the blood-brain barrier, Acta Neurol. Scand. 72:125 (1985).
19. M. P. Remler, W. H. Marcussen, and J. Tiller-Borsich, The late effects of radiation on the blood-brain barrier, Int. J. Radiation Oncology Biol. Phys. 12: 1965 (1986).
20. W. F. Caveness, Experimental observations: delayed necrosis in normal monkey brain, In "Radiation Damage to the Nervous System. A Delayed Therapeutic Hazard," H. A. Gilbert and A. R. Kagan, eds., Raven Press, New York (1980).

21. A. Keyeux, D. Ocrymowicz-Bemelmans, and A. A. Charlier, Radiation late effect on the blood-brain barrier (BBB) permeability and the antipyrine (AP) distribution volumes in the rat brain, Int. J. Radiat. Biol. 51:751 (1987).
22. M. S. Edwards, V. A. Levin, and A. Byrd, Quantitative observations in the subacute effects of x-irradiation on brain capillary permeability: Part II. Int. J. Radiation Oncology Biol. Phys. 5:1633 (1979).
23. H. Nakasaki, G. Brunhart, T. L. Kemper, and W. F. Caveness, Monkey brain damage from radiation in the therapeutic range, J. Neurosurg. 44:3 (1976).
24. V. A. Levin, H. T. D. Landahl, and M. A. Freeman-Dove, The application of brain capillary permeability coefficient measurements to pathological conditions and the selection of agents which cross the blood-brain barrier, J. Pharmacok. and Biopharm. 4:499 (1976).
25. P. N. Plowman, J. Fuentos, and A. N. Harnett, Early radiation swelling remains a problem in the management of pediatric brain tumors, Br. J. Radiol. 60:931 (1987).
26. R. G. Fairchild and V. P. Bond, New compounds for neutron capture therapy (NCT) and their significance, Strahlentherapie. 160:764 (1984).
27. A. H. Soloway, F. Alam, and R. F. Barth, Future boronated molecules for neutron capture therapy, in "Workshop on Neutron Capture Therapy," R. G. Fairchild and V. P. Bond, eds., Brookhaven National Laboratory, Upton, New York (1986).
28. J. W. Hopewell and C. M. A. Young, Changes in the microcirculation of normal tissues after irradiation, Int. J. Radiation Oncology Biol. Phys. 4:53 (1978)
29. H. F. Moustafa and J. W. Hopewell, Late functional changes in the vasculature of the rat brain after local x-irradiation, Br. J. Radiol. 53:21 (1980).
30. H. S. Reinhold and G. H. Buisman, Repair of radiation damage to capillary endothelium, Br. J. Radiol. 48:727 (1975).
31. J. F. Llena, G. Cespedes, A. Hirano, H. M. Zimmerman, E. H. Feiring, and D. Fine, VAscular alterations in delayed radiation necrosis of the brain, Arch. Pathol. Lab. Med. 100:531 (1976).
32. H. D. Thames and J. H. Hendry, "Fractionation in Radiotherapy," Taylor and Francis, London (1987).

IMPLICATIONS OF GENOTYPIC AND MICROENVIRONMENTAL HETEROGENEITY FOR THE CURE OF SOLID TUMORS BY NEUTRON CAPTURE THERAPY

Sara Rockwell

Department of Therapeutic Radiology
Yale University School of Medicine
333 Cedar Street, New Haven, CT 06510

There is increasing evidence for genotypic, phenotypic, and microenvironmental heterogeneity within solid tumors in experimental animals and in humans. This heterogeneity influences the response of the tumors to treatment with radiation, cytotoxic drugs, hyperthermia, and immunotherapy, and may also influence the efficacy of neutron capture therapy. This paper reviews the data on heterogeneity in solid tumors and considers the implications of these data for curative NCT.

GENOTYPIC HETEROGENEITY

Genetically distinct subpopulations can be identified in some human and animal tumors on the basis of karyotypes, DNA contents, or the presence of genetic markers.[1-7] In some tumors, different subpopulations may be present in different areas of the tumor; in other tumors, the cells may be intermixed. In some cases, the subpopulations reflect a progressive evolution to a more aggressive malignancy, while in others distinct subpopulations appear to exist in a state of stable equilibrium throughout a relatively long period in the natural history of the cancer.[1,3,4,5]

The phenotypic characteristics of the cells in different subpopulations may influence their responses to treatment. This is exemplified by the drug-resistant subpopulations[5,8] which become evident during cancer chemotherapy and may comprise the predominant cell populations in the relapsing neoplasm. The efficacy of cytotoxic drugs may be circumvented by a number of genetic changes, including mutations which alter drug uptake or efflux rates (e.g. pleiotropic drug resistance), mutations which alter the structure or function of an enzyme critical to the cytotoxic action of a antimetabolite or to the activation of a prodrug, or changes in the level of a critical enzyme through gene amplification.[8-10] Genetic differences between tumor cell subpopulations could influence the uptake and accumulation of some boronated compounds through similar mechanisms. Other mutations which alter the fixation or repair of DNA damage can alter the response of cells to both drugs and radiation. Human and rodent tumors have been observed that contain identifiable subpopulations with intrinsically different sensitivities to radiation, hyperthermia, and cancer chemotherapeutic drugs.[1-5,7]

More subtle genotypic differences between tumor cell subpopulations are also important in chemotherapy and may be important in NCT. Some tumors contain malignant subpopulations which differ in their cell cycle times, proportion of quiescent cells, and patterns of cell loss. This genetically determined proliferative heterogeneity would become important if the uptake, processing, or retention of a boronated compound varied with the proliferative status of the cell. Heterogeneity in the expression of specific metabolic pathways in a relatively well-differentiated tumor can result in heterogeneity in the accumulation and efficacy of cytotoxic compounds targeted *via* these pathways. For example, the variation in melanogenesis within individual melanomas has limited the clinical utility of certain cytotoxic agents targeted through the melanogenic pathway; the possible implications of such heterogeneity for NCT of melanoma using targeted boronated compounds are being examined by several investigators.[11,12] Subpopulation differences in the structure or expression of cell surface antigens or cell membrane receptors[1,6] can limit the homogeneity of the distribution of compounds targeted through the use of antibodies or of molecules targeted to specific receptors. The distribution problems to be anticipated in targeting boronated compounds would be similar to those which have been encountered with cytotoxins or radioactive isotopes targeted by these approaches.

Genotypic heterogeneity within solid tumors theoretically could lead to heterogeneous distributions of boronated compounds. It is difficult to study the effects of genotypic heterogeneity using *in vitro* systems, transplanted rodent tumors, or human tumor cell lines xenografted into immune-deficient mice, because virtually all of these model tumor lines have been deliberately cloned or heavily selected by repeated serial passage to produce genetically uniform cell populations.[13-15] Detailed studies of the microscopic distribution of the boronated compounds within human neoplasms and within autochthonous (spontaneous or induced) tumors in animals will be necessary to assess the importance and therapeutic implications of genotypic heterogeneity for NCT.

MICROENVIRONMENTAL HETEROGENEITY

Microenvironmental heterogeneity also occurs in solid tumors.[16-18] The rapid growth of malignant cells, relative to the vasculature, may lead to the development of avascular areas with chronic perfusion deficits, and ultimately to the development of avascular necrosis. The environment of cells in these chronically unperfused areas is different from that of cells in well-perfused areas.[16] The cells may be subjected to chronic, moderate, or severe hypoxia and to chronic deficiencies in glucose, nutrients, and metabolic precursors. Use of anaerobic metabolism, chronic deficiencies in energy metabolism, and limited removal of catabolites may produce an acidic microenvironment. The extracellular pH in poorly-perfused areas containing viable, metabolizing cells can be lower than that in (non-metabolizing) necrotic areas. The intracellular pH of cells in poorly-perfused areas also may be perturbed, as hypoxia and deficiencies in energy metabolism compromise the ability of cells to maintain a normal intracellular pH in an acidic extracellular milieu.[17] As hypoxia, nutrient deficiencies, and low extracellular pH can all inhibit cell proliferation, it is not surprising that poorly-perfused regions of solid tumors contain large numbers of quiescent cells blocked in various phases of the cell cycle, as well as proliferating cells traversing the cell cycle unusually slowly.[16] These cells retain their clonogenic potential and will resume rapid proliferation if their environment improves - they cannot be ignored if cancer therapy is to be curative. The unusual metabolic and proliferative characteristics of cells in these deficient microenvironments may alter the accumulation of some boronated compounds.

The perfusion deficits _per se_ may contribute to heterogeneity in the distribution of some boronated compounds. There is growing evidence that many organic dyes, metabolic precursors, and cancer chemotherapeutic agents penetrate poorly into non-perfused areas of solid tumors.[16-22] There is also evidence that the efficacy of some cytotoxic anticancer drugs against solid tumors is limited by their inability to reach the viable cells of poorly perfused areas.[16-18,21] Chronic infusion of drugs does not always circumvent this problem, especially when penetration is limited by the fact that the active agent is destroyed or scavenged by cellular metabolic reactions, in a process analogous to the utilization of O_2 which leads to hypoxia in poorly-perfused areas.

Transient perfusion deficits also occur within solid tumors. These appear to reflect the transient variations in blood flow through individual tumor blood vessels which have been demonstrated by microscopic cinematography techniques.[23] Studies of hemoglobin saturation in tumor samples confirm that tumors in animals and humans contain blood vessels which are not actively perfused.[24,25] Temporal variations in the perfusion of tumor tissue with dyes,[22] temporal fluctuations in local tumor pH and pO_2,[17,24,25] and temporal variations in pyridine nucleotide fluorescence[26] all have been observed in solid tumors. These occur in areas of tumor which histologically appear to contain patent blood vessels and to be composed of "healthy" malignant cells with normal proliferative and metabolic characteristics. Different blood vessels, and therefore different regions of the tumor, may be affected at different times. The effects of transient perfusion variations on the delivery of injected compounds will be similar to the effects of chronic perfusion deficits if the availability of the compound in the circulating blood is of very short duration. If the duration of availability of the compound is long relative to the duration of the transient perfusion deficits (e.g. as with a prolonged infusions of drug or multiple drug treatments), these variations in perfusion would not lead to absolute deficits in the delivery of drug to any one area or set of areas, but rather to decreased average delivery of the compound and lower drug concentrations in many areas of the tumor.

Microenvironmental heterogeneity within solid tumors may lead to heterogeneity in the distribution, uptake, and retention of boronated compounds, because of the perfusion deficits _per se_ and also because of the perturbed environment, metabolic characteristics, and proliferative status of the cells in unperfused regions. It is critical that high levels of boron be obtained in these cells, which are unusually resistant to radiation and to many cytotoxic drugs used in cancer chemotherapy.[16-18] These cells are radioresistant primarily because of hypoxia. For low LET radiations, the D_0's for severely hypoxic cells are approximately 3 times greater than the D_0's for aerobic cells (i.e. the OER = 3). These cells therefore are extremely resistant to the low LET components of the radiation given during NCT. Although the OER for neutrons is somewhat lower (~1.5), hypoxic cells are still relatively resistant to neutrons. The low OER of the very high LET radiations associated with NCT effectively eliminates the radioprotection associated with hypoxia.[27] Achieving high boron compounds in the poorly perfused areas will increase the radiosensitivity of these cells by decreasing the OER, as well as by increasing the local radiation dose.

IMPLICATIONS OF HETEROGENEITY

The genetic and microenvironmental heterogeneity within a solid tumor could create difficulties in obtaining uniform, high distributions of ^{10}B throughout its volume. Uniform distributions are essential if tumors are to be controlled through NCT. The reason for this is illustrated on Fig. 1. "Partial responses", and "complete responses" often are used as indicators of tumor response in cancer chemotherapy. Although these effects require that large numbers of tumor cells be killed, they actually reflect relatively small changes in the surviving fraction of the tumor cells and represent only the beginning of the survival curve for the tumor cells. To cure a tumor, the surviving fraction must be reduced to a value so low that it is improbable that any clonogenic tumor cells remain. This value depends upon the number of clonogenic cells in the tumors; it has been estimated for experimental rodent tumors that the surviving fraction must be reduced to approximately 10^{-9}. Even a small number of resistant cells will compromise the probability of reaching this surviving fraction and curing a tumor with a radiation dose that can be tolerated by dose-limiting normal tissues.

A somewhat analogous situation has been analyzed, modeled, and studied extensively by those assessing the importance of hypoxic cells in determining the radiation response of solid rodent tumors. Data on a large number of experimental rodent tumors showed that even small numbers of hypoxic cells (<1%) can produce demonstrable and statistically significant effects on the survival curves of the tumor cell, the growth of recurrent tumors, and the dose of radiation necessary to cure the tumors.[16] Fischer[28] calculated that if the proportion of radioresistant hypoxic cells in a tumor is 1 in 10^6, a tumor recurring after a radiation dose near the TCD_{50} is as likely to arise from a hypoxic cell as from an aerobic cell. If the hypoxic fraction is $>10^{-6}$, recurrences will arise primarily from the hypoxic cell population. It is notable that it is essentially impossible to detect a hypoxic fraction of this magnitude by any technique which requires sampling and characterization of microscopic tumor specimens

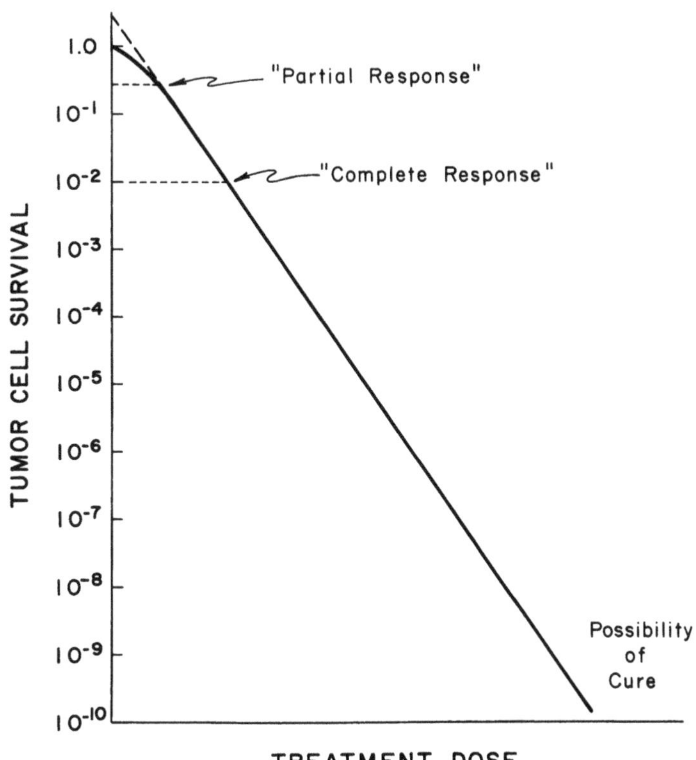

Fig. 1. Relationship between tumor cell survival, tumor response, and tumor cure.

or by any technique which examines the average characteristics of tumor cells within a macroscopic volume of tumor.

If this analogy pertains to NCT, it implies an extremely stringent requirement for the adequate distribution of ^{10}B throughout the tumor cells: if even a very small subpopulation of tumor cells fails to accumulate ^{10}B, either because of their intrinsic characteristics or because of their location or environment, these cells will compromise the efficacy of the treatment in producing tumor cure. It will not be sufficient to obtain high boron levels in most of the tumor cells, or even in the vast majority of the tumor cells; rather, it will be necessary to ensure that not one cell in a million remains untreated. Obtaining adequate distribution of ^{10}B throughout the tumor, while simultaneously ensuring adequate differential between ^{10}B levels in the tumor cells and in the critical cells of normal tissues within the irradiated field, provides one of the major challenges which must be met if NCT is to be effective in curing cancer.

REFERENCES

1. G.H. Heppner, and B.E. Miller, Tumor heterogeneity: Biological implications and therapeutic consequences, Cancer Metast. Rev. 2:5 (1983).
2. G.H. Heppner, Tumor heterogeneity, Cancer Res. 44:2259 (1984).
3. G.H. Heppner, Tumor subpopulation interactions, in: "Tumor Cell Heterogeneity", A.H. Owens, D.S. Coffey, and S.B. Baylin, eds., Academic Press, Inc., NY (1982).
4. D.L. Dexter, E.N. Spremulli, Z. Fligiel, J.A. Barbosa, R. Vogel, A. VanVoorhees, and P. Calabresi, Heterogeneity of cancer cells from a single human colon carcinoma, Am. J. Med. 71:949 (1981).
5. W-K.A. Yung, J.R. Shapiro, and W.R. Shapiro, Heterogeneous chemosensitivities of subpopulations of human glioma cells in culture, Cancer Res. 42:992 (1982).
6. J.C. Hager, and G.H. Heppner, Heterogeneity of expression and induction of mouse mammary tumor virus antigens in mouse mammary tumors, Cancer Res. 42:4325 (1982).
7. E.K. Rofstad, and T. Brustad, Differential responses to radiation and hyperthermia of cloned cell lines derived from a single human melanoma xenograft, Int. J. Radiat. Oncol. Biol. Phys. 10:857 (1984).
8. V. Ling, Genetic basis of drug resistance in mammalian cells, in: "Drugs and Human Resistance in Neoplasms," N. Bruckovsky and J.H. Goldie, eds., CRC Press, Boca Raton, FL (1983).
9. J.H. Goldie, and A.J. Coldman, The genetic origin of drug resistance in neoplasms: Implications for systemic therapy, Cancer Res. 44:3643 (1984).
10. G.L. Rice, C. Hoy, and R.T. Schimke, Transient hypoxia enhances the frequency of dihydrofolate reductase gene amplification in

Chinese hamster ovary cells, Proc. Natl. Acad. Sci. USA 83:5978 (1986).
11. J.A. Corderre, These Proceedings.
12. Y. Mishima, These Proceedings.
13. S. Rockwell, Maintenance of tumor systems and appropriate treatment techniques for experimental tumors, in: "Rodent Tumors in Experimental Cancer Therapy," R.F. Kallman, ed., Pergamon Press, NY (1987).
14. G.G. Steel, V.D. Courtenay, and M.J. Peckham, The response to chemotherapy of a variety of human tumour xenografts, Br. J. Cancer 47:1 (1983).
15. E.K. Rofstad, Human tumour xenografts in radiotherapeutic research, Radiother. Oncol. 3:35 (1985).
16. J.E. Moulder, and S. Rockwell, Tumor hypoxia: Its impact on cancer therapy, Cancer Metast. Rev. 5:313 (1987).
17. K.A. Kennedy, Hypoxic cells as specific drug targets for chemotherapy, Anti-Cancer Drug Design 2:181 (1987).
18. K.A. Kennedy, B.A. Teicher, S. Rockwell, and A.C. Sartorelli, The hypoxic tumor cell: A target for selective cancer chemotherapy, Biochem. Pharm. 29:1 (1980).
19. R.J. Goldacre, and B. Sylven, On the access of blood-borne dyes to various tumour regions, Br. J. Cancer 16:306 (1962).
20. D.C. Rowe-Jones, The penetration of cytotoxins into malignant tumours, Br. J. Cancer 22:155 (1968).
21. P.E. Noker, L. Simpson-Herren, and S.D. Wagoner, Heterogeneity of response of mammary adeno carcinoma 16/C (MamAd 16/C) to Melphalan (L-Pam) (NSC 8806), Proc. Am. Assoc. Cancer Res. 26:338 (1985).
22. D.J. Chaplin, P.L. Olive, and R.E. Durand, Intermittent blood flow in a murine tumor, Cancer Res. 47:597 (1987).
23. H.S. Reinhold, B. Blachiewicz, and A. Berg-Blok, Reoxygenation of tumours in sandwich chambers, Europ. J. Cancer 15:481 (1979).
24. W. Mueller-Klieser, P. Vaupel, R. Manz, and W.A. Grunewald, Intracapillary oxyhemoglobin saturation in malignant tumors in humans, Int. J. Radiat. Oncol. Biol. Phys. 7:1397 (1981).
25. P. Vaupel, R. Manz, W. Mueller-Klieser, and W.A. Grunewald, Intracapillary HbO_2 saturation in malignant tumors during normoxia and hyperoxia, Microvas. Res. 17:181 (1979).
26. M. Gosalvez, R.G. Thurman, B. Chance, and H. Reinhold, Regional variation in the oxygenation of mouse mammary tumours in vivo demonstrated by fluorescence of pyridine nucleotide, Br. J. Radiol. 45:510 (1972).
27. R.G. Fairchild, and V.P. Bond, Current status of ^{10}B-neutron capture therapy: Enhancement of tumor dose via beam filtration and dose rate, and the effects of these parameters on minimum boron content: A theoretical evaluation, Int. J. Radiat. Oncol. Biol. Phys. 11:831 (1985).
28. J.J. Fischer, S. Rockwell, and D.F. Martin, Perfluorochemicals and hyperbaric oxygen in radiation therapy, Int. J. Radiat. Oncol. Biol. Phys. 12:95 (1986).

STATUS REPORT ON THE DEVELOPMENT OF A SPALLATION NEUTRON SOURCE FOR NEUTRON CAPTURE THERAPY (NCT)

H. Conde, E. Grusell, B. Larsson, E. Ramstrom,
T. Ronnqvist, H. Sornsuntisook, S. Villa*,
J .Crawford, H. Reist**, B. Dahl, N.G. Sjostrand***,
and G. Russel****

*Department of Radiation Sciences, Box 535
Uppsala University
S-75121 Uppsala, Sweden

**Paul Scherrer Institute
Villigen, Switzerland

***Department of Reactor Physics
Chalmers University of Technology
Goteborg, Sweden

****Los Alamos National Laboratory
Los Alamos, NM

INTRODUCTION

The eventual aim of the present study is to construct an accelerator-based intermediate-energy neutron source that would permit irradiation of neoplasms in the central nervous system by an intermediate-energy fluence rate of at least 10^9 $n \cdot cm^{-2} \cdot s^{-1}$ in fields of 4-8 cm in diameter. The accelerator should be of a moderate size to permit accommodation in a hospital environment. In the first instance, a prototype source has to be designed that could be conveniently tested in a laboratory dedicated to radiation research, such as the Paul Scherrer Institute (PSI), where the measurements here reported were performed.

A tentative strategy is to accept a dose fraction due to neutrons above the energy range usually considered for intermediate-energy neutron therapy. This would, in fact, mean that the boron neutron capture dose in the target area would be of the same order of magnitude as the absorbed fast neutron dose. The radiobiological motivation would be that the latter dose fraction would be responsible for part of the therapeutically useful dose. Indeed, fast neutron therapy is an accepted therapeutic modality. The practical consequence of such a strategy would be that filtration of the moderated neutron beam would not be required.

The clinical interests beyond this Swedish-Swiss joint collaboration are primarily focused on the treatment of vascular malformations in the central nervous system. In a longer perspective, the treatment of malignant brain tumors is given priority over other malignancies considered, such as melanomas and colorectal carcinomas. The biomedical research program conducted in parallel with this study has been presented in a review paper given at the present workshop.[1]

The work on the project has so far been devoted to studies of different moderator materials and configurations in combination with neutron production by 72 MeV protons stopped in heavy materials. The aim has been to optimize the performance of a neutron source for NCT. The required characteristics are firstly that the bulk of the neutrons should have an energy between 1-100 keV and secondly that the dose of the moderated beam should be of the order of $10^{13} \cdot n/cm^2$ delivered in a time of approximately 3 hours.

Water Moderator

Neutron transport calculations, using Monte Carlo methods, were made both at the Institute for Reactor Physics, Chalmers University of Technology, and at the Department of Physical Biology, Uppsala University. Evaluations were made of different water moderators surrounding a spallation neutron source. The neutron production by 72 MeV protons stopped in a copper block, as measured by Broome.[2], was used as input to the calculations of the neutron transport through the moderator. Excellent agreement was obtained between the calculations and measurements made in the same geometry at the 72 MeV Injector I cyclotron at PSI/SIN. The results have been reported in two papers.[3,4]

Calculations of the neutron production from 72 MeV protons stopped in copper and tungsten were made at Los Alamos National Laboratory using the code HETC. Recently, measurements were made at the Svedberg Laboratory in Uppsala of the neutron output from 72 MeV proton stopped in copper and lead. Data handling is in progress. The results of both investigations indicate an increase of the neutron output going from copper to tungsten or lead.

The results from the studies of different water moderators show a relatively large contribution of fast neutrons (> 500 keV) and gamma rays in the beam. The quotient of the number of fast neutrons ($N_f, E_n > 500$ keV) to the number of epithermal neutrons (N_{eth}, 10 keV > E_n > 1 keV) was measured to be 3.0 and the quotient of the number of gamma rays (N_γ, $E_\gamma > 600$ keV) to the number of epithermal neutrons was 7. This observation became an incentive to look for altenative moderator options.

Iron and Graphite Moderator

Monte Carlo calculations were made in Uppsala on spherical iron moderators (diameters ranging from 40 to 150 cm) with and without a cover of about 10 cm of graphite. The results indicate a very efficient slowing down by the iron of the fast neutrons to an energy of about 1-2 MeV. A further moderation to keV-energies was obtained by adding graphite outside the iron sphere.

The iron and graphite moderation option was studied experimentally at the 72 MeV Injector I cyclotron at PSI/SIN on August 29-September 2, 1988. The neutrons were produced by 72 MeV protons stopped in a tungsten block. The moderator consisted of an iron block (40 cm x 60 cm x 60 cm) with and without an outside graphite shield (13 cm). The moderated neutrons were measured by time-of-flight using a Li-glass detector while the fast neutrons (> 0.5 MeV) were measured with a liquid scintillator (NE213). The gamma-ray flux was measured with a Na-I crystal. A special measurement was made of the very fast neutrons ($E_n > 10$ MeV) in two different angles (0° and 90°) to the incoming proton beam with the liquid scintillator.

The neutron field in plastic phantoms (20 cm x 20 cm x 20 cm) was mapped with different foil detectors: Au-foils with and without Cd-shield, TLD for gamma-ray and neutron detection, boron track detectors and detector films (NEUTRAK) for slow and fast neutrons. The phantoms were placed in the moderated neutron field which was generated by the pure iron cube but also by the iron cube plus graphite.

The results from the experiment will be checked against calculations utilizing the input neutron spectrum for tungsten calculated by G. Russel, and Monte Carlo transport calculations (MCNP) with the exact material and geometry of the moderator. The neutron cross sections needed for the transport calculations of the high energy neutrons ($E_n > 20$ MeV) will be calculated from the preequilibrium code ALICE.

At present, the only available result from the measurement is the thermal neutron field determination in the plastic phantom with the Au-foil activation method. The preliminary result of the thermal neutron dose for an integrated proton beam of 1 mC (100 nA for about 3 h) is:

Depth in Phantom	Moderation configuration	Thermal Neutron Fluence
2 cm	Iron	7×10^{10} n/cm^2
5 cm	Iron	4×10^{10} n/cm^5
5 cm	Iron + Graphite	2×10^{10} n/cm^2
10 cm	Iron	1×10^{10} n/cm^2
10 cm	Iron + Graphite	2×10^9 n/cm^2

Thus, if one assumes a beam current of 100 μA a dose of 2×10^{13}n/cm^2 is obtained at 5 cm depth in 3 h with fully moderated neutrons (iron + graphite).

CONCLUSIONS

The final evaluation of the experimental results, and the definite calculations, still remain to be done. It is likely, however, that the continued study would lead to a design of a spallation source based on protons from a cyclotron of a size corresponding to installations already in use for hospital-based fast neutron therapy. When the present study has been finalized, a decision has to be made whether a prototype source, intended for pre-therapeutic biomedical tests at Paul Scherrer Institute, would be based on the iron/carbon moderation option. The preliminarily calculated neutron fluence would be adequate for both adjuvant neutron capture therapy[4] and neutron capture therapy *per se*, at the assumed proton beam current of 100 μA. As a working hypothesis, no filtration would be required, as the fast neutron components present would contribute a useful component to the absorbed radiation dose.

REFERENCES

1. B. Larsson, Neutron capture therapy in support of other radiation treatment, this volume.
2. T. A. Broome, D. R. Perry, and G. B. Stapleton, Particle distribution around a copper beam stop for 72 MeV protons, *Health Phys.* 44:487 (1983).
3. H. Conde, C. B. Pettersson, O. Sornsuntisook, L. Thuresson, N. G. Sjoestrand, and J. Crawford, Intermediate-energy neutrons for NCT. Status report on production and properties, *in:* "Proc. 2nd Int. Symp. on Neutron Capture Therapy", H. Hatanaka and M. Hiroshi, eds., Nishimura, Niigata, Japan (1986).

4. H. Conde, E. Grusell, B. Larsson, C. B. Petterson, L. Thuresson, J. Crawford, H. Reist, B. Dahl, and N. G. Sjoestrand, Time of flight measurements of the energy spectrum of neutrons emitted from a spallation source and moderated in water, Nucl. Instr. and Methods A261:587 (1987).

UPTAKE OF BORON INTO HUMAN GLIOMAS OF ATHYMIC MICE AND INTO SYNGENEIC CEREBRAL GLIOMAS OF RATS AFTER INTRACAROTID INFUSION OF SULFHYDRYL BORANES

D. D. Joel, D. N. Slatkin, P. L. Micca,
M. M. Nawrocky, T. Dubois and C. Velez

Medical Department
Brookhaven National Laboratory
Upton, New York 11973

INTRODUCTION

Effective boron neutron capture therapy (BNCT) of brain tumor will be dependent upon the use of boron-transport agents that give adequate levels of ^{10}B in tumor tissue but low boron concentrations in blood and normal brain.[1] Several ^{10}B-transport agents are being studied in animals, however, only the sulfhydryl borane monomer ($Na_2B_{12}H_{11}SH$) is currently used (in Japan) for the treatment of human malignant gliomas.[2] Our studies show that after the administration of the sulfhydryl borane dimer ($Na_4B_{24}H_{22}S_2$) tumor boron concentrations are significantly higher than those obtained following the administration of equal amounts of boron as monomer.[3,4] This report presents preliminary results on: a) the uptake of monomer and dimer in tumors arising from a human malignant glioma-derived cell line inoculated subcutaneously in athymic (nude) mice; and b) the comparison of intracarotid and intravenous infusion of monomer and dimer on the resultant boron concentrations in cerebral gliomas of rats.

METHODS

Nude Mouse-Human Glioma Model

Six male 5-to 8-week old athymic mice (nu/nu genotype, NIH Swiss background) were used as tumor hosts. The human malignant glioma-derived cell line U-87 MG, originally established by Ponten et al.,[5] was obtained from American Type Culture Collection (Rockville, Maryland) and maintained in culture at our laboratory. Two subcutaneous tumors were initiated in each mouse by the inoculation of 2.5×10^6 cells suspended in 50 μl of culture medium. About 4 weeks later, when tumors weighed between 500 and 800 mg, each mouse was implanted intraperitoneally with an osmotic pump (Model 2001, ALZA Corp., Palo Alto, California) filled with an aqueous solution of monomer or dimer containing about 60 mg ^{10}B/ml. Three or four days later the mice were euthanized and samples of tumor, blood, liver and brain were taken for ^{10}B analysis. The ^{10}B remaining in the osmotic pumps was also measured to provide an assessment of total ^{10}B delivered intraperitoneally.

Rat Glioma Model

An N-nitrosomethylurea-induced[6] rat glioma cell line (GS-9L) maintained in culture was used to produce solid tumors by intracerebral and subcutaneous inoculation. Using aseptic techniques the scalp was incised and a 0.5 mm burr hole made in the skull at a point 3 mm to the left of the midline and 1 mm anterior to the coronal suture. One μl of a glioma cell suspension containing 10^7 cells/ml (10^4 cells injected) was injected, using a 27 gauge needle fitted with a Teflon collar, into the left frontal lobe to a depth of 3-4 mm. Two subcutaneous tumors were initiated by the injection of 5-8 μl of the same cell suspension. Nineteen to twenty-one days later the rats were anesthetized and the left common carotid artery was exposed at its bifurcation. Infusion of sulfhydryl boranes via the internal carotid artery was accomplished by the retrograde insertion of a silastic rubber cannula into the external carotid artery with the tip of the cannula secured near the bifurcation. For intravenous infusion, a silastic rubber cannula was inserted into the anterior facial vein with the tip of the cannula secured near that vein's entrance into the external jugular vein. Continuous infusions were done following recovery from anesthesia using small animal infusion swivels (Harvard Apparatus, South Natick, MA) with spring tethers and calibrated syringe pumps.

Sulfhydryl Borane Solutions and Borane Analysis

The Cs salt of ^{10}B-enriched $[B_{12}H_{11}SH]^{2-}$ (Callery Chemical Company, Pittsburgh, PA) was converted to the Na salt by ion exchange on a 100-200 mesh Dowex 50W-X8 column.[3] The dimer was prepared as previously described.[7] Briefly, $Cs_2B_{12}H_{11}SH$ was oxidized to $Cs_4B_{24}H_{11}S_2$ using o-iodosobenzoic acid, and converted to the sodium salt by ion-exchange. Thin layer chromatography was used to assay the purity of the preparations.[3] For animal perfusions, solutions were made isotonic with sodium chloride and sterilized althrough 0.22 μm diameter pore membrane-filters. To minimize oxidation the solutions were refrigerated and aliquoted daily.

Boron concentrations in blood and tissue samples weighing 0.3-1.0 g were analyzed by gamma spectroscopy, measuring 478 keV photons from the $^{10}B(n,\gamma)^{7}Li$ reaction.[8]

RESULTS AND DISCUSSION

The average boron concentration in subcutaneous rat gliomas following the slow infusion of dimer was nearly double that observed after the similar administration of the same amount of boron as monomer.[4] Although the uptake of boron following infusion of monomer has been studied in human malignant gliomas[2,9,11] similar information is not available for the dimer. Since the nude mouse-human glioma model has been used extensively for studies of brain tumor therapy,[10] we used this tumor model to compare boron uptake following the slow infusion of monomer and dimer.

As shown in Table 1, the concentrations of boron in subcutaneous gliomas of human origin were significantly higher in mice that were infused with dimer than in mice infused with monomer. However, boron concentrations in gliomas of human origin growing in athymic mice were lower than the tumor boron levels obtained when equivalent doses of monomer or dimer were infused into rats bearing syngeneic gliomas.[4] A similar variance was evident in the comparison of liver boron concentrations. These findings suggest a fundamental difference between rats and mice in the rates of metabolism, transport and tissue exchange of the sulfhydryl boranes.

For BNCT of human malignant gliomas in Japan, ^{10}B is introduced into the tumor during a 1-2 hour intraarterial (carotid or vertebral artery) infusion of ^{10}B-enriched monomer at a dose range of 30-80 mg ^{10}B per kg body weight. The average tumor boron concentration 11 to 16 hours after infusion was 22 μg ^{10}B/g (summarized by Sweet[9]). To our knowledge no animal study comparing intracarotid and intravenous infusions of either monomer or dimer has been published. Table 2 presents such data from preliminary experiments in which rats bearing cerebral gliomas were given monomer or dimer via intracarotid infusion. A dose of 50 μg ^{10}B/gbw as dimer was administered either via the carotid artery (Rats 1-3) or intravenously (Rats 4-6) over a 24-hour period. These rats were euthanized immediately after infusion. There was no significant difference between cerebral tumor boron concentrations following intravenous and intracarotid infusion.

Table 1. ^{10}B Concentrations in Tissues of Six Male Athymic (nude) Mice Bearing Subcutaneous Tumors.[a]

Mouse	Sulfhydryl Borane	^{10}B Dose (μg B/gbw)	Days of Infusion	Tissue Boron Concentration (μg $^{10}B/g$) Blood	Liver	Brain	Tumor
1	Monomer	167	3	3.1	9.6	1.5	2.6
2	Monomer	133	4	4.3	9.0	0.2	2.1
3	Monomer	50	4	1.5	9.6	0.9	1.8
		Average		[3.4]	[13.4]	[1.2]	[2.9]
4	Dimer	207	3	5.6	46.3	1.5	10.4
5	Dimer	101	4	6.2	44.6	0.1	9.0
6	Dimer	102	4	7.7	47.7	1.7	9.3
		Average		[6.9]	[48.0]	[1.1]	[9.8]

[a]The tumors were initiated from a human glioma-derived cell line following the intraperitoneal infusion of monomer or dimer. The average concentrations in square brackets are extrapolated linearly to the mean boron dose administered to the six mice; i.e., to 127 μg ^{10}B per gram body weight (gbw).

Furthermore, in Rats 1-3, the indirectly perfused subcutaneous tumor contained essentially the same level of boron as did the corresponding cerebral tumor. All tumors in these six rats had in excess of 20 μg ^{10}B/g which is considered to be the minimum level necessary for BNCT.

In Rats 7-13, the infusion time was reduced to 2 hours thereby approximating the administration schedule used by Hatanaka[2] in BNCT of human malignant glioma. When dimer was infused via the carotid artery at a dose of 50 μg ^{10}B/gbw, three rats died during the infusion period and a fourth rat (Rat 7, Table 2) died 25 min after termination of the infusion. The extremely high level of boron in the cerebral tumor, as compared to the subcutaneous tumor, in Rat 7 suggested that rapid intracarotid infusion may be advantageous. In one rat (Rat 8), the dose of dimer was reduced to 30 μg ^{10}B/gbw with no apparent toxicity. However, when this animal was euthanized 2 hours after infusion, the boron concentration in the cerebral tumor was essentially the same as in the subcutaneous tumor. Intravenous administration of 50 μg ^{10}B/gbw as dimer, even when infused in a 1-hour period (D. Joel, unpublished observation), was not lethal.

Sulfhydryl borane monomer was clearly less toxic than dimer. Intracarotid infusion of 50 μg ^{10}B/gbw was well tolerated in the three rats that were euthanized 15 min (Rat 10) and 2 hours (Rats 11 and 12) post-infusion. A fourth rat (Rat 13) was administered 30 μg ^{10}B/gbw for comparison with Rat 8. In all four rats infused with monomer the boron concentrations in the cerebral tumors were slightly higher than the boron concentration in the corresponding subcutaneous tumors. Although the tumor boron levels immediately after infusion were high (Rat 10), by 2 hours post-infusion the boron concentration in all tumors had fallen below 20 μg/g. This finding is consistent with previously published[4] observations, indicating that the post-infusion decrease in tumor boron concentration is significantly more rapid for monomer than for dimer.

CONCLUSIONS

These preliminary studies clearly show that boron concentrations in gliomas of human origin are greater following the administration of the sulfhydryl borane dimer than those obtained from the administration of equal amounts of boron as monomer.

Table 2. ^{10}B Concentrations in Tissues Following Intracarotid and Intravenous Infusions of Monomer or Dimer.

Rat	^{10}B Dose[1] μg/gbw	Route,[2] Compound	Infusion[3] Time, Hours	Boron Concentration, μg $^{10}B/g$				
				Blood	Right Cerebrum	Left Cerebrum	Subcutaneous[4] Tumor	Cerebral[5] Tumor
1	50	IC,D	24(0)	33.0	0.4	--	22.7	25.0
2	50	IC,D	24(0)	21.2	1.1	--	23.3	23.9
3	50	IC,D	24(0)	21.3	1.2	--	21.9	21.3
4	50	IV,D	24(0)	29.7	0.5	--	21.9	24.2
5	50	IV,D	24(0)	29.5	1.0	--	20.8	24.5
6	50	IV,D	24(0)	30.5	1.3	--	41.9	34.9
7	50	IC,D	2(0.40)	66.5	9.1	--	35.1	170.0
8	30	IC,D	2(2.00)	29.6	1.1	2.0	23.5	25.8
9	50	IV,D	2(1.00)	43.8	1.1	--	36.4	33.9
10	50	IC,M	2(0.25)	64.2	1.0	3.1	28.6	32.6
11	50	IC,M	2(2.00)	27.2	2.4	6.7	11.9	15.4
12	50	IC,M	2(2.00)	15.5	0.3	3.0	6.2	12.0
13	30	IC,M	2(2.00)	7.0	0.4	1.9	6.3	8.1

[1]Boron dose - micrograms (μg) ^{10}B per gram body weight (gbw).
[2]IC - intracarotid; IV - intravenous; D - dimer; M = monomer.
[3]The hours in parenthesis represent the time between the end of infusion and euthanasia.
[4]The two subcutaneous tumors (right and left flank) were combined and analyzed as one sample.
[5]Cerebral tumor was located in the left cerebrum.

Although additional work needs to be done, these data do not provide strong support for intracarotid rather than intravenous administration of the sulfhydryl boranes, particularly in view of the risks associated with intraarterial infusions in humans. The unilateral intracarotid infusion of dimer may be particularly hazardous since a rapidly adminstered dose of 50 $\mu g\ ^{10}B/gbw$ (a boron dose equivalent to that given humans as monomer[2]) was promptly lethal to rats.

ACKNOWLEDGEMENTS

The rat glioma cell line (GS-9L) was kindly supplied by Victor Hatcher, Montefiore Medical Center, Bronx, NY. We thank S. Iwai and E. Medina for their technical assistance and G. Jackson for typing and assembling this transcript. Work was performed under Contract No. DE-AC02-76CH000016 with the U.S. Department of Energy.

REFERENCES

1. W. H. Sweet and J. J. Javid, The possible use of neutron capturing isotopes such as boron-10 in the treatment of neoplasms. I. Intracranial Tumors, Neurosurgery 9:200 (1952).
2. H. H. Hatanaka. Clinical experience of boron neutron capture therapy for malignant brain tumors, in "Proc. First Int. Symp. Neutron Capture Therapy," R. G. Fairchild and G. L. Brownell, eds., BNL 512730, Brookhaven National Laboratory, Upton, New York (1983).
3. D. Slatkin, P. Micca, A. Forman, D. Gabel, L. Wielopolski, and R. Fairchild, Boron uptake in melanoma, cerebrum and blood from $Na_2B_{12}H_{11}SH$ and $Na_4B_{24}H_{22}S_2$ administered to mice, Biochem. Pharmacol. 35: 1771 (1986).
4. D. Joel, D. Slatkin, R. Fairchild, P. Micca, and M. Nawrocky, Pharmacokinetics and tissue distribution of the sulfhydryl boranes (monomer and dimer) in glioma-bearing rats, in "Proc. Third Int. Symp. on Neutron Capture Therapy," Strahlentherap. Onkologie; Urban & Vogel, GmbH, Munich (in press).
5. J. Ponten and E. H. Macintyre, Long-term culture of normal and neoplastic human glia, Acta Path. Microbiol. Scand. 74:465 (1968).
6. H. H. Schmidek, S. L. Nielsen, A. L. Schiller, and J. Messer. Morphological studies of rat brain tumors induced by N-nitrosomethylurea, J. Neurosurg. 34:335 (1971).

7. G. R. Wellum, E. I. Tolpin, A. H. Soloway, and A. Kaczmarczyk. Synthesis of μ-disulfido-bis (undecahydro-closo-dodecaborate) (4-) and of a derived free radical. Inorg. Chem. 16:2120 (1977).
8. R. G. Fairchild, D. Gabel, B. H. Laster, D. Greenberg, W. Kiszenick, and P. L. Micca, Microanalytical techniques for boron analysis using the $^{10}B(n,\gamma)^{7}Li$ reaction. Med. Phys. 50:56 (1986).
9. W. H. Sweet, Medical aspects of boron-slow neutron capture therapy, in "Workshop on Neutron Capture Therapy," R. G. Fairchild and V. P. Bond, eds., Brookhaven National Laboratory, Upton, New York (1986).
10. S. C. Schold, H. S. Friedman and D. D. Bigner, Therapeutic profile of the human glioma line D-54 mg in athymic mice, Cancer Treatment Reports 71: 849 (1987).
11. G. C. Finkel, C. E. Poletti, R. G. Fairchild, D. N. Slatkin, and W. H. Sweet, Distribution of ^{10}B after Na_2-$^{10}B_{12}H_{11}SH$ infusion into a patient with malignant astrocytoma: implications for boron neutron capture therapy. Neurosurgery, in press (1989).

TOXICITIES OF $Na_2B_{12}H_{11}SH$ AND $Na_4B_{24}H_{22}S_2$ IN MICE

Paul G. Marshall, Marilyn E. Miller,
Stanley Grand*, Peggy L. Micca**,
and Daniel N. Slatkin**

Division of Hematological Research
Memorial Hospital
Pawtucket, RI 02860

*Department of Pathology
John T. Mather Memorial Hospital
Port Jefferson, NY 11777

**Medical Department
Brookhaven National Laboratory
Upton, NY 11973

INTRODUCTION

The sodium salt of the anionic icosahedral borane ($B_{12}H_{11}SH^{2-}$)[1,2] is used clinically in Japan[3,4] as a ^{10}B transport agent for boron neutron capture therapy [BNCT] of brain tumors. Although the dimer of that borane has greater affinity to a transplanted murine melanoma and to a transplanted rat glioma than does the parent monomer, the toxicity of the dimer has been cited[5] as a factor that might limit its usefulness for BNCT clinically. Thus, it was considered appropriate to assess the relative severity of the toxic effects of the monomer and the dimer in mice.

METHODS

Osmotic pumps with capacities of ~0.24 ml and pumping rates of ~1.0 μl/hr [Alza Corp., Palo Alto, California; Model 2001] were implanted under ether anesthesia through a ~1.0 cm incision in the left lower quadrant of the abdominal wall into the peritoneal cavities of ~8-10-week-old virgin female CF_1

Swiss albino mice (Charles River Breeding Labs, Cambridge, MA) for infusion of an aqueous solution of the monomer (BSH) or dimer (BSSB) form of a sulfhydryl borane[6,7]. The mice were observed daily for overt signs of toxicity and weighed regularly at intervals of several days (Tables 1 and 4).

Hemoglobin was measured and leukocytes were enumerated in anticoagulated whole blood (Tables 2 and 5). Lymphocytes, monocytes and granulocytes were counted in randomly selected samples of 100 leukocytes on one Giemsa-stained air-dried blood smear from each mouse (Table 3). Chemical and enzymatic analyses were performed on plasma from these blood samples (Table 7). Concentrations of urea nitrogen and creatinine indicated renal function. Aspartate aminotransferase, alanine aminotransferase and alkaline phosphatase concentrations in plasma indicated the severity of hepatocellular damage. Mitoses and hepatocyte macronuclei were counted by light microscopy in 4.0 mm^2 of one 5-μm-thick section per mouse cut from paraffin-embedded formalin-fixed liver tissue and stained with hematoxylin and eosin (Table 6). These counts were measures of the rapidity of hepatocellular regeneration five days after cessation of borane infusion.

The Wilcoxon Two-Sample test[8] was used to compare measures of toxicity non-parametrically in different experimental groups of mice. A short computer program for this test (Table 8) was written using the version of BASIC for a portable minicomputer (Texas Instruments, Lubbock, TX; Model CC-40).

RESULTS

The behavior of borane-infused mice was not obviously different from that of mice that were infused in other ways (Tables 1-6: H_2O alone; histamine + H_2O; cyclophosphamide + H_2O). Statistical analyses of Table 1 with the Wilcoxon Two-Sample test[8] indicate that weight loss was several percent more in BSSB-infused than in BSH-infused animals three days after osmotic pump implantation, but not 7 or 12-14 days after implantation. When a similar experiment was followed for a longer time (77 days after implantation), weight loss was slightly greater in BSSH-infused mice until day 16, but not thereafter (Table 4).

Neither numbers of leukocytes nor concentrations of hemoglobin in blood were affected by BSH or BSSB (Tables 2,3 and 5). The slightly higher average hemoglobin concentration on Day 3 (Table 2) and the slightly greater leukocyte count on Day 77 (Table 5) after BSSB-pump than BSH-pump implantation are

Table 1. Mouse Body Weights and Changes in Weight. Changes in Whole-Body Weights of Mice Either During 2 Weeks Following Intraperitoneal Implantation of 9-day Osmotic Pumps Containing a Solution of $Na_2B_{12}H_{11}SH$ (BSH) or $Na_4B_{24}H_{22}S_2$ (BSSB) in Water or Containing Water Alone, or During 2 Weeks Following Sham-Infusion.

Exp't.	Treatment	Mouse No.	Borane Dose (mgB/gbw)	Preinfusion Wt. (g) (Day 0)	Percent of Day 0 Weight[a] Day 3	Day 7	Day 12	Day 14
I	BSH,H_2O	1	0.22	28.5	94	94	99	--
	in IP pump,	2	0.23	28.5	95	99	106	--
	Anesthesia,	3	0.22	26.9	90	95	100	--
	Abdominal	4	0.23	27.8	89	97	96	--
II	incision.	1	0.22	24.8	89	90	--	98
		2	0.18	29.1	91	83	--	98
		3	0.17	34.9	91	87	--	91
		4	0.21	27.6	93	87	--	96
		[Average]	$[0.21]_8$	$[28.5]_8$	$[92]_8$[b]	$[92]_8$	--	$[98]_8$ --
I	BSSB,H_2O	1	0.21	26.6	93	94	102	
	in IP pump,	2	0.21	26.5	88	94	94	
	Anesthesia,	3	0.24	24.6	89	96	108	
	Abdominal	4	0.22	25.7	88	94	100	
II	incision.	1	0.19	30.2	83	78	--	94
		2	0.21	28.7	92	92	--	103
		3	0.20	29.3	83	79	--	95
		4	0.16	30.0	89	79	--	--
		[Average]	$[0.21]_8$	$[27.7]_8$	$[88]_8$[b]	$[88]_8$	--	$[99]_7$ --

(continued)

Table 1 (cont.)

Exp't.	Treatment	Mouse No.	Borane Dose (mgB/gbw)	Preinfusion Wt. (g) (Day 0)	Percent of Day 0 Weight[a] Day 3	Day 7	Day 12	Day 14
I	H_2O in	1	--	26.8	89	94	101	--
	IP pump,	2	--	25.1	96	101	108	--
	Anesthesia,	3	--	28.2	86	88	93	--
	Abdominal	4	--	26.1	102	105	104	--
	incision.	5	--	27.4	93	96	97	--
V		1		22.0	84	104	--	114
		2		22.1	87	98	--	112
		3		22.1	86	97	--	108
		4		21.0	94	100	--	107
		5		23.5	93	99	--	115
		[Average]		$[24.5]_{10}$	$[91]_{10}$	$[98]_{10}$	--$[106]_{10}$	--
II	Anesthesia,	1	--	29.4	96	86		95
	Abdominal	2	--	25.8	91	81	--	96
	incision,	3	--	27.2	96	85	--	96
	No pump.	4	--	26.2	94	87	--	95
		[Average]		$[27.1]_{4}$	$[94]_{4}$	$[85]_{4}$	$[96]_{4}$	
I	Pump inserted	1	--	27.4	97	97	100	
	IP, promptly removed. Double anesthesia.	2	--	26.8	100	103	108	
I	No anesthesia.	1	--	25.5	100	98	105	
	No incision.	2	--	25.1	102	98	105	

[a]Whole body weights of mice are corrected for original dry weights of osmotic pumps.
[b]Percents indicated by superscripts b are significantly different by the Wilcoxon Two-Sample Test[8] at the 90% confidence level.

Table 2. Changes in Blood Leukocyte Counts and in Hemoglobin Concentrations in Blood of Mice Either During 2 weeks After Intraperitoneal Implantation of 9-day Osmotic Pump Containing a Solution of BSH, BSSB in Water or Containing Water Alone, or During 2 Weeks After a Sham-Infusion.

Exp't.	Mouse No.	Treatment	Borane Dose mgB/gbw	Blood Leukocyte Concentration $x10^3$ cells/mm^3			Blood Hemoglobin Concentration g/dl		
				Day 3	Day 7	Day 12[a]	Day 3	Day 7	Day 12[a]
I	1	BSH,H_2O	0.22	8.8	8.0	10.0	14.0	12.5	14.4
	2	in IP pump	0.23	4.9	6.8	6.5	14.5	14.9	14.7
	3	Anesthesia,	0.22	7.6	7.5	5.4	16.2	12.6	14.5
	4	Abdominal	0.23	9.7	10.1	9.4	14.7	15.6	15.3
II	1	incision.	0.22	7.3	10.6	4.6	14.4	12.5	15.6
	2		0.18	7.2	12.0	9.6	13.8	13.8	14.4
	3		0.17	7.3	10.7	5.7	14.0	13.4	14.5
	4		0.21	4.2	11.8	9.0	12.2	12.8	13.1
[Average]			$[0.21]_8$	$[7.1]_8$	$[9.7]_8$	$[7.5]_8$	$[14.2]_8$[b]	$[13.5]_8$	$[14.6]_8$
I	1	BSSB,H_2O	0.21	5.6	10.1	7.8	15.6	14.4	14.4
	2	in IP pump	0.21	6.5	9.2	3.3	16.1	13.5	14.2
	3	Anesthesia,	0.24	8.0	16.5	5.0	16.9	12.9	14.4
	4	Abdominal	0.22	2.6	12.0	4.1	14.6	12.7	13.6
II	1	incision.	0.19	9.6	16.0	9.1	15.7	13.5	15.1
	2		0.21	8.3	6.6	7.1	13.9	12.7	13.9
	3		0.20	6.0	10.7	8.4	15.2	14.6	15.0
	4		0.16	8.2	11.6	--	14.6	14.6	--
[Average]			$[0.21]_8$	$[6.9]_8$	$[11.6]_8$	$[6.4]_7$	$[15.3]_8$[b]	$[13.6]_8$	$[14.4]_7$
I	1	H_2O in IP	--	5.7	10.4	3.3	14.0	13.7	13.6
	2	pump	--	11.9	12.5	3.8	13.2	14.4	13.0
	3	Anesthesia,	--	5.6	12.6	4.9	12.5	14.1	14.0
	4	Abdominal	--	6.8	5.9	4.9	12.1	14.0	15.1
	5	incision.	--	7.5	12.9	8.6	14.3	13.6	15.6

(continued)

Table 2 (cont.)

Exp't.	Mouse No.	Treatment	Borane Dose mgB/gbw	Blood Leukocyte Concentration $x10^3$ cells/mm^3			Blood Hemoglobin Concentration g/dl		
				Day 3	Day 7	Day 12[a]	Day 3	Day 7	Day 12[a]
V	1			10.8	23.3	21.0	--	13.1	13.8
	2			9.2	13.1	16.5	--	15.0	14.9
	3			9.7	13.5	13.1	--	14.1	14.6
	4			5.1	11.1	16.2	--	15.0	14.9
	5			7.9	10.3	10.1	--	15.7	14.2
	[Average]			$[8.0]_{10}$	$[12.6]_{10}$	$[10.2]_{10}$	$[13.2]_5$	$[14.3]_{10}$	$[14.3]_5$
II	1	Anesthesia, Abdominal	--	8.2	13.6	13.9	15.3	14.1	15.3
	2	incision.	--	7.3	11.6	4.2	13.5	14.4	15.3
	3	No pump.	--	8.1	10.9	4.1	14.5	15.7	15.7
	4		--	8.4	10.9	5.0	14.5	14.2	16.8
	[Average]			$[8.0]_4$	$[11.8]_4$	$[6.8]_4$	$[14.5]_4$	$[14.6]_4$	$[15.8]_4$
I	1	IP pump	--	7.9	8.4	4.6	16.1	14.2	15.3
	2	inserted then removed in < 1 hour. Anesthesia twice.	--	6.5	4.8	5.2	14.1	13.3	16.8
I	1	No anesthesia,	--	8.9	11.7	2.9	15.2	16.6	15.8
	2	No incision. Mice caged and tested as above.		9.8	8.7	3.5	14.6	14.6	16.1

[a]In experiment II, entries are averages of concentrations on days 10 and 14.
[b]Concentrations indicated by superscript b are significantly different by the Wilcoxon Two-Sample test[8] at the 90% confidence level.

Table 3. Changes in Differential Leukocyte Counts in Blood of Mice During 2 Weeks After Intraperitoneal Implantation of 9-day Osmotic Pump Containing a Solution of BSH, BSSB in Water, Water Alone, or After Sham-Infusion. The Table Shows the Number of Cells per 100 Leukocytes.

Exp't.	Mouse No.	Treatment	Lymphocytes Day 3	Lymphocytes Day 7	Lymphocytes Day 12[a]	Neutrophils Day 3	Neutrophils Day 7	Neutrophils Day 12[a]	Monocytes, Eosinophils Day 3	Monocytes, Eosinophils Day 7	Monocytes, Eosinophils Day12[a]
I	1	BSH, H_2O.	85	74	55	15	14	44	0, 0	9, 3	1, 0
	2	Anesthesia.	93	80	53	7	19	41	0, 0	1, 0	3, 3
	3	IP pump.	79	70	60	19	25	30	1, 0	5, 0	6, 4
	4		94	71	63	3	25	36	3, 0	4, 0	0, 1
II	1		72	67	62	27	27	28	1, 0	6, 0	10, 0.5
	2		64	52	80	34	45	20	0, 2	2, 1	0.5, 0
	3		76	64	75	21	26	18	1, 2	10, 0	7, 0.5
	4		50	58	53	50	41	41	0, 0	1, 0	6, 0.5
	[Average]		$[77]_8$	$[67]_8$	$[63]_8$	$[22]_8$	$[28]_8$	$[32]_8$			
I	1	BSSB, H_2O.	88	75	64	12	19	30	0, 0	5, 1	1, 5
	2	Anesthesia.	92	47	61	8	47	34	0, 0	5, 1	1, 4
	3	IP pump.	77	40	49	21	55	47	2, 1	2, 2	2, 2
	4		87	66	45	11	31	51	2, 1	3, 0	3, 1
II	1		60	60	68	40	38	28	0, 0	2, 0	4, 0.5
	2		76	55	60	23	43	35	0, 1	2, 0	5, 0.5
	3		70	49	63	29	47	30	0, 1	4, 0	8, 0
	4		76	79	--	20	18	--	3, 1	2, 1	-, -
	[Average]		$[78]_8$	$[59]_8$	$[59]_7$	$[21]_8$	$[37]_8$	$[36]_7$			
I	1	H_2O only.	95	62	60	5	32	38	0, 0	6, 0	0, 2
	2	Anesthesia.	95	25	92	5	65	7	0, 0	6, 0	1, 0
	3	IP pump.	83	76	78	16	18	20	0, 1	5, 1	0, 2
	4		94	76	79	6	24	19	0, 0	0, 0	1, 1
	5		83	80	71	13	13	27	4, 0	6, 0	0, 2
	[Average]		$[90]_5$	$[64]_5$	$[76]_5$	$[\ 9]_5$	$[30]_5$	$[22]_5$			

(continued)

Table 3 (cont.)

Exp't.	Mouse No.	Treatment	Lymphocytes Day 3	Lymphocytes Day 7	Lymphocytes Day 12[a]	Neutrophils Day 3	Neutrophils Day 7	Neutrophils Day 12[a]	Monocytes, Eosinophils Day 3	Monocytes, Eosinophils Day 7	Monocytes, Eosinophils Day12[a]
II	1	Abdominal	66	68	84	33	29	15	0, 1	1, 2	2, 0
	2	incision	83	80	72	17	18	20	0, 0	2, 1	7.5, 0.5
	3	under anesthesia.	80	85	74	20	14	25	0, 0	1, 0	1.5, 0
	4	No pump.	85	87	60	12	10	34	2, 1	3, 0	6, 0.5
	[Average]		[79]4	[80]4	[73]4	[21]4	[18]4	[24]4			
I	1	IP pump	89	66	71	8	28	28	3, 0	5, 1	0, 1
	2	inserted then removed within < 1 hour. Anesthesia twice.	82	79	85	16	17	14	2, 0	4, 0	0, 1
II	1	No anesthesia.	87	81	86	8	15	11	5, 0	3, 1	1, 2
	2	No incision.	95	62	86	5	34	13	0, 0	3, 1	0, 1

[a]In experiment II, entries are averages of counts on days 10 and 14.

Table 4. Changes in Whole-Body Weights of Mice During 77 Days After Intraperitoneal Implantation of a 9-day Osmotic Pump Containing a Solution of BSH, BSSB, Cyclophosphamide or Histamine in Water or Containing Water Alone.

Exp't.	Treatment	Mouse Number	Dose (mg B/gbw)	Preinfusion Weight (g) Day 0	Percent of Day 0 Weight[a] Day 5	Day 16	Day 22	Day 29	Day 53	Day 77
III	BSH, H_2O in IP pump. Anesthesia. Abdominal incision.	1	0.24	24.8	88	97	112	106	114	132
		2	0.26	22.7	94	102	104	109	128	137
		3	0.26	23.0	90	94	110	123	140	140
		4	0.52	22.6	91	98	105	108	130	136
		5	0.54	22.1	101	107	113	117	132	141
		6	0.51	23.3	87	97	100	105	127	136
	[Average]	6	[0.39]	[23.1]	[92][b]	[99][c]	[107]	[111]	[129]	[137]
III	BSSB, H_2O in IP pump. Anesthesia. Abdominal incision.	1	0.31	23.0	83	97	118	121	134	150
		2	0.21	24.2	79	88	96	106	120	134
		3	0.62	23.0	78	97	84	126	138	147
		4	0.68	20.8	87	89	111	113	129	133
		5	0.61	23.1	76	78	109	99	118	129
	[Average]	5	[0.49]	[22.8]	[81][b]	[90][c]	[104]	[113]	[128]	[139]
III	H_2O only in IP pump. Anesthesia. Abdominal incision.	1	--	22.8	83	88	105	104	128	134
		2	--	21.6	90	96	113	116	135	151

(continued)

Table 4 (cont.)

Exp't.	Treatment	Mouse No.	Dose (mg B/gbw)	Preinfusion Weight (g) Day 0	Percent of Day 0 Weight[a] Day 5	Day 16	Day 22	Day 29	Day 53	Day 77
			(mg/gbw)							
III	Cyclophosphamide,	1	0.41	23.1	90	92	113	113	124	128
	H_2O	1	0.40	24.0	89	97	101	108	119	133
		3	0.39	24.3	94	95	114	115	120	141
			(μmol/gbw)							
III	Histamine,	1	5.0	23.9	88	94	92	105	122	133
	H_2O	2	5.5	21.8	91	98	109	106	131	141
		3	4.8	24.8	90	92	112	117	130	136

[a]Whole-body weights of mice corrected for original dry weights of osmotic pumps.
[b,c]Percents indicated by superscript b or c are significantly different by the Wilcoxon Two-Sample test[8] at the 90% confidence level.

Table 5. Changes in Blood Leukocyte Counts and Hemoglobin Concentrations in Blood of Mice During 77 Days After Intraperitoneal Implantation of a 9-day Osmotic Pump Containing a Solution of BSH, BSSB, Cyclophosphamide or Histamine in Water, or Containing Water Alone.

Exp't.	Treatment	Mouse No.	Dose (mg B/gbw)	Preinfusion Weight (g)	Blood Leukocyte, Blood Hemoglobin Concentrations (10^3 cells/mm^3, g/dl)					
				Day 0	Day 5	Day 16	Day 22	Day 29	Day 53	Day 77
III	BSH,H_2O	1	0.24	24.8	6.8,16.1	8.3,14.9	12.9,13.9	15.6,13.7	9.7,13.8	5.7,--
	in IP pump.	2	0.26	22.7	10.0,15.7	12.6,16.4	20.7,16.3	12.2,15.5	9.0,15.0	8.6,--
	Anesthesia.	3	0.26	23.0	4.0,15.0	7.3,16.9	7.8,15.1	9.2,12.7	6.4,11.8	6.4,--
	Abdominal	4	0.52	22.6	7.8,13.8	7.6,14.2	8.9,16.2	10.8,12.4	10.0,15.6	4.8,--
	incision.	5	0.54	22.1	6.8,17.2	9.2,15.1	5.2,14.0	9.2,15.4	12.8,13.4	5.2,--
		6	0.51	23.3	4.8,16.5	11.0,17.3	9.9,16.8	7.6,15.9	11.0,13.4	5.6,--
	[Average]	6	[0.39]	[23.1]	[6.7,15.7]	[9.3,15.8]	[10.9,15.4]	[10.8,14.3]	[9.8,13.8]	[6.1,--]
III	BSSB,H_2Oin	1	0.31	23.0	6.2,14.4	9.8,15.6	7.8,15.1	9.4,15.1	7.4,14.5	9.2,--
	IP pump.	2	0.21	24.2	6.5,17.9	12.9,15.6	9.4,15.2	10.0,14.3	8.3,15.1	9.9,--
	Anesthesia.	3	0.62	23.0	6.8,14.2	14.4,14.4	10.4,15.7	12.0,14.3	8.0,16.0	13.4,--
	Abdominal	4	0.68	20.8	6.1,16.1	5.5,15.9	11.8,15.0	8.9,15.3	8.6,15.4	10.4,--
	incision.	5	0.61	23.1	12.8,19.3	15.6,14.8	10.1,16.2	8.4,15.9	7.8,14.4	8.2,--
	[Average]	5	[0.49]	[22.8]	[7.7,16.1]	[11.6,15.3]	[9.9,15.4]	[9.7,15.0]	[8.0,15.1]	[10.2,--]
III	H_2O only in	1	--	22.8	7.2,17.2	13.3,17.2	10.0,15.3	9.5,16.7	5.8,14.3	5.2,--
	IP pump.	2	--	21.6	6.2,16.3	19.9,16.5	12.6,15.2	10.0,15.5	9.3,15.5	10.8,--
	Anesthesia.									
	Abdominal									
	incision.									

(continued)

Table 5 (cont.)

Exp't.	Treatment	Mouse No.	Dose (mg B/gbw)	Preinfusion Weight (g)	Blood Leukocyte, Blood Hemoglobin Concentrations (10^3 cells/mm^3, g/dl)					
				Day 0	Day 5	Day 16	Day 22	Day 29	Day 53	Day 77
			(mg/gbw)							
III	Cyclophos-	1	0.41	23.1	5.6,14.2	6.9,14.6	7.4,14.1	9.8,13.1	5.2,14.1	7.0,--
	phamide,	2	0.40	24.0	6.8,16.1	16.8,14.5	10.8,15.3	9.0,14.9	10.0,15.1	7.6,--
	H_2O	3	0.39	24.3	6.7,15.8	13.4,15.7	5.1,13.0	10.4,15.9	7.8,15.2	10.1,--
			(μmol/gbw)							
III	Histamine,	1	5.0	23.9	3.6,17.0	9.1,16.2	9.0,13.6	6.6,14.5	8.8,16.0	11.6,--
	H_2O	2	5.5	21.8	8.9,16.5	16.1,16.6	13.4,17.0	6.8,15.8	7.0,15.5	4.4,--
		3	4.8	24.8	10.3,13.6	7.7,16.2	19.8,15.5	8.3,16.4	12.2,15.1	8.4,--

Table 6. Quantitative Indices of Hepatic Regeneration (Counts of Hepatocyte Macronuclei, Counts of Mitotic Liver Cells) Enumerated in ~5 μm-thick Sections of Liver from Mice 14 Days After Intraperitoneal Implantation of 9-day Osmotic Pump Containing a Solution of BSH, BSSB or Cyclophosphamide in Water or 14 Days After Sham Operation. The Sections were Stained with Hematoxylin and Eosin. For Convenience of Morphometry, One "Macronuclear Hepatocyte" Represents Either a Single Hepatocyte Nucleus that Measures >20 μm in Greatest Diameter or Two Contiguous Hepatocyte Nuclei, Apparently in the Same Hepatocyte, the sum of the Diameters of Which Measures >20 μm.

Exp't.	Treatment	Mouse number	Dose (mgB/gbw)	% Day 0 Weight at Day 14	Liver section area examined (mm^2)	Total Mitoses	Liver section area examined (mm^2)	Total Macronuclear hepatocytes	Number in liver sections mm^{-2}: Mitotic cells	Number in liver sections mm^{-2}: Macronuclear hepatocytes
II	BSH, H_2O	1	0.22	98	4.0	1	2.0	23		
	in IP pump	2	0.18	98	4.0	0	2.0	5		
	Anesthesia,	3	0.17	91	4.0	36	2.0	19		
	Abdominal	4	0.21	96	4.0	1	2.0	14		
	incision						[Average]		[2.4]	[7.6]
II	BSSB, H_2O	1	0.19	94	4.0	2	2.0	14		
	in IP pump	2	0.21	103	4.0	20	2.0	13		
	Anesthesia,	3	0.20	95	4.0	6	2.0	10		
	Abdominal									
	incision						[Average]		[2.3]	[6.2]
II	Anesthesia,	1	--	95	4.0	0	2.0	7		
	Abdominal	2	--	96	4.0	0	2.0	10		
	incision. No	3	--	96	4.0	0	2.0	3		
	pump	4	--	95	4.0	0	2.0	10		
							[Average]		[0.0]	[3.8]

(continued)

Table 6 (cont.)

Exp't.	Treatment	Mouse number	Dose (mgB/gbw)	% Day 0 Weight at Day 14	Liver section area examined (mm^2)	Total Mitoses	Liver section area examined (mm^2)	Total Macronuclear hepatocytes	Number in liver sections mm-2: Mitotic Cells	Number in liver sections mm-2: Macronuclear hepatocytes
			(μg/gbw)							
II	Cyclophos-phamide	1	9	93	4.0	0	2.0	4		
	H_2O in IP pump	2	80	125	4.0	0	2.0	3		
	Anesthesia, Abdominal incision							[Average]	[0]	[2]

Table 7. Concentrations of Plasma Constituents that Indicate Renal Function (Urea Nitrogen; Creatinine) and the Structural Integrity or Membrane Permeability of Liver Cells (Aspartate Aminotransferase, AST; Alanine Aminotransferase, ALT; Alkaline Phosphatase, ALP) in the Blood of Normal Mice and Mice 3-10 Days After Intraperitoneal Implantation of 9-day Osmotic Pumps Containing a Solution of BSH or BSSB in Water.

					Concentration in Serum				
Exp't.	Treatment	Mouse No.	Days After Pump Insertion	Borane dose (mgB/gbw)	Urea-N (mg/dl)	Creatinine (mg/dl)	AST (U/l)	ALT (U/l)	ALP (U/l)
IV	BSH, H_2O in IP Pump	1	3	0.047	25.3	0.33	144	18	119
		2	3	0.045	23.6	0.32	206	30	24
		3	3	0.043	23.1	0.25	403	42	1
		4	6	0.101	27.5	0.41	317	50	75
		5	6	0.077	27.5	0.35	201	13	43
		6	6	0.078	31.4	0.35	349	46	5
		7-9[a]	10	0.139	29.6	0.27	292	33	53
[Average]				$[0.076]_7$	$[26.9]_7$	$[0.33]_7$	$[273]_7$	$[33]_7$	$[29]_7$
IV	BSSB, H_2O in IP Pump	1	3	0.048	22.3	0.39	273	54	107
		2	3	0.047	27.4	0.38	317	34	136
		3	3	0.043	19.9	0.38	529	55	92
		4	6	0.081	26.7	0.41	363	46	130
		5	6	0.081	23.0	0.35	547	102	135
		6	6	0.079	18.1	0.33	718	59	112
		7-8[a]	10	0.151	27.1	0.30	741	86	123
[Average]				$[0.076]_7$	$[23.5]_7$	$[0.36]_7$	$[498]_7$	$[62]_7$	$[119]_7$

(continued)

Table 7 (cont.)

Exp.	Treatment	Mouse Number	Days After Pump Insertion	Borane dose (mgB/gbw)	Concentration in Serum: Urea-N (mg/dl)	Creatinine (mg/dl)	AST (U/l)	ALT (U/l)	ALP (U/l)
IV	None	1	--	--	3.7[b]	0.46	67	21	122
		2	--	--	27.6	0.38	118	42	244
		3	--	--	33.2	0.43	59	22	208
		4	--	--	28.3	0.41	82	28	217
		5	--	--	30.0	0.36	127	62	234
		6	--	--	25.5	0.38	94	34	122
		7	--	--	25.7	0.41	82	37	207
		8	--	--	26.2	0.38	49	4[b]	111
		9	--	--	29.3	0.40	95	40	223
		10	--	--	24.5	0.26	164	20	148
		11	--	--	28.3	0.42	72	18	84
[Average]					$[27.9]_{10}$	$[0.39]_{11}$	$[92]_{11}$	$[32]_{10}$	$[175]_{11}$

[a]Entries represent average values from unequal numbers of mice euthanized 10 days after pump insertion.

[b]Outlying value omitted from calculations of averages.

Table 8. Program Wilcoxon. Computer program (BASIC) that computes the sum, T1, of the rank numbers assigned to the first (L=1) of two samples of values from any undetermined, continuous distribution when the first sample is compared by the ranks of the relative magnitudes of its constituent values with those of a second sample (L=2) from the same, unknown form of continuous distribution. N(1) and N(2) are the numbers of values in the first and second samples, respectively. This program automatically takes into account values of equal magnitude within a sample or between the two samples. For each level of significance, a Wilcoxon Two-Sample Test table[8] lists intervals of "rank sum" values, T1, for which the mean values of the two distributions are not significantly different. These intervals are tabulated as functions of N(1), N(2) and T1.

```
 10 DIM W(3,100),N(2),C(3)
 20 FOR L = 1 TO 2:INPUT " # IN SERIES" &STR$(L)& " = ";
    N(L):FOR I = 1 TO N(L)
 30 INPUT "SERIES" &STR$(L)& ",#" &STR$(I)& " = " ;W(L,I)
 40 NEXT I:FOR K = 1 TO N(L)-1:X = W(L,K):FOR J = K + 1 TO N(L)
 50 IF W(L,J) < = W(L,K)THEN W(L,K) = W(L,J):W(L,J) = X:X =
    W(L,K)
 60 NEXT J:NEXT K:NEXT L:P = N(1):Q = N(2):S = P + Q:T = 0
 70 FOR I = 1 TO P: PRINT I:PAUSE .1
 80 FOR J = 1 TO Q:IF W(1,I) <= W(2,J)THEN 110
 90 IF J = Q THEN W(2,Q + 1) = W(1,I):W(3,Q + 1) = W(1,I)
100 NEXT J:Q = J:NEXT I:GOTO 130
110 FOR K = Q + 1 TO J + 1 STEP -1:W(2,K) = W(2,K-1):W(3,K) =
    W(3,K-1)
120 NEXT K:W(2,J) = W(1,I):W(3,J) = W(1,I):J = Q:GOTO 100
130 FOR I = 1 TO S:PRINT I:PAUSE .1:IF W(3,I) = 0 THEN 150
140 IF W(3,I) = W(2,I) THEN R = I:GOTO 160
150 NEXT I:DISPLAY BEEP AT(1) USING 200; T:PAUSE:END
160 FOR K = 3 TO 2 STEP -1:C(K) = 0
170 FOR J = 1 TO S:IF W(3,I) = W(K,J) THEN C(K) = C(K) + 1:M = J
180 NEXT J:NEXT K:IF C(3) = C(2) THEN 190 ELSE R = (2*M-C(2) +
    1)/2
190 T = T + R: GOTO 150
200 IMAGE RANK SUM T1 = ######.#
```

barely significant statistically. There was little difference in the rates of liver regeneration five days after cessation of borane infusion between BSH- and BSSB-treated mice (Table 6, Day 14), although aspartate and alanine aminotransferase levels in plasma indicate more active hepatocellular damage in the BSSB-treated animals (Table 7). Apparent depression of plasma alkaline phosphatase activity was observed in borane-treated mice, but we did not exclude the possibility that this resulted from non-specific inactivation of an assay reagent by the borane anion.

DISCUSSION

Mice were infused intraperitoneally for 9 days with the sodium salt of either the monomer $(B_{12}H_{11}SH)^{2-}$ or the dimer $(B_{24}H_{22}S_2)^{4-}$ form of an icosahedral mercaptoborane in doses ranging from 160 to 680 μgB/g body weight. Neither of these boranes affected leukocyte numbers or hemoglobin concentrations in the blood but each was hepatotoxic, the dimer more so than the monomer. There was histopathologic evidence of liver regeneration at similar rates five days after infusion of monomer and dimer. Although only the monomer is used now as a ^{10}B-transport agent for BNCT of brain tumors, the dimer can be considered a candidate ^{10}B-transport agent for BNCT because of its greater affinity for tumor tissue than that of the monomer and because its toxicity to the liver, although more severe, seems to be not much more prolonged than that of the monomer.

Higher doses of BSH and BSSB can be tolerated by mice than was thought previously (Table 4: BSH mice numbers 4, 5 and 6; BSSB mice numbers 3, 4 and 5). Moreover the hepatotoxicity to mice of BSSH, although more marked than that of BSH, apparently is reversible nearly as fast as that of BSH. These results suggest a need for studies of BSH and BSSB toxicity by slow infusion into larger experimental mammals using doses of up to several hundred micrograms per gram of body weight (gbw) and for clinical studies of the comparative pharmacokinetics of trace doses of ^{10}B-labeled BSH and BSSB in patients with malignant glioma.

We speculate that BSH and BSSB, if infused slowly over a period of several days, may also be tolerated by glioma-bearing patients when administered to deliver total boron doses of several hundred micrograms per gram of body weight. Such infusions may be useful for boron neutron capture therapy of malignant gliomas.

ACKNOWLEDGEMENTS

We thank B. Armstrong, G. Jackson, J. Pastore, E. L. Roche and A. L. Ruggiero for technical assistance. This work was supported in part under Contract No. DE-AC02-76CH00016 with the U.S. Department of Energy.

REFERENCES

1. W. H. Knoth, J. C. Sauer, D. C. England, W.R. Hertler and E.L. Muetterties, Chemistry of Boranes. XIX. Derivative chemistry of $B_{10}H_{10}^{-2}$ and $B_{12}H_{12}^{-2}$, J. Am. Chem. Soc. 86:3973 (1964).
2. A. H. Soloway, H. Hatanaka and M. A. Davis, Penetration of brain and brain tumor. VII. Tumor-binding sulfhydryl boron compounds, J. Med. Chem. 10:714 (1967).
3. Neutron Capture Therapy, ed. H. Hatanaka, Nishimura Co., Ltd., Niigata 951, Japan (1986).
4. Workshop on Neutron Capture Therapy, R. G. Fairchild and V. P. Bond, eds., Brookhaven National Laboratory, Upton, New York, BNL-51994 (1986).
5. A. H. Soloway, F. Alam and R. F. Barth, Workshop on Neutron Capture Therapy, R. G. Fairchild and V. P. Bond, eds., Brookhaven National Laboratory, Upton, BNL-51994, pp. 162-172 (1986).
6. G. R. Wellum, E. I. Tolpin, A. H. Soloway and A. Kaczmarczyk, Synthesis of μ-Disulfido-bis (undecahydro-closo-dodecaborate)(4-) and of a derived free radical, Inorg. Chem. 16:2120 (1977).
7. D. Slatkin, P. Micca, A. Forman, D. Gabel, L. Wielopolski and R. Fairchild, Boron uptake in melanoma, cerebrum and blood from $Na_2B_{12}H_{11}SH$ and $Na_4B_{24}H_{22}S_2$ administered to mice, Biochem. Pharmacol. 35, 1771 (1986).
8. Geigy Scientific Tables, 8th Edition, Vol. 2, ed. C. Lentner, Ciba-Geigy, Basle, 1982, p. 156.

PARTICIPANTS

ALLEN, Barry J.
Australian Nuclear Science and Technology Organization
Lucas Heights Research Labs
Menai 2234 N.S.W. Australia

ACKERMANN, Arlene L.
New Technology Development Projects
EG & G Idaho, Inc.
P.O. Box 1625
Idaho Falls, Idaho 83415

ALAM, Fazul
Ohio State University
School of Medicine
450 West 10th Avenue
Columbus, Ohio 43210

ARCHAMBEAU, John O.
Director, Radiation Research
Loma Linda University Medical Center
P. O. Box 2000
11234 Anderson Street
Loma Linda, California 92354

ARCHIBALD, George
Idaho Area Office
U. S. Department of Energy
EG & G Idaho, Inc.
Idaho Falls, Idaho 83415

ATKINS, Harold L.
Department of Radiology
School of Medicine
Health Sciences Center
State University of New York
Stony Brook, New York 11794

BARTH, Rolf F.
Department of Pathology
Ohio State University
4170 Graves Hall
333 W. Tenth Avenue
Columbus, Ohio 43210

BELLOWS, Jerry L.
Brookhaven Area Office
Department of Energy
Upton, New York 11973

BENDER, Michael A.
Medical Department
Brookhaven National Laboratory
Upton, New York 11973

BLUME, Martin
Director's Office
Brookhaven National Laboratory
Upton, New York 11973

BOND, Victor P.
Medical Department
Brookhaven National Laboratory
Upton, New York 11973

BORG, Donald C.
Medical Department
Brookhaven National Laboratory
Upton, New York 11973

BRUGGER, Robert M.
Research Reactor Facility
University of Missouri
Columbia, Missouri 65211

CHANANA, Arjun D.
Medical Department
Brookhaven National Laboratory
Upton, New York 11973

CHO, Paul
Human Health and Assessments
Office of Health and Environmental Research (GTN)
U. S. Department of Energy
19901 Germantown Road, ER-73
Germantown, Maryland 20874

CODERRE, Jeffrey A.
Medical Department
Brookhaven National Laboratory
Upton, New York 11973

COLE, Donald W.
Office of Health and Environmental Research
U. S. Department of Energy
19901 Germantown Road, ER-73
Germantown, Maryland 20874

CRONKITE, Eugene P.
Medical Department
Brookhaven National Laboratory
Upton, New York 11973

DILMANIAN, F. Avraham
Medical Department
Brookhaven National Laboratory
Upton, New York 11973

DORN, Ronald V., III
Mountain States Tumor Inst.
151 East Bannock
Boise, Idaho 83712

DURRANT, Keith R.
Oxfordshire Health Authority
The Department of Radiotherapy and Oncology
The Churchill Hospital
Headington, Oxford, OX3 7LJ
England, United Kingdom

FAIRCHILD, Ralph G.
Medical Department
Brookhaven National Laboratory
Upton, New York 11973

FEINENDEGEN, Ludwig W.
Institut fur Medizin
Der Kerforschungsanlage Julich GmbH
Postfach 1913
D-5170 Julich 1
West Germany

FIARMAN, Sidney
Medical Department
Brookhaven National Laboratory
Upton, New York 11973

GABEL, Detlef
Universitat Bremen
Fachbereich Chemie
Postfach 330 440
D-2800 Bremen 33,
West Germany

GAHBAUER, Reinhard A.
Division of Radiation Oncology
The Ohio State University
450 West 10th Avenue
Columbus, Ohio 43210

GLASS, John D., Jr.
Medical Department
Brookhaven National Laboratory
Upton, New York 11973

GOLDHABER, Maurice
Director's Office
Brookhaven National Laboratory
Upton, New York 11973

GOODMAN, Joseph H.
Room N 935 Doan Hall
Ohio State University Hospital
Radiation/Oncology
410 W. 10th Avenue
Columbus, Ohio 43210

GRAHAM, Bernard W.
EG & G Idaho
Idaho National Engineering Lab
Idaho Falls, Idaho 83415

GRIEBENOW, Merle L.
New Technol. Development Proj.
EG & G Idaho, Inc.
P.O. Box 1625
Idaho Falls, Idaho 83415

HARKNESS, William
Department of Neurosurgery
Radcliffe Infirmary
Oxford OX2 6HE
England, United Kingdom

HARLING, Otto
Mass. Institute of Technology
Nuclear Reactor Laboratory
138 Albany Street
Cambridge, Massachusetts 02139

HOPEWELL, John
Churchill Hospital
Old Road
Headington, Oxford OX3, 7LJ
Oxford, England, United Kingdom
HUDIS, Jerome
Vice President and Secretary
Associated Universities, Inc.
Brookhaven National Laboratory
Upton, New York 11973

IWAI, Junichi
Medical Department
Brookhaven National Laboratory
Upton, New York 11973

JOEL, Darrel D.
Medical Department
Brookhaven National Laboratory
Upton, New York 11973

KABALKA, George
Department of Chemistry
University of Tennessee
Knoxville, Tennessee 37916
KAHL, Stephen B.
School of Pharmacy
Department of Pharmaceutical Chemistry
University of California
San Francisco, California 94143
KALEF-EZRA, John A.
Medical Department
Brookhaven National Laboratory
Upton, New York 11973
KAMEN, Yakov
Medical Department
Brookhaven National Laboratory
Upton, New York 11973
KINNE, Gerald C.
Director's Office
Brookhaven National Laboratory
Upton, New York 11973

LARSSON, Borje
Gustav Werner Institute
Box 531 - S-75121
Uppsala, Sweden

LASTER, Brenda H.
Medical Department
Brookhaven National Laboratory
Upton, New York 11973
LASTER, Marvin
Brookhaven Area Office
U.S. Department of Energy
Upton, New York 11973

MADOC-JONES, Hywel
Dept. of Radiation Oncology
New England Medical Center
750 Washington Street
Boston, Massachusetts 02111
MARANO, Stephen R.
EG & G Idaho, Inc.
P.O. Box 1625
Idaho National Engineering Lab
Idaho Falls, Idaho 83415
MAUSNER, Leonard F.
Medical Department
Brookhaven National Laboratory
Upton, New York 11973
McCALMONT, Samuel
Callery Chemical Company
P.O. Box 429
Pittsburgh, Pennsylvania 15230
McGREGOR, J.
Department of Neurosurgery
Ohio State University
410 West 10th Avenue
Columbus, Ohio 43210
MEEK, Allen G.
Chairman, Associate Professor
Dept. of Radiation Oncology
University Hospital
Stony Brook, New York 11794
MICCA, Peggy L.
Medical Department
Brookhaven National Laboratory
Upton, New York 11973
MISHIMA, Yutaka
Professor and Chairman
Department of Dermatology
Director, The Insitute of Cancer Neutron Therapy
Kobe U. School of Medicine
5-1 Kusunoki-Cho 7-Chome, Chuo-Ku
Kobe 650, Japan

MIURA, Michiko
Medical Department
Brookhaven National Laboratory
Upton, New York 11973
MOSS, Richard L.
HFR Division
Joint Research Center
Petten Establishment
1755 ZG Petten
The Netherlands
MONHART, Jane
Brookhaven Area Office
U.S. Department of Energy
Upton, New York 11973

NAWROCKY, Marta
Medical Department
Brookhaven National Laboratory
Upton, New York 11973

PACKER, Samuel
Department of Ophthalmology
North Shore U. Hospital
Manhasset, New York 11030
POPENOE, Edwin A.
Medical Department
Brookhaven National Laboratory
Upton, New York 11973

REINSTEIN, Lawrence E.
Dept. of Radiat. Oncology, L-2
University Hospital
Stony Brook, N. Y. 11794-7028
RYABUKHIN, Yuri
Radiation Scientist
Prevention of Environmental Pollution
Div. of Environmental Health
World Health Organization
1211 Geneva 27
Switzerland
ROBERTSON, James S.
Director, Human Health and Assessments
Office of Health and Environmental Research
U.S. Department of Energy
19901 Germantown Road, ER-73
Germantown, Maryland 20874

ROCKWELL, Sara
Dept. of Therapeutic Radiology
Yale School of Medicine
333 Cedar Street
New Haven, Conn. 06510-8040
RORER, David C.
Reactor Division
Brookhaven National Laboratory
Upton, New York 11973
RUSSELL, John L., Jr.
Theragenics Corporation
900 Atlanta Drive, N.W.
Atlanta, Georgia 30318
SAMIOS, Nicholas P.
Director
Brookhaven National Laboratory
Upton, New York 11973
SETLOW, Richard B.
Director, Life Sciences
Brookhaven National Laboratory
Upton, New York 11973
SLATKIN, Daniel N.
Medical Department
Brookhaven National Laboratory
Upton, New York 11973
SOLOWAY, Albert H.
Dean, College of Pharmacy
Ohio State University
500 West 12th Avenue
Columbus, Ohio 43210
SPICKARD, John H.
EG & G Idaho
Idaho National Engineering Lab
Idaho Falls, Idaho 83415
SRIVASTAVA, Suresh C.
Medical Department
Brookhaven National Laboratory
Upton, New York 11973
SWEET, William H.
Ambulatory Care Center
312 Mass. General Hospital
15 Parkman Street
Boston, Massachusetts 02114

TOVARYS, Frantisek
Neurosurgical Clinic
Charles University
U vojenske nemocnice 1200
169 00 Praha 6,
Czechoslovakia

TYSON, George W.
Chairman & Associate Professor
Department of Neurosurgery
State University of New York
Stony Brook, New York 11794

WAMBERSIE, Andre
Catholic University of Louvain
Medical Faculty
Avenue Hippocrate 54
B-1200
Brussels, Belgium

WEBER, David A.
Medical Department
Brookhaven National Laboratory
Upton, New York 11973

WHEELER, Floyd
EG & G Idaho, Inc.
Idaho National Engineering Lab
Idaho Falls, Idaho 83415

WIELOPOLSKI, Lucian
Dept. of Radiation Oncology
University Hospital
Stony Brook, New York 11794

WOODHEAD, Avril D.
Technical Information Division
Brookhaven National Laboratory
Upton, New York 11973

ZAMENHOF, Robert C.
Dept. of Therapeutic Radiology
Tufts University
New England Medical Center
171 Harrison Avenue
Boston, Massachusetts 02111

INDEX

GPSR Compliance
The European Union's (EU) General Product Safety Regulation (GPSR) is a set of rules that requires consumer products to be safe and our obligations to ensure this.

If you have any concerns about our products, you can contact us on

ProductSafety@springernature.com

In case Publisher is established outside the EU, the EU authorized representative is:

Springer Nature Customer Service Center GmbH
Europaplatz 3
69115 Heidelberg, Germany

www.ingramcontent.com/pod-product-compliance
Ingram Content Group UK Ltd.
Pitfield, Milton Keynes, MK11 3LW, UK
UKHW051130260726
13967UKWH00010B/2972
* 9 7 8 1 4 6 8 4 5 6 2 3 3 *